Berries and Cancer Prevention

Gary D. Stoner · Navindra P. Seeram
Editors

Berries and Cancer Prevention

Springer

Editors
Gary D. Stoner, Ph.D
Department of Medicine
Medical College of Wisconsin
Milwaukee, WI 53226, USA

Navindra P. Seeram, Ph.D
Department of Biomedical and
Pharmaceutical Sciences
University of Rhode Island
Kingston, RI 02881, USA

ISBN 978-1-4419-7553-9
e-ISBN 978-1-4419-7554-6
DOI 10.1007/978-1-4419-7554-6
Springer New York Dordrecht Heidelberg London

Printed on acid-free paper

Springer is part of Springer Science+Business Media (www.springer.com)

Preface

Among colorful fruits, berries and their derived products command an overwhelming and rapidly growing body of scientific data to support their ability to prevent, delay and potentially treat certain types of human cancers. Given that the worldwide incidence of cancer is rapidly increasing, intervention with foodstuffs, such as berries and berry formulations, provide an attractive strategy to cancer prevention. Like many other fruits, berries contain micro- and macronutrients such as vitamins, minerals, and fiber. However, berries also contain a multitude of plant secondary metabolites (phytochemicals) that exhibit a diverse array of chemical structures. It has become apparent that multiple berry constituents, through additive, complementary, and/or synergistic interactions, exhibit chemopreventive effects superior to any single component alone.

This book provides focused and timely discussions on berries and cancer. The chapters presented here are collected from a multi-disciplinary team of international researchers. Thus, the fifteen chapters are organized into four sections. The first section consists of three chapters, examining the overall theme of berry composition, bioavailability, metabolism and biological effects. The second section examines the antioxidant effects of berry components which are presented in a single chapter. The third section, groups eight chapters which examine the chemopreventive effects of berries and berry components in animal model systems. The fourth and last section comprises three chapters that individually discuss cancer prevention studies with berries and berry formulations in human subjects. We think this collection of writings is the first of many to come in the future regarding the role of berries and their components as preventative agents for cancer.

We thank all authors for their contributions towards making this book a success. Also, Sophia O. Tolliver for her invaluable assistance in coordinating this project.

Milwaukee, WI, USA — Gary D. Stoner
Kingston, RI, USA — Navindra P. Seeram

Contents

Contributors

Vaqar Mustafa Adhami Department of Dermatology, University of Wisconsin, Madison, WI 53706, USA

Amit Agrawal Department of Otolaryngology, The Ohio State University College of Medicine, Columbus, OH 43210, USA

Harini Aiyer James Graham Brown Cancer Center, University of Louisville, Louisville, KY 40202, USA; Department of Surgery, University of Louisville, Louisville, KY 40202, USA

Mark Arnold Department of Surgery, The Ohio State University College of Medicine, Columbus, OH 43210, USA

Tongjian Cai Nelson Institute of Environmental Medicine, New York University School of Medicine, Tuxedo, NY 10987, USA

Bruce C. Casto Division of Environmental Health Sciences, College of Public Health, The Ohio State University, Columbus, OH 43210, USA

Yeon Tae Chung Department of Pathology, Northwestern University Feinberg School of Medicine, Chicago, IL 60611, USA

Steven K. Clinton Division of Hematology and Oncology, The Ohio State University College of Medicine, Columbus, OH 43210, USA

Amy Exum Department of Epidemiology and Public Health, Miller School of Medicine, University of Miami Sylvester Cancer Center, Miami, FL 33136, USA

Wendy Frankel Department of Pathology, The Ohio State University College of Medicine, Columbus, OH 43210, USA

M. Monica Giusti Department of Food Science and Technology, The Ohio State University, Columbus, OH 43210, USA

Gayle M. Gordillo Division of Plastic Surgery, Davis Heart Lung Research Institute, The Ohio State University, Columbus, OH 43212, USA

Ramesh Gupta James Graham Brown Cancer Center, University of Louisville, Louisville, KY 40202, USA; Department of Pharmacology and Toxicology, University of Louisville, Louisville, KY 40202, USA

Chuanshu Huang Nelson Institute of Environmental Medicine, New York University School of Medicine, Tuxedo, NY 10987, USA

Pu Jing Institute of Food and Nutraceutical Science, School of Agriculture and Biology, Shanghai Jiao Tong University, Shanghai 200240, P.R. China

Naghma Khan Department of Dermatology, University of Wisconsin, Madison, WI 53706, USA

Thomas J. Knobloch Division of Environmental Health Sciences, College of Public Health, The Ohio State University, Columbus, OH 43210, USA

Laura A. Kresty Department of Epidemiology and Public Health, Miller School of Medicine, University of Miami Sylvester Cancer Center, Miami, FL 33136, USA

Haonan Li Department of Pathology, Northwestern University Feinberg School of Medicine, Chicago, IL 60611, USA

Jie Liao Department of Pathology, Northwestern University Feinberg School of Medicine, Chicago, IL 60611, USA

Susan R. Mallery Division of Oral Maxillofacial Surgery, Pathology and Anesthesiology, College of Dentistry, The Ohio State University, Columbus, OH 43210, USA

Edward Martin Department of Surgery, The Ohio State University College of Medicine, Columbus, OH 43210, USA

Hasan Mukhtar Department of Dermatology, University of Wisconsin, Madison, WI 53706, USA

Catherine C. Neto Department of Chemistry and Biochemistry, University of Massachusetts Dartmouth, North Dartmouth, MA 02747, USA

Tatiana Oberyszyn Department of Pathology, The Ohio State University, Columbus, OH 43201, USA

Dennis Pearl Department of Statistics, The Ohio State University, Columbus, OH 43210, USA

Srivani Ravoori James Graham Brown Cancer Center, University of Louisville, Louisville, KY 40202, USA

Christine Sardo Comprehensive Cancer Center, The Ohio State University College of Medicine, Columbus, OH 43210, USA

Claire M. Seguin Comprehensive Cancer Center, The Ohio State University College of Medicine, Columbus, OH 43210, USA

Chandan K. Sen Department of Surgery, Davis Heart Lung Research Institute, The Ohio State University, Columbus, OH 43212, USA

Gary D. Stoner Department of Medicine, Medical College of Wisconsin, Milwaukee, WI 53226, USA

Meng Tong Division of Oral Maxillofacial Surgery, Pathology and Anesthesiology, College of Dentistry, The Ohio State University, Columbus, OH 43210, USA

Li-Shu Wang Comprehensive Cancer Center, The Ohio State University College of Medicine, Columbus, OH 43210, USA

Shiow Y. Wang Genetic Improvement of Fruits and Vegetables Lab, US Department of Agriculture, ARS, Beltsville, MD 20705, USA

Christopher M. Weghorst Division of Environmental Health Sciences, College of Public Health, The Ohio State University, Columbus, OH 43210, USA

Allison Yang Department of Pathology, Northwestern University Feinberg School of Medicine, Chicago, IL 60611, USA

Guang-Yu Yang Department of Pathology, Northwestern University Feinberg School of Medicine, Chicago, IL 60611, USA

Bree Zeyzus-Johns Department of Epidemiology and Public Health, Miller School of Medicine, University of Miami Sylvester Cancer Center, Miami, FL 33136, USA

WanYing Zhang Department of Pathology, Northwestern University Feinberg School of Medicine, Chicago, IL 60611, USA

Part I
Berry Composition, Bioavailability, Metabolism and Biological Effects

Chapter 1
Contribution of Berry Anthocyanins to Their Chemopreventive Properties

Pu Jing and M. Monica Giusti

Abstract Interest in berry fruits has intensified worldwide because of the multiple health-promoting phytochemicals present. Anthocyanins represent a major class of phytochemicals present in most colorful berries, and are of interest to nutritionists because of their postulated health benefits, as well as to food processors because of their colorful character and their use as natural colorants. This chapter presents an overview of the role of anthocyanins in the chemoprotective effects of berries. We will review incidence of anthocyanins in berries, their chemistry and concentration, as well as the reported literature regarding *in vitro* and *in vivo* chemoprotective studies, structure/chemoprotection relationship, bioavailability, and the interaction of berry anthocyanins with other phytochemicals. The data presented suggests that anthocyanins play a major role in the chemoprotective effects of many berry fruits.

Keywords Berry · Anthocyanin · Concentration · Structure · Chemoprevention · Bioavailability · Interaction effect · Structure-bioactivity relationship

1 Introduction

Berries are popularly consumed in North America both in fresh or frozen forms and in a variety of processed foods such as yogurts, beverages, jams, canned fruits, jellies, et al. Recently, interest in berry fruits has intensified around the world because of the multiple health-promoting phytochemicals found in berries. Berry extracts are being commercialized as nutraceuticals and as dietary supplements to meet consumers' demands.

M.M. Giusti (✉)
Department of Food Science and Technology, The Ohio State University, Columbus, OH 43210, USA
e-mail: giusti.6@osu.edu

G.D. Stoner, N.P. Seeram (eds.), *Berries and Cancer Prevention*,
DOI 10.1007/978-1-4419-7554-6_1, © Springer Science+Business Media, LLC 2011

Anthocyanins represent one of major phytochemicals present in most colorful berries and are of interest to nutritionists because of their postulated health benefits, as well as to food processors because of their colorful character as a natural alternative to the use of synthetic dyes. This chapter will present an overview of the incidence of anthocyanins in berries, their chemistry and concentration, as well as the reported literature regarding in vitro and in vivo chemoprotective studies, structure/chemoprotection relationship, bioavailability, and the interaction of berry anthocyanins with other phytochemicals.

2 Incidence of Anthocyanins in Berries

Anthocyanins are responsible for most of the wonderful orange-red, red, purple, blue and even some deep black colors in berries. Visual appearance of fresh and processed berries is the first factor influencing acceptability and quality perception regarding flavor and texture by consumers. Anthocyanin-rich berries and anthocyanin pigments from berry fruits have been suggested as potential chemoprotective agents, and a large and growing body of evidence from in-vitro cell culture studies, in-vivo animal model tumor systems, as well as human epidemiological studies. However, color appearance and cancer preventive properties are closely associated with the concentration of the pigments as well as their chemical structures. Therefore, accurate data about anthocyanin content and distribution in berry fruits are important. The most commonly consumed berry fruits in North America include strawberries, blueberries, cranberries, red raspberries, blackberries, and black raspberries (Strik, 2007). In the following sections, we will discuss the types and concentration of anthocyanins in those berries and in other less common berries of growing interest.

2.1 Types of Anthocyanins Found in Berries

Anthocyanins belong to the class of flavonoid compounds and are commonly known as plant polyphenols. The anthocyanin pigments consist of two or three main chemical units: the flavylium ring or aglycone base (anthocyanidin), sugars, and sometimes acylating groups. Anthocyanidins present the basic structure of a C6-C3-C6 carbon skeleton typical of flavonoids. They are polyhydroxy and polymethoxy derivatives of 2-phenylbenzoprylium or flavylium salts, differing in the number and position of their hydroxyl and methoxyl groups on the B ring (Fig. 1.1). There are 27 known anthocyanidins present in nature (Andersen and Jordheim, 2005), however, only six (cyanidin, pelargonidin, peonidin, delphinidin, petunidin, and malvidin) are commonly found in berries (Giusti and Jing, 2007). One of the unusual anthocyanidin structures found in berries was a 4-substituted aglycone, recently found in strawberries (*Fragaria* × *ananassa* Duch.), a 5-carboxypryanopelargonidin 3- *O*- ß-glucopyranoside, although present only in small concentrations (Andersen et al., 2004).

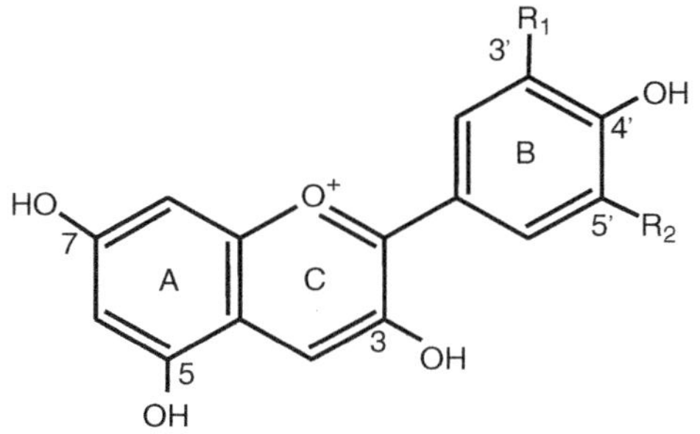

Pelargonidin	R_1=H	R_2=H
Cyanidin	R_1=OH	R_2=H
Delphinidin	R_1=OH	R_2=OH
Peonidin	R_1=OCH_3	R_2=H
Petunidin	R_1=OCH_3	R_2=OH
Malvidin	R_1=OCH_3	R_2= OCH_3

Fig. 1.1 Chemical structures of anthocyanidins commonly found in berries

Anthocyanidins rarely occur in their free form in nature because of their high reactivity. Anthocyanins are mainly glycosylated with one or more sugar moieties that enhance their stability and solubility (Harborne, 1979; Clifford, 2000; Giusti and Wrolstad, 2003). The most common sugar moieties found attached to the aglycone is glucose (Table 1.1), followed by galactose, rhamnose, xylose, arabinose. Anthocyanins can be glycosylated with one or more sugar units, typically up to 3, with some rare exceptions. The C_3-hydroxyl position of the C-ring is the primary place for glycosylation, followed by the C_5 position of the A ring (Fig. 1.1). Less common sites of glycosylations are the C_7 position, and in rare cases, glycosylation has been reported on the B ring.

Although not common in berries, some anthocyanins may be acylated. Acylated anthocyanins have acids attached to the sugar moiety, either aliphatic (such as acetic or malonic) acids or aromatic (such as *p*-coumaric or caffeic) acids. Acylated anthocyanins have been reported in boysenberries and marionberries.

Different combinations of types and numbers of sugars and/or acids attached to the different type of aglycons lead to a wide range of different anthocyanins found in berries. However, the most predominant berry anthocyanin is cyanidin-3-glucoside. The anthocyanin composition in berries (Table 1.1) has been used as a botanical tool for taxonomic classification of plants, as the anthocyanin profile tends to be characteristic of a plant, similar to a fingerprint. Anthocyanin profiles vary largely among different species but tend to remain quite similar within the same species. Some profiles are rather simple, such as the cases of strawberry, where 80–90% of the pigment composition is just one pigment, pelaronidin-3-glucoside. Other berries are characterized for their complex anthocyanin profiles, such as *Vaccinium corymbosum* commonly known as highbush blueberries that exhibit 5 of the different aglycones (cy, dp, pt, mv and pn), 3 different glycosylating sugars (glu, gal, and ara), and also exhibit some acylated derivatives of these anthocyanins – the acetylated monoglycosides. The most widespread anthocyanin in berries is cyanidin 3-glucoside. Differential anthocyanin profiles can be also used for the detection of adulteration in specific commodities of berry fruit products.

Table 1.1 Anthocyanins composition in common berries

Scientific name	Common name	Anthocyanin composition	References
Caprifoliaceae			
Sambucus canadensis L.	Common elderberry	**Cy 3-(6″-*p*-coumaryl-2″-xyl)-(1→2)glc-5-glc**; Cy 3-sam-5-glc; Cy 3,5-diglc; Cy 3-sam; Cy 3-glu; Cy 3-(6″-*p*- coumaryl -2-xyl)-glu-5-glu; Cy 3-(6″-*p*-coumaryl-2″-xyl)- (1→2)glc	Inami et al. (1996)
Sambucus nigra L.	Elderberry	**Cy 3-sam;Cy 3-glc**; Cy 3-sam-5-glc; Cy 3,5-diglc;Cy 3-rut; Pg 3-glc; Pg 3-sam	Inami et al. (1996), Wu et al. (2004)
Elaeocarpaceae			
Aristotelia chilensis (Mol.) Stuntz	Maquei/macqui	Dp 3-sam-5-glc; Dp 3-glc; Dp 3,5-diglc; Dp 3-sam; Cy 3-sam-5-glc; Cy 3-glc; Cy 3,5-diglc; Cy 3-sam	Escribano-Bailón et al. (2006)
Ericaceae			
Vaccinium angustifolium Aiton	Lowbush blueberry	Dp 3-gal; Dp 3-glc; Cy 3-gal; Dp 3-ara; Cy 3-glc; Pt 3-gal; Cy 3-ara; Pt 3-glc; Pn 3-gal; Pt 3-ara; Pn 3-glc; Mv 3-gal;	Wu and Prior (2005)
Vaccinium arctostaphylos L.	Caucasian whortleberry	Dp 3-glc; Pt 3-glc; Mv 3-glc	Nickavar and Amin (2004)
Vaccinium ashei Reade cv. Tifblue	Rabbiteye blueberry/ smallflower blueberry	Dp-3-gal; Dp-3-glc; Cy-3-gal; Dp-3-ara; Cy-3-glc; Pt-3-gal; Pt-3-glc; Pn-3-gal; Pt-3-ara; Mv-3-gal; Mv-3-glc; Pn-3-ara; Mv-3-ara	Prior et al. (2001)
Vaccinium corymbosum cv. Bluecrop	Highbush blueberry	Dp 3-gal; Dp 3-glc; Cy 3-gal; Dp 3-ara; Cy 3-glc; Pt 3-gal; Cy 3-ara; Pt 3-glc; Pn 3-gal; Pt 3-ara; Mv 3-gal; Mv 3-glc; Pn 3-ara; Mv 3-ara; Dp 3-(acetyl)-glc; Pt 3-(acetyl)-glc; Mv 3-(acetyl)-glc	Cho et al. (2004)
Vaccinium macrocarpon Aiton.	American cranberry	**Cy 3-gal; Cy 3-ara; Pn 3-gal; Pn 3-ara**; Cy 3-glc; Pt 3-gal **Cy 3-gal; Cy 3-ara; Pn 3-gal; Pn 3-ara**; Cy 3-glc; Pn 3-glc; Dp 3-gal; Dp 3-glc	Prior et al. (2001) Huopalahti et al. (2000)

Table 1.1 (continued)

Scientific name	Common name	Anthocyanin composition	References
Vaccinium membranaceum Douglas ex Torr.	Thinleaf huckleberry	Dp 3-gal; Dp 3-glc; Dp 3-ara; Cy 3-gal; Cy 3-glc; Pt 3-gal; Cy 3-ara; Pt 3-glc; Pn 3-gal; Pt 3-ara; Mv 3-gal; Pn 3-glc; Pn 3-ara; Mv 3-glc; Mv 3-ara	Lee et al. (2004)
Vaccinium myrtillus L.	Bilberry/Whortleberry	**Dp 3-glc; Cy 3-gal; Cy 3-ara; Pt 3-glc; Mv 3- glc; Dp 3-gal; Dp 3-ara; Pt 3-gal; Pt 3-ara; Mv 3-gal; Mv 3-ara**; Pn 3-gal; Pn 3-ara	Kähkönen et al. (2003)
		Cy 3-ara; Cy 3-gal; Cy 3-glc; Dp 3-ara; Dp 3-gal; Dp 3-glc; Pt 3-ara; Pt 3-gal; Pt 3-glc; Pn 3-gal; Pn 3-glc; Mv 3-ara; Mv 3-gal; Mv 3- glc; Pn 3-ara	Dugo et al. (2001)
Vaccinium ovatum Pursh	California huckleberry	Dp 3-gal; Dp 3-glc; Dp 3-ara; Cy 3-gal; Cy 3-glc; Pt 3-gal; Cy 3-ara; Pt 3-glc; Pn 3-gal; Pt 3-ara; Mv 3-gal; Pn 3-glc; Pn 3-ara; Mv 3-glc; Mv 3-ara	Lee et al. (2004)
		Cy 3-glc; Pn 3-glc; Cy 3-gal; Cy 3-ara; Dp 3-glc; Pn 3-glc; Pn 3-ara; Pt 3-glc; Mv 3-glc	Andersen (1989)
Vaccinium oxycoccus L.	Small Cranberry	Cy 3-gal; Cy 3-glc; Cy 3-ara; Pn 3-gal; Pn 3-glc; Pn 3-ara; Dp 3-glc; Dp 3-gal	Huopalahti et al. (2000)
Vaccinium uliginosum L.	Bog blueberry/Bog whortleberry	**Mv 3-glc; Mv 3-ara; Mv 3-gal; Dp 3-glc; Dp 3-ara; Dp 3-gal; Cy 3-glc; Cy 3-ara; Cy 3-gal; Pt 3-glc; Pt 3-ara; Pt 3- gal: Pn 3-glc**; Pn 3-ara; Pn 3-gal	Andersen (1987)
Vaccinium vitis-idaea L.	Lingonberry/mountain cranberry/cowberry	**Cy 3-gal; Cy 3-ara; Cy 3-glc**; Dp 3-glc	Andersen (1985), Kähkönen et al. (2003)
Grossulariaceae			
Ribes uva-crispa	Gooseberry	**Cy 3-glc, Cy 3-rut, Cy 3-(6″-** *p*- coumaryl)**-glc**; Pn 3-glc; Pn 3-rut; Cy 3-xyl; Cy 3-(6″-caffeoyl)-glc	Wu et al. (2004)

Table 1.1 (continued)

Scientific name	Common name	Anthocyanin composition	References
Ribes nigrum	Black currant	**Dp 3-glc; Dp 3-rut; Cy 3-glc; Cy 3-rut**; Pt 3-glc; Pg 3-glc; Pt 3-rut; Pn 3-glc; Dp 3-xyl; Pg 3-rut; Pn 3-rut; Cy 3-xyl; Pt 3-(6″-*p*-coumaryl)-glc; Cy 3-(6″- *p*-coumaryl)-glc	Kähkönen et al. (2003), Wu et al. (2004), Slimestad et al. (2005)
Ribes × *Pallidum*	Red currant	Cy 3-(2″-glc)-rut; Cy 3-sam; Cy 3-glc; Cy 3-(2″-xyl)-rut; Cy 3-rut	Maatta et al. (2003)
Ribes rubrum cv. Red lake	Cultivated currant	Cy 3-(xyl)-rut; Cy 3-rut; Cy 3-sam; Dp 3-sam; Cy 3-soph; Cy 3-(glc)-rut; Cy 3-glc	Goiffon et al. (1991), Wu et al. (2004)
Lauraceae			
Laurus nobilis L.	Sweet bay	**Cy 3-glc; Cy 3-rut**; Pn 3-glc; Pn 3-rut	Longo and Vasapollo (2005)
Moraceae			
Morus nigra L.	Mulberry	Cy 3-soph; **Cy 3-glc; Cy 3-rut**; Pg 3-glc; Pg 3-rut	Dugo et al. (2001)
Myrtaceae			
Eugenia umbelliflora O.Berg	Baguaçu	Dp 3-glc; Cy 3-glc; Pt 3-glc; Pg 3-glc; Pn 3-glc; Mv 3-glc	Kuskoski et al. (2003)
Rhamnaceae			
Rhamnus alaternus L.	Italian buckthorn	**Dp 3-rut; Pt-3-rut; Cy 3-rut**; Pn 3-rut; Mv 3-rut; Pg 3-rut	Longo et al. (2005)
Rosaceae			
Amelanchier alnifolia Nutt.	Saskatoon	Cy-3,5-diglc; **Cy-3-gal; Cy-3-glc; Cy-3-ara; Cy-3-xyl** **Cy 3-gal; Cy 3-glc; Cy 3-ara; Cy 3-xyl**; Pg 3-ara; Pg 3-gal	Bakowska-Barczak and Kolodziejczyk (2008) Oszmianski and Sapis (1988), Wu et al. (2004)

Table 1.1 (continued)

Scientific name	Common name	Anthocyanin composition	References
Fragaria × ananassa D. cv. Camarosa.	Strawberry	**Pg 3-glc**; Pg 3- rut; Pg 3-ara; Pg 3-(malonyl)-glc; Pg 3-acetyl-glc; Pg 3-(succinyl)-glc; Cy 3-glc; Cy 3-rut; Cy 3-(malony)-glc-5-glc; 5-carboxypryanopelargonidin 3-glc	Fiorini (1995), Lopes-da-Silva et al. (2002), Andersen et al. (2004), Maatta-Riihinen et al. (2004)
Rubus glaucus Benth.	Andes berry	Cy 3-sam; Cy 3-glc; Cy 3-xylorutinoside, Cy 3-rut; Pg 3-glc; Pg 3-rut	Garzón et al. (2009)
Rubus idaeus L cv. Glen Ample.	Red raspberry	Cy-3-soph; Cy-3-(2″–glc)-(1→2)rut; Cy-3-glc; Pg-3-soph; Cy-3-rut; Pg-3-(2 ″-glc)- (1→2)rut; Pg-3-glc; Pg-3-rut	Mullen et al. (2002)
Rubus laciniatus	Cutleaf blackberry/ Evergreen blackberry	Cy 3-glc; Cy 3-ara; Cy 3-(6″-malonyl)-glc	Wada and Ou (2002)
Rubus occidentalis L.	Black raspberry	**Cy 3-glc; Cy 3-sam; Cy 3-(xyl)-rut; Cy 3-rut**; Pg 3-rut	Tian et al. (2006)
Rubus spp.	Blackberry	Cy 3-gal; Cy 3-glc; Cy 3-ara; Cy 3-xyl; Mv 3- glc; Pg 3-glc	Dugo et al. (2001)
Rubus ursinus	Marionberry	Cy 3-(6″-*p*-coumaryl)-glc; Cy 3-(6″-malonyl)-glc	Wada and Ou (2002)
Rubus ursinus × idaeus	Boysenberry	Cy 3-(6″-*p*-coumaryl)-glc-5-glc; Cy 3-glc Cy 3-soph; Cy 3-glc-rut; Cy 3-glc; Cy 3-rut	Wada and Ou (2002) McGhie et al. (2002)

Individual anthocyanins in bold font are major components in anthocyanin profile.
Abbreviations: Cyanidin (Cy); Delphinidin (Dp); Pelargonidin (Pg); Peonidin (Pn); Petunidin (Pt); Malvidin (Mv); Arabinoside (ara); Diglcuoside (diglc); Galactoside (gal); Glucoside (glc); Xyloside (xyl); Diglucoside (diglc); Rutinoside (rut); Sambubioside (sam); Sophoroside (soph).
Adapted from Giusti and Jing (2007) with updated information.

2.2 Anthocyanin Concentration in Berries

Anthocyanin concentration in berries can be affected by many different factors: the species, cultivar, growing conditions and maturity are all factors that will affect anthocyanin content in the fruit. Quantitative data presented on Table 1.2 is a summary of available literature and measured for the most part on mature, ready to eat berries, grown under typical commercial conditions. For instance, anthocyanin concentration in black chokeberries (*Aronia melanocarpa* [Michx] Elliot) reached up to 1458 mg/100 g fresh weight (Wu et al., 2004), whereas anthocyanins are not detectable in berries such as red currant (*Ribes* × *Pallidum cv.* White Duch) (Maatta-Riihinen et al., 2004) and gooseberry (*Ribes uva-crispa* cv. Careless) (Wu et al., 2004). Berries known for their typical high concentration of anthocyanins are black raspberries, blackberries and chokeberries. Recently, a berry from the South American Andes has been reported to present anthocyanins in concentrations up to 7% of dry fruit weight. Within the same species, anthocyanin content may differ with cultivars, as well as growing seasons and conditions. The same cultivar even has different values of anthocyanin concentration mainly due to analytic technology applied in different literatures. Researchers from different groups reported that anthocyanins concentration of black currant (*Ribes nigrum* cv. Ojebyn) varied several fold from 165 to 412 mg/g fresh weight (FW). Except differences of growing location and conditions, the reported anthocyanin content of black currant (*Ribes nigrum* cv. Ojebyn) was affected by the extraction method used, evaluation assays (colormetric method or HPLC analysis), anthocyanin equivalents or standards used for quantification (Kampuse et al., 2002; Moyer et al., 2002; Kähkönen et al., 2003; Maatta et al., 2003; Maatta-Riihinen et al., 2004). In Table 1.2, the anthocyanin content of berries is marked clearly by quantitative analytic assays (pH differential method or HPLC method) and equivalents or standards (cyanidin 3- glucoside, cyanidin 3-galactoside, pelargonidin 3- glucoside, malvidin 3- glucoside, delphinidin 3- glucoside, etc.). Increased concentration of anthocyanins in berries intensifies their color and occasionally very high concentration results in a very dark color with berries appearing "black" despite the fact that the pigments are indeed red to purple, such as in the case of blackberries, black raspberries and black chokeberries.

3 Anthocyanin Chemoprotective Effects: In Vitro Studies

Anthocyanins have been shown to exhibit anticarcinogenic activity against multiple cancer cell types in vitro, and the mechanism of action seems to be rather complex. Interest in the health benefits of these compounds derives from finding of their potent antioxidant capacity. Many studies have tried to determine the contribution of berry anthocyanins to the reduced incidence of chronic diseases associated with fruit and vegetable consumption. However, there have been multiple mechanisms of action proposed for anthocyanin compounds, and it is likely that more than one mechanism is taking place at a time.

Table 1.2 Anthocyanins concentration in common berries

Scientific name	Common name	Cultivar	Anthocyanins (mg/100 g FW)	References
Caprifoliaceae				
Sambucus nigra L.	Elderberry	n.s.[a]	*332*[b,c];**1374**[b,d,e]	Maatta-Riihinen et al. (2004), Wu et al. (2004)
Elaeocarpaceae				
Aristotelia chilensis (Mol.) Stuntz	Maquei/macqui	n.s.	138[b,f]	Escribano-Bailón et al. (2006)
Empetraceae				
Empetrum nigrum L.	Black crowberry	n.s.	409[b,c]	Maatta-Riihinen et al. (2004)
E. nigrum ssp. Hermaphroditum		n.s.	768[b,c]	Maatta-Riihinen et al. (2004)
Ericaceae				
Vaccinium angustifolium Aiton	Lowbush blueberry	*Blomidin*, **Lowbush**[g]	*91*, **95–180**[h,i]	Prior et al. (1998)
		Brunsweick	208[h,i]	Moyer et al. (2002)
		Cumberland	*103*[h,i]; **164**[h,i,e]	Prior et al. (1998), Connor et al. (2002)
		Fundy	*192*[h,i]; **234**[h,i]	Prior et al. (1998), Connor et al. (2002)
		Michigan lowbush, N70127, GR V.a, N7068, N70249, **N70145**	*128*, 174, 186, 202, 205, **209**[h,i]	Connor et al. (2002)
		n.s.	*170*[h,i]; **230**[h,j]	Prior et al. (2001), Kalt et al. (1999)

Table 1.2 (continued)

Scientific name	Common name	Cultivar	Anthocyanins (mg/100 g FW)	References
Vaccinium ashei Reade	Rabbiteye blueberry/smallflower blueberry	*Bluegem*, CVAC 200.003, CVAC 1161.001, **CVAC 1170.001**	*242*, 383, 484, **515**[h,i]	Moyer et al. (2002)
		Tifblue	*87-154*[h,i]; **220**[h,i]	Prior et al. (1998), (2001)
		Brightwell, Climax, **Little Giant**	*62-162*, 91, **187**[h,i]	Prior et al. (1998)
Vaccinium constablaei Gray	Mountain highbush blueberry	*N8426*, N8428, **N87014**	*168*, 211, **290**[h,i]	Connor et al. (2002)
Vaccinium corymbosum L	Highbush blueberry (northern high)	Aino	147[b,c]	Maatta-Riihinen et al. (2004)
		Bluecrop	*84*[h,i]; 93[h,i]; 120[h,i] **141**[h,j]	Moyer et al. (2002), Prior et al. (1998), Connor et al. (2002), Kalt et al. (1999)
		N70218, Bounty, B6, Nelson, B11, B1-1, B10, N86161, **Friendship**	*139*, 169, 181, 188, 190, 223, 240, 375, **383**[h,i]	Connor et al. (2002)
		Duke	*127*[h,i]; 173[h,i]; **274**[h,i]	Prior et al. (1998), Moyer et al. (2002), Connor et al. (2002)
		G-224, **Brigitta Blue**	*91*, **103**[h,i]	Moyer et al. (2002)
		Jersey	*101-116*[h,i]; **197**[h,i]	Prior et al. (1998), Connor et al. (2002)
		Croatan, Rancocas, **Rubel**	*118*, 141, **235**[h,i]	Prior et al. (1998)
Vaccinium corymbosum L	Highbush blueberry (southern high)	*Reveille*, O'Neal, Blue ridge, Bladen, **Cape fear**, **Pender**	*63*, 93, 110, 131, **157**, **157**[h,i]	Prior et al. (1998)
		Summit, G-344, Summit II, CVAC 24.001, CVAC 1057.001, CVAC 45.001, CVAC 25.001, CVAC 35.001; CVAC 23.001, **CVAC 5.00**	*73*, 101, 119, 224, 239, 279, 303, 304, 322, **430**[h,i]	Moyer et al. (2002)

Table 1.2 (continued)

Scientific name	Common name	Cultivar	Anthocyanins (mg/100 g FW)	References
Vaccinium constablaei × *Vaccinium ashei*	n.a.[k]	*MN494, 515, 676,* Chippewa, Patriot, Northsky, MN496, Northblue, MN455, MN61, MN497, R2P4, Polaris, St. Cloud, MN84, Bluetta, MN449, Noththcounty, Northland, Bluegold, N86158, MN452, **GR2**	*1, 1, 1,* 114, 156, 158, 162, 164, 165, 176, 194, 199, 202, 202, 210, 211, 214, 217, 240, 249, 280, 341, **428**[h,i]	Connor et al. (2002)
Vaccinium macrocarpon Aiton.	American cranberry	Ben lear	*25*[h,l]; **32**[h,i]	Wang and Stretch (2001), Zheng and Wang (2003)
		Cropper, Pilgrim, Stevens, Howes, Wilcox, #35, Franklin, Early black, **Crowley**	*20*, 21, 23, 24, 24, 29, 54, 63, **66**[h,l]	Wang and Stretch (2001)
		n.s.	360[h,i]	Prior et al. (2001)
Vaccinium membranaceum Douglas ex Torr.	Thinleaf huckleberry	n.s.	*116-153*[a,i]; **167**[h,i]	Moyer et al. (2002), Lee et al. (2004)
Vaccinium myrtilloides Michx.	Canadian blueberry/ Velvet-leaf blueberry	CVAC 19.001	298[h,i]	Moyer et al. (2002)
		N69180, **N70239**	*218*, **259**[h,i]	Connor et al. (2002)
Vaccinium myrtillus L.	Bilberry/Whortleberry	n.s.	*300*[h,i]; 600[b,d]; **808**[b,c]	Prior et al. (1998), Kähkönen et al. (2003), Maatta-Riihinen et al. (2004)

Table 1.2 (continued)

Scientific name	Common name	Cultivar	Anthocyanins (mg/100 g FW)	References
Vaccinium ovalifolium Sm.	Black huckleberry/ Oval-Leaf Blueberry	n.s.	266[h,i]	Moyer et al. (2002)
Vaccinium oxycoccus L.	Small Cranberry	n.s.	*78*[h,i]; **86**[b,c]	Andersen (1989), Maatta-Riihinen et al. (2004)
Vaccinium parvifolium Smith	Red huckleberry	n.s.	34[h,i]	Moyer et al. (2002)
Vaccinium uliginosum L.	Bog blueberry/Bog whortleberry	n.s.	*256*[b,j]; **261–432**[b,c]	Andersen (1987), Maatta-Riihinen et al. (2004)
Vaccinium vitis-idaea L.	Lingonberry/mountain cranberry/cowberry	Amberland	*45*[h,i]; **96**[h,i]	Zheng and Wang (2003), Wang et al. (2005)
		Sanna and Sussi	49–69[h]	Saario (2000)
		Sanna, Erntedank, Scarlett, Erntesegen, Koralle, European red, Red pearl, Splendor, Ida (8726-8), Koralle-German, **Sussi**	*31*, 38–57, 41, 52–57, 54–87, 55, 55–62, 56–60, 63, 64, **92**[h,i]	Wang et al. (2005)
		n.s.	68[b,d]	Kähkönen et al. (2003)
Grossulariaceae				
Ribes uva-crispa L.	Gooseberry	*Careless*, Dan's Mistake, **Lancashine**, **Whinham**	*0*, 2, **10**, **10**[b,d]	Wu et al. (2004)
		Hinnonmaki's yellow, **Hinnonmaki's red**	*0*, **24**[b,c]	Maatta-Riihinen et al. (2004)

Table 1.2 (continued)

Scientific name	Common name	Cultivar	Anthocyanins (mg/100 g FW)	References
Ribes grossularia × *Ribes oxyacanthoides*	Gooseberry hybrids	Captivator	14[h,i]	Moyer et al. (2002)
Ribes nidigrolaria Bauer	Jostaberries	n.s.	43–89[h,i]	Moyer et al. (2002)
Ribes nigrum L.	Black currant	Baldwin	*153*[h,i]; **186**[h,i]	Benvenuti et al. (2004), Moyer et al. (2002)
		Beloruskaja sladkaja	*157*[h,i]; **165**[h]	Moyer et al. (2002), Kampuse et al. (2002)
		Ben Alder	*240*[h]; **562**[b,d]	Kampuse et al. (2002), Wu et al. (2004)
		Ben Lomond	*206*[h,i]; 261[h,i]; **574**[b,d]	Benvenuti et al. (2004), Moyer et al. (2002), Wu et al. (2004)
		Ben Nevis	*252*[h,i]; **587**[b,d]	Moyer et al. (2002), Wu et al. (2004)
		Ojebyn	*165*[h,i]; 180[h]; 236[b,d]; 301[b,c]; **412**[b,c]	Moyer et al. (2002), Kampuse et al. (2002), Kähkönen et al. (2003), Maatta et al. (2003), Maatta-Riihinen et al. (2004)
		Tsema	*180*[h,i]; **261**[h,i]	Moyer et al. (2002), Benvenuti et al. (2004)
		Titania	*281*[h,i]; **360**[b,d]	Moyer et al. (2002), Wu et al. (2004)
		Lentjai, Stella II, Sanjuta, Selechens kaja, Viuchiai, Pileniai, Vernisaz, Joniniai, Almiai, Chornij kenravr, **Laimiai**	*96*, 165, 172, 173, 188, 205, 221, 226, 242, 253, **267**[h]	Kampuse et al. (2002)
		Silvergieters, Tenah, Noir De Bourgogne, **Burga**	*202*, 224, 229, **281**[h,i]	Benvenuti et al. (2004)

Table 1.2 (continued)

Scientific name	Common name	Cultivar	Anthocyanins (mg/100 g FW)	References
		Slitsa, Hystawneznaja Minaj smyriov, Ben conan, Alagan, Kantata, Risager, Wassil, Kantata 50, Pinot deboir, Polar, Blackdown, Neosyspujastaja, Kosmiczeskaja, Coronet Boskoop, Nikkala XI, Nikkala XI, Dosz siberjoczk, Kirovchanka Tunnaja, Willoughby, Strata, Crusader, Silvergieters, Zwarte, **Consort**	*128*, 156, 158, 162, 169, 180, 181, 199, 207, 208, 213, 216, 220, 220, 221, 231, 240, 257, 257, 259, 263, 275, 275, 298, 319, 346, **411**[h,i]	Moyer et al. (2002)
		Ukraine, **Ben tirran**	*323*, **452**[b,d]	Wu et al. (2004)
		n.s.	350[i]	Lister et al. (2002)
Ribes odoratum Wendland	Buffalo currant	Crandall	273[h,i]	Moyer et al. (2002)
Ribes × Pallidum	Red currant	Red Dutch	*18*[b,c]; **21**[b,c]	Maatta et al. (2003), Maatta-Riihinen et al. (2004)
		White Dutch	0[b,c]	Maatta-Riihinen et al. (2004)
Ribes rubrum L.	Cultivated currant	*Rosetta*, Red lake, **Rotet**	*22*, 23, **34**[h,i]	Benvenuti et al. (2004)
Myrtaceae				
Eugenia umbelliflora O.Berg	Baguaçu	n.s.	342[b,m]	Kuskoski et al. (2003)
Rosaceae				
Amelanchier alnifolia Nutt.	Saskatoon	n.s.	139[b,i] (conversion from 562 mg/100 g on dry weight)	Hosseinian and Beta (2007)

Table 1.2 (continued)

Scientific name	Common name	Cultivar	Anthocyanins (mg/100 g FW)	References
		Smokey, Pearson, Lee2, Pembina, Parkhill, Success, Quaker, Honeywood, Forestburg, Pasture, Thiessen, Lee8, Regent, Northline, Lee3, Martin, **Nelson**	190, 190, 195, 199, 200, 204, 205, 253, 266, 274, 275, 276, 291, 293, 320, 342, **382**[b,m]	Bakowska-Barczak and Kolodziejczyk (2008)
Aronia melanocarpa (Michx.) Elliot	Black chokeberry	Nero	461[h,i]	Benvenuti et al. (2004)
		Viking	842[b,c]	Maatta-Riihinen et al. (2004)
		Albigowa, Dabrowice, Egerta, Kutno, Nero, Nowa wies	440–574	Strik et al. (2003)
		n.s.	*307–631*; 428 [h,i]; 481 [b,l]; 750–950; **1480** [b,d]	Strigl et al. (1995), Zheng et and Wang (2003), Slimestad et al. (2005), Kaack and Kuhn (1992), Wu et al. (2004)
Grataegosorbus mitschurinii	Sweet rowanberry	Granatnaja	88[b,c]	Maatta-Riihinen et al. (2004)
Fragaria × *ananassa* D.	Strawberry	Allstar	*22*[h,i]; **23**[h,n]	Meyers et al. (2003), Wang and Lin (2000)
		Earliglow	*28*[h,i]; **45**[h,n]	Meyers et al. (2003), Wang and Lin (2000)
		Kent	8[h,j]	Kalt et al. (1999)
		Polka	42[h,n]	Klopotek et al. (2005)
		Campineiro, Toyonoka, Pajaro, Oso Grande, Dover, **Mazi**	*13*, 19, 21, 42, 52, **55**[h,n]	Cordenunsi et al. (2002)
		Latestar, Delmarvel, Red Chief, Mohawk, Lester, **Northeaster**	*25*, 26, 29, 32, 36, **39**[h,n]	Wang and Lin (2000)
		Sable, Jewel, Annapolis, Sparkle, Mesabi, **Evangelien**	*37*, 38, 39, 41, 44, **47**[h,i]	Meyers et al. (2003)

Table 1.2 (continued)

Scientific name	Common name	Cultivar	Anthocyanins (mg/100 g FW)	References
Prunus spinosa L.	Blackthorn	n.s.	54[b,c]	Maatta-Riihinen et al. (2004)
Rubus caucasicus Focke	n.a.	n.s.	33[h,i]	Deighton et al. (2000)
Rubus coreanus Miq.	n.a.	n.s.	11–34[h,i]	Deighton et al. (2000)
Rubus Cyri Juz	n.a.	n.s.	143[h,i]	Moyer et al. (2002)
Rubus fruticosus L.	Shrubby Blackberry	*Darrow,* Hull thornless, Black satin, Chester, Smoothstem, Black diamond, **Thornless Boy Sembes**	*67*, 69, 75, 76, 87, 119, **127**[h,i]	Benvenuti et al. (2004)
Rubus glaucus Benth.	Andes berry	n.s.	45	Garzón et al. (2009)
Rubus idaeus L.	Red raspberry	*Glen Ample*, Veten	*37*, **57**[h,i]	Haffner et al. (2002)
		Glen Lyon	39[h,i]	Deighton et al. (2000), Haffner et al. (2002)
		Nova	44[h,j]	Kalt et al. (1999)
		Anne, Kiwigold, Goldie, **Heritage**	< *1*, 3, 5, **58**[h,l]	Liu et al. (2002)
		Canby, Sentry, Autumn Bliss, **Summit**	*45*, 53, 75, **100**[h,i]	Wang and Lin (2000)
		Tulameen, Chilliwack, Comox, **Willamette**	*28–44*, 52–59, 63, **72**[h,l]	Burrows and Moore (2002)
		Zvjozdocka, Skromnica, Bulgarskij rubin, Rubin brjanskij, Norna, **Zuravlik**	*21*, 26, 29, 35, 42, **66**[h]	Kampuse et al. (2002)
		September, Sumner	29–41[h,i]	Benvenuti et al. (2004)
		n.s.	*28–75*[b,l]; **65**[h,i]	McGhie et al. (2002), Wada and Ou (2002)

Table 1.2 (continued)

Scientific name	Common name	Cultivar	Anthocyanins (mg/100 g FW)	References
Rubus laciniatus	Cutleaf or Evergreen blackberry	n.s.	91[h,i]	Wada and Ou (2002)
Rubus occidentalis L.	Black raspberry	Earlysweet	464[h,i]	Moyer et al. (2002)
		Jewel	*197*[h,i]; **607**[h,i]	Wang and Lin (2000), Moyer et al. (2002)
		Munger	627 h,i	Moyer et al. (2002)
		n.s.	*145–536*[h,l]; **589**[h,i]	McGhie et al. (2002), Wada and Ou (2002)
Rubus spp.	Blackberry	Chester thornless	153[h,i]	Wang and Lin (2000)
		Choctaw	*100–101*[h,j]; **114**[h,i]	Clark et al. (2002), Perkins-Veazie and Kalt (2002)
		Hull thornless	172[h,i]	Wang and Lin (2000)
		Navado	*111–185*[h,j]; **136**[h,i]	Clark et al. (2002), Perkins-Veazie and Kalt (2002)
		Shawnee	*122–128*[h,j]; **139**[h,i]	Clark et al. (2002), Perkins-Veazie and Kalt (2002)
		Triple Grown	*108 -176*[h,j]; **134**[h,i]	Clark et al. (2002), Wang and Lin (2000)
		APF-12, APF-8, A-1689, Chickasaw, A-1817, A-1942, Apache, A-1857, Kiowa, A-1963, A-2049, A-1960, A-1859, A-2005, **A-1905**	*72*, 85, 107, 113–124, 116, 121, 130, 131, 131–363, 132, 139, 143, 166, 175, **1208–1221**[h,j]	Clark et al. (2002)

Table 1.2 (continued)

Scientific name	Common name	Cultivar	Anthocyanins (mg/100 g FW)	References
Rubus ursinus	Marionberry	n.s.	*62–105*[h,i]; **155**[h,i]	Deighton et al. (2000), Wada and Ou (2002)
	Pacific dewberry	*G4-19*, **G4 bulk**	*206*, **211**[h,i]	Moyer et al. (2002)
Rubus ursinus × *idaeus*	Boysenberry	n.s.	*131*[h,i]; **210**[i]	Wada and Ou (2002), Lister et al. (2002)

[a]n.s.: none specified.
[b]HPLC method.
[c]Quantification based upon representative anthocyanidins as standards.
[d]Quantification based on representative anthocyanins as standards (Dp 3-glucoside, Cy 3-glucoside, Pt 3-glucoside, Pg 3-glucoside, Pn 3-glucoside, and Mv 3-glucoside).
[e]The same cultivar has different values of anthocyanin concentration mainly due to analytic technology applied in different literatures. The value of anthocyanin concentration in bold font is highest whereas the italic font being lowest in this cultivar or none-specified cultivars while the corresponding references are cited in same order.
[f]Quantification only based upon Dp 3-glucoside as standard.
[g]The value of anthocyanin concentration in bold font is highest whereas the italic font being lowest among the group of cultivars from the same literature and the corresponding cultivar shows the same front as its value of anthocyanin concentration.
[h]pH differential method.
[i]Quantification only based upon Cy 3-glucoside as standard.
[j]Quantification only based upon Mv 3-glucoside as standard.
[k]n.a.: none available.
[l]Quantification only based upon Cy 3-galactoside as standard.
[m]Quantification based upon extinction coefficients and molecular weights of every representative anthocyanin.
[n]Quantification only based upon Pg 3-glucoside as standard.
Adapted from Giusti and Jing (2007) with updated information.

3.1 Antioxidative Activity

Oxidative stress induced by free radicals causes DNA damage, including base mutation, single- and double-strand breaks, DNA cross-linking, chromosomal breakage and rearrangement. Those oxidative modifications at oncogenes, tumor-suppressing genes and DNA-repair genes may lead to carcinogenesis (Poulsen et al., 1998). The phenolic structure of anthocyanins is responsible for their high antioxidant activity as scavengers of reactive oxygen species (ROS), metal chelators and protein binders. Berry extracts or juices have been shown to exhibit high antioxidant capacity in numerous studies. In cell culture systems, berry anthocyanin extracts as well as pure anthocyanins have shown antioxidant activities on colon (Renis et al., 2008), intestinal (Elisia et al., 2007), endothelial (Youdim et al., 2000), liver (Shih et al., 2007), lung (Zhang et al., 2005), breast (Olsson et al., 2004; Singletary et al., 2007), leukemic (Dai et al., 2009), and brain cells (Hogan et al., 2010). The reported mechanisms for those cell culture systems could be categorized as directly scavenging ROS (Singletary et al., 2007), increasing the oxygen absorbing capacity of cells (Youdim et al., 2000), stimulating activation of phase II enzymes through antioxidant response element pathway (Shih et al., 2007; Singletary et al., 2007), developing anthocyanin-DNA copigmentation complex possible against oxidative damage of DNA (Sarma and Sharma, 1999), reducing the formation of DNA adducts (Jung et al., 2006; Singletary et al., 2007), and chelating metals and binding proteins (Kong et al., 2003; Dreiseitel et al., 2008). On the contrary, anthocyanidins produced ROS, showing pro-oxidant activities, as apoptosis inducers in HL-60 cells instead of the antioxidant activities of anthocyanidins in the inhibition of TPA-induced cell transformation in mouse skin JB6 cells (Hou et al., 2003, 2004b). In later studies, anthocyanins were found to induce apoptosis through reactive oxygen species-mediated mitochondrial pathway (Hou et al., 2005a; Feng et al., 2007).

3.2 Detoxification Activity

Carcinogens are activated by phase I enzymes and inactivated by phase II enzymes through a process called detoxification. The products from a typical phase I reaction are usually more reactive molecules than the parent molecules. If these reactive molecules are not further metabolized by phase II enzymes, they may react with DNA and develop DNA adducts, inducing carcinogenesis. Phase II enzymes include glutathione-S-transferases, UDP-glucuronosyl-transferase, Quinone reductase and others.

Concord grape juice, rich in anthocyanins, significantly inhibited in vivo mammary (7,12-dimethylbenz[a]anthracene) DMBA-DNA adduct formation by 34 and 56%, partially explained by highly increased liver activity of the phase II metabolizing enzyme (glutathione S-transferase) (Jung et al., 2006). Treatment of anthocyanins on rat liver Clone 9 cells demonstrated positive effects on elevating the antioxidant capacity by activating expression of phase II enzymes (glutathione reductase, glutathione peroxidase, and glutathione S-transferase) and promoting activity of NAD(P)H: quinone oxidoreductase (Shih et al., 2007). Therefore, Shih et al. (2007) concluded that the molecular mechanism was associated with the activation of antioxidant response elements upstream of genes that regulate the expression of phase II detoxification enzymes. However, the crude extracts, anthocyanin and proanthocyanidin fractions of four *Vaccinium* species (lowbush blueberry, bilberry, cranberry, and lingonberry) were not found to be highly active to induce quinone reductase (QR) that belongs to phase II detoxification enzymes while the ethyl acetate extracts were active QR inducers in vitro (Bomser et al., 1996).

3.3 Antiproliferation

One of the hallmarks of cancer is their acquired ability of over-proliferation (Evan and Vousden, 2001). The antiproliferative effects of berry anthocyanin-rich extracts and pure anthocyanins from variable berries have been studied on multiple cancer cell types. Among the berries studied are raspberry (*Rubus idaeus* L.) (Han et al., 2005; Liu et al., 2002; Olsson et al., 2004), strawberry (*Fragaria* × *ananassa* Duch,) (Sun et al., 2002; Meyers et al., 2003), black chokeberry (*Aronia melon-carpa* E) (Olsson et al., 2004; Zhao et al., 2004), black currant (*Ribes nigrum* L.) (Olsson et al., 2004), lingonberry (*Vaccinium vitis-idae* L.) (Olsson et al., 2004), bilberry (*Vaccinium myrtillus* L.) (Katsube et al., 2003; Zhao et al., 2004), cranberry (*Vaccinium macrocarpon* Ait.) (Sun et al., 2002; Seeram et al., 2004), blueberry (*Vaccinium corymbosum* L.) (Olsson et al., 2004; Seeram et al., 2006).

Although difficult to compare due to the differences in the experimental approaches, it can be observed that different species and cultivars of berries show different cell antiproliferative activity. The ethanol anthocyanin-rich extract from bilberry was found to be more effective than those from lowbush blueberry (*Vaccinium angustifolium*), highbush blueberry (*Vaccinium corymbosum*), cranberry, raspberry, strawberry, black currant, red currant (*Ribes sativum*), cowberry (*Vaccinium vitis-idaea*), etc (Katsube et al., 2003). In this study, the bilberry anthocyanin-rich extract inhibited the growth of HL60 cells and HCT116 cells by 84 and 97% respectively at 4 mg dry wt/mL. Different cultivars of blueberries were also tested for their inhibitory effects on HT-29 and CaCo-2 cells. As a result, the cultivar Briteblue showed the highest potential inhibition than Tifblue and Powderblue (Yi et al., 2005).

Selective carcinoma cell antiproliferation of anthocyanins has been shown in a few studies. Several studies have shown that the inhibition of cell proliferation by anthocyanins or anthocyanin-rich extracts was more pronounced on carcinoma cells than on immortalized normal cells. Zhao et al. (2004) found that anthocyanin-rich extracts inhibited the growth of HT29 cells with little or no effects on normal colonic cell growth when added to the media in the same concentrations. In another study, flavonoid fractions of a red grape wine showed their selective cytotoxicity on MCF-7 cells with relatively low effect towards normal human mammary epithelial cells (HMEC) and non-tumorigenic MCF-10A cells (Hakimuddin et al., 2004).

Hakimuddin et al. (2004) proposed that the mechanism was related to the interference of flavonoids with calcium second messenger function since the efficiency of cell antiproliferation by flavonoid fractions was associated with their inhibition of calcium and calmodulin-promoted phosphodiesterase activity. Stoner and coworkers (2008) found that the ethanol extract of black rasberries selectively inhibited the growth and stimulated apoptosis of a tumor rat esophageal epithelial cells but not the low tumorigenic precursor line. They also found that the uptake of anthocyanins was 100-fold higher in the highly tumorigenic cells than in the low tumorigenic precursor line and remained at steady state levels for 12 h (Wang and Stoner, 2008).

The mechanisms behind those chemopreventive effects of anthocyanins need to be considered at the molecular level. Anthocyanin inhibition of cancer cell growth involve blockage of various stages of the cell cycle, which are related to variable cell cycle regulator proteins (p53, p21, p27, cyclin D1, cyclin A, etc.) (Malik et al., 2003; Martin et al., 2003; Chen et al., 2005). For instance, the human HT-29 colon cancer cells treated with anthocyanin-rich extract from chokeberries (*Aronia meloncarpa* E.) showed a blockage at G1/G0 and G2/M phases of the cell cycle through an increased expression of the p21WAF1 and p27KIP1 genes and decreased expression of cyclin A and B genes (Malik et al., 2003).

Besides targeting cell cycle arrest, inhibition of cancer cell growth could also be evaluated by blocking other signal transduction pathways such as epidermal growth factor receptor (EGFR) and the mitogen activation protein kinases (MAPK). The transcription factor activator protein 1 (AP-1) plays an important role in carcinogenesis by activating transcription of genes involved in cell proliferation (Angel and Karin, 1991).

Lingonberry anthocyanin extracts effectively targeted signaling transduction pathways by blocking phosphorylation of the MAPK signaling members ERK1, ERK2 p38, and MEK1/2 induced by either 12-O-tetradecanoylphorbol-13-acetate or ultraviolet-B and as a result suppressed the activation of AP-1 and nuclear factor-κB (NF-κB) in JB6 mouse epidermal cells (Wang et al., 2005). In another study, anthocyanidins contributed to the inhibition of tumorigenesis by blocking activation of the MAPK pathway (Hou et al., 2004).

3.4 Apoptosis Induction

In addition to the uncontrolled cell proliferation, resistance to apoptosis (programmed cell death) is another important hallmark of cancer cells. Therefore, both proliferation and apoptosis of cells are critical points to target for chemoprevention of fruits and vegetables (Evan and Vousden, 2001). Anthocyanin-rich extracts from berries or pure anthocyanins have exhibited as inducers of apoptosis in variable premalignant and malignant cells in vitro (Katsube et al., 2003; Fimognari et al., 2004; Chen et al., 2005; Shih et al., 2005; Seeram et al., 2006; Yi et al., 2006; Feng et al., 2007; Hafeez et al., 2008).

Hou et al. (2005) found that delphinidin 3-sambubioside induced apoptosis in human leukemia cells through a reactive oxygen species (ROS)-mediated mitochondrial pathway. In another study, cyanidin-3-rutinoside isolated from the black raspberry induced apoptosis selectively towards HL-60 cells in a dose- and time-dependent manner through ROS-dependent activation of p38 MAPK and JNK, which contributed to cell death by activating the mitochondrial pathway without cytotoxic effects on normal cells (Feng et al., 2007).

Cyanidin-3-glucoside induced apoptosis in two human leukemia cell lines through modulation of p53 and bax protein expression (Fimognari et al., 2004). Cyanidin 3-glucoside and peonidin 3-glucoside induced caspase-3 activation, chromatin condensation, and cell death (Chen et al., 2005). The occurrence of apoptosis induced by malvidin was confirmed in human gastric adenocarcinoma cells by apoptotic bodies formation, caspase-3 activation and poly(ADP-ribose) polymerase proteolysis (Shih et al., 2005). Delphinidin treatment of PC3 prostate carcinoma cells resulted in a dose-dependent induction of apoptosis and cells arrest in G2-M phase. This induction of apoptosis appeared to be related to activation of caspases (Hafeez et al., 2008).

3.5 Anti-inflammatory Effects

Inflammatory cells are implicated in the tumor microenvironment and play a crucial role in tumor development and progression (Balkwill and Mantovani, 2001). The microenvironment of many human cancers is rich in cytokines, chemokines, and inflammatory enzymes.

Anthocyanins exhibit their anti-inflammation effect largely through targeting NF-κB pathway and cycloxygenase-2 (COX-2) gene (Hou et al., 2004). Anthocyanin-rich extracts from berries and pure anthocyanins exhibited inhibition of the mRNA and/or protein expression of NF-κB and COX-2 in multiple cell types (Seeram et al., 2001; Huang et al., 2002; Hou et al., 2005; Reddy et al., 2005; Rodrigo et al., 2006; Bovin et al., 2007).

3.6 Anti-angiogenic Activity

Angiogenesis is another key regulator for cancer progression which is defined as new blood vessel formation. Vascular endothelial growth factor (VEGF) is a key stimulator of angiogenesis. VEGF is another target to prevent or treat many cancers (Padhani et al., 2005; Sandler, 2005; Fox, 2006; Yance and Sagar, 2006). Wild blueberry, bilberry, raspberry seeds, and strawberry suppressed significantly both H_2O_2- and TNF-alpha-induced VEGF expression by human keratinocytes in the following order: wild blueberry > raspberry seed > strawberry > bilberry and wild blueberry > bilberry > raspberry seed > strawberry (Roy et al., 2002). The anthocyanin-rich extract of black raspberries showed inhibitory effect on VEGF expression through inhibition of the phosphoinositide 3-kinase/Akt pathway in JB6 cells (Huang et al., 2006).

3.7 Anti-invasiveness

Tumor metastasis is the most important cause of cancer death and various treatment strategies have targeted preventing the occurrence of metastasis. The degradation of basement membrane collagen by proteolysis is an early and critical invasion event. Matrix metalloproteinases (MMP) and plasminogen activators responsible for regulating basement membrane degradation, as well as their inhibitors, have been studied for anthocyanin anti-invasive activity (Chen et al., 2006a, b; Coates et al., 2007). The cyanidin 3-rutinoside/3-glucosides extracted from mulberry (*Morus alba* L) exhibited an inhibitory effect on the migration and invasion of a human lung cancer cell line through decreasing the expressions of MMP-2 and urokinase-plasminogen activator (u-PA) in a dose-dependent manner and enhancing the expression of tissue inhibitor of matrix metalloproteinase-2 (TIMP-2) and plasminogen activator inhibitor (PAI) (Chen et al., 2006a). In a similar study by Chen et al. (2006), major anthocyanins extracted from black rice, peonidin 3-glucoside and cyanidin 3-glucoside, inhibited the invasion of SKHep-1 cells. This effect was associated with a reduced expression of MMP-9 and u-PA.

4 In Vivo Chemoprotective Studies

4.1 Animal Studies

Anthocyanin-rich extracts, as well as pure anthocyanins, have shown relatively more effective chemoprevention towards tumorigenesis at directly accessible targets such as gastrointestinal tract (oral, esophagus, colon, etc.) and skin, than other sites in animal models suggesting that the low absorption into the plasma limits their ability to exert protective effects on tissues that require delivery of nutrients through the blood.

4.1.1 Colon Cancer

Freeze-dried black raspberries were found to reduce azoxymethane (AOM)-induced aberrant crypt foci (ACF), colon tumors, and the level of urinary 8-hydroxy-2′-deoxyguanosine (8-OHdG) in male F344 rats (Harris et al., 2001). The chemoprotective activity of anthocyanin-rich extracts from bilberry, chokeberry, and grape was investigated by assessing multiple biomarkers of colon cancer in male F344 rats treated with AOM. Total ACF were reduced significantly in colon tissues of rats receiving a diet enhanced with bilberry, chokeberry, and grape compared with the control group. The number of large ACF was also reduced in bilberry and chokeberry diet groups. Rats fed with bilberry/grape anthocyanin-rich diets had lower COX-2 mRNA expression of gene. A significant reduction in fecal bile acids was observed and the levels of urinary 8-hydroxyguanosine were similar among rats fed different diets. Protective roles of anthocyanin-rich extracts from those fruits were shown in colon carcinogenesis and multiple mechanisms of action appear to be involved (Lala et al., 2006). The possible chemopreventive effects of berry fruits (blueberries, blackberries, and cranberries) were compared with other fruit types (plums, mangoes, pomegranate, and watermelon) on AOM-induced ACF in F344 male rats (Boateng et al., 2007). Among these fruits, blueberry and pomegranate contributed the most significant reductions in the formation of AOM-induced ACF.

Anthocyanins have also been shown to inhibit the development of cancer in animals with hereditary predisposition to cancer. Cyanidin 3-glucoside, the most abundant anthocyanin in berries, was investigated for the colorectal adenoma formation in Apc^{Min} mice. Ingestion of cyanidin 3-glucoside reduced adenoma load dose-dependently. After supplementation of 0.3% of cyanidin 3-glucoside in the diet for 12 weeks, adenoma numbers were decreased by 45% compared to controls, suggesting that it could be a potential chemopreventive agent for human colorectal cancer (Cooke et al., 2006).

4.1.2 Esophageal Cancer

Freeze-dried strawberries, freeze-dried black raspberries and freeze-dried blueberries were fed to F-344 rats in the diets before repeatedly treating with N-nitrosomethylbenzylamine (NMBA) (Carlton et al., 2001; Kresty et al., 2001; Aziz et al., 2002). At 30 weeks, strawberries and black raspberries were found to significantly inhibit NMBA-induced esophageal tumor multiplicity in a dose-dependant manner in the rat esophagus. In a post-initiation study, animals fed 5 and 10% freeze-dried strawberries and freeze-dried black raspberries in the diet after NMBA treatment significantly reduced tumor multiplicity by 38 and 31% for strawberries, 62 and 43 % for black raspberries (Carlton et al., 2001; Kresty et al., 2001). Blueberries did not inhibit the initiation and progression of NMBA-induced tumorigenesis in the rat esophagus (Aziz et al., 2002). A significant decrease in O^6-methylguanine adducts was observed in the esophageal DNA of animals fed with strawberries or black raspberries (Carlton et al., 2001; Kresty et al., 2001), but not with blueberries (Aziz et al., 2002). Both freeze-dried strawberries and black raspberries appear to possess bioactive compounds for potential inhibition of both initiation and promotion/progression during NMBA-induced esophageal tumorigenesis. In a follow up study, both the anthocyanin-rich fraction and the ellagitannins-rich residue of black raspberries effectively reduced NMBA-induced tumors in the rat esophagus, suggesting anthocyanins and ellagitannins appear to be important for the chemopreventive effects of berries (Stoner et al., 2007).

4.1.3 Other Cancers

The available data on the prevention of oral, skin, lung, and prostate cancers by anthocyanins in animal models is summarized alternately since there are relatively fewer studies reported in the literature for them than for colorectal and esophageal cancers.

Freeze-dried black raspberries (FBR) at 5 and 10% in the diets were fed to male Syrian Golden hamsters for 2 weeks prior to treatment with 0.2% 7,12-dimethylbenz(a) anthracene in dimethylsulfoxide and were found to reduce significantly the tumor formation in the oral cavity (Casto et al., 2002).

Pretreatment to SKH-1 hairless mouse skin with delphinidin inhibited UVB-mediated apoptosis and markers of DNA damage such as cyclobutane pyrimidine dimers and 8-OHdG suggested that delphinidin exhibited a photochemopreventive effect in the animal model (Afaq et al., 2006). Cyanidin 3-glucoside treatment decreased the number of non-malignant and malignant skin tumors induced by 12-O-tetradecanolyphorbol-13-acetate (TPA) in 7, 12-dimethylbenz[a]anthracene-initiated mouse skin (Ding et al., 2006). Cyanidin 3-glucoside was reported to reduce the size of A549 tumor xenograft growth and significantly inhibited metastasis in nude mice, whereas the mechanisms behind the inhibition is related to inhibition of migration and invasion of A549 tumor cells (Ding et al., 2006).

Delphinidin has also been investigated for possible prostate cancer chemoprevention. Delphinidin administration (2 mg, i.p injection, thrice weekly) to athymic nude mice implanted with PC3 cells significantly inhibited tumor growth together with a significant decrease in the expression of NF-κB/p65, Bcl2, Ki67, and proliferating cell nuclear antigen in delphinidin-treated mouse tumors (Hafeez et al., 2008).

4.2 Human Studies

Although the information is still limited, available information indicates that dietary intake of anthocyanins or anthocyanin-rich food can protect against different cancers, mainly of the gastrointestinal tract in human subjects, largely through their protection from oxidative DNA damage. A summary of the available data on the prevention of cancer in human studies by anthocyanins from berries follows.

A study by Thomasset and coworkers (2009) showed that 25 colorectal cancer patients received a standardized anthocyanin-rich extract from bilberry at doses from 0.5 to 2.0 g anthocyanins daily for 7 days. As a result, the proliferation in the tumor tissue of treated patients was decreased by 7% compared with preintervention values. The low dose caused a small but non-significant reduction in circulating insulin-like growth factor (IGF)-1 concentrations (Thomasset et al., 2009).

An anthocyanin/polyphenol-rich fruit juice has been shown to reduce oxidative DNA damage and increase glutathione level during intervention compared to the control group who consumed a corresponding polyphenol-depleted juice (Weisel et al., 2006).

Black raspberries contain high levels of anthocyanins and the chemoprevention of lyophilized black raspberries (LBRs) has been discussed previously towards oral, esophageal, and colon carcinogenesis in animal models. In a clinical study, interim results showed that daily consumption of LBRs for 6 months promoted reductions in the urinary excretion of two oxidative stress markers (8-epi-prostaglandin F2alpha and 8-hydroxy-2′-deoxyguanosine) in Barrett's esophagus patients (Kresty et al., 2006). Another study from the same laboratory was conducted on colon caner chemoprevention of black raspberry. Fifty subjects with colorectal cancer and/or polyps consumed LRBs daily for 2–4 weeks before the surgery. Biopsies of normal and tumor/polyp tissues are collected for biomarker analysis before and after berry treatment. Their results showed that proliferation and angiogenesis biomarkers during the colon cancer development were reduced significantly by the berry treatment, whereas apoptosis was enhanced (Stoner et al., 2008).

However, epidemiological studies in humans have not shown that anthocyanin consumption could reduce cancer risks in humans as discussed by Stoner and coworkers (Wang and Stoner, 2008).

5 Impact of Anthocyanin Chemical Structure on Their Chemoprotective Properties

Anthocyanin chemopreventive activity appears to be affected by their chemical structures (Koide et al., 1997; Kamei et al., 1998; Yoshimoto et al., 2001; Zhang et al., 2005). However, anthocyanin structure/function relationships are not well understood. In addition, impact of anthocyanin structures on their biological activities was dependant on experimental models (Koide et al., 1997; Yoshimoto et al., 2001; Zhang et al., 2005), which complicated the enigma of structure-bioactivity relationship.

Since anthocyanidins are relatively simple in chemical structure (Fig. 1.1) and likely absorbed in GI tract due to their relative hydrophilic character, they are the primary targets to clarify the structure/function relationship of anthocyanins. Pure anthocyanidins were tested for different inhibition towards the growth of HL60 and HCT116 cell lines. Their antiproliferation effects were followed in an order: malvidin > delphinidin > peonidin > cyanidin > pelargonidin in HL60 cells, whereas delphinidin > cyanidin > peonidin > pelargonidin > malvidin in HCT116 cells (Katsube et al., 2003). Delphinidin and malvidin showed the greatest cell antiproliferation in HL60 and HCT116, respectively. Those two types of aglycons have been reported for their biological activity and relative mechanisms.

Delphinidin, owning three hydroxyl groups on the B ring in the molecular structure, also showed the greatest chemopreventive activity in other studies. The ortho-dihydroxyphenyl structural property was proposed to be critical for their activity. Meiers et al. (2001) found that cyanidin and delphinidin, not malvidin, exerted great inhibitory effect on the growth of human vulva carcinoma cell line A431 in vitro by suppressing EGFR and blocking downstream signaling cascades (Meiers et al., 2001). Delphinidin inhibited cell growth in uterine carcinoma (HeLa S3 cells) and colon adenocarcinoma cells (CaCo-2 cells) through a reduction of cells in G1 phase, inducing apoptosis (Lazze et al., 2004). In another study, six anthocyanidins were also evaluated on inhibition of TPA-induced JB6 mouse epidermal cell transformation and AP-1 transcription activity in an order: dephinidin > petunidin > cyanidin >> pelargonidin > malvidin > peonidin (Hou et al., 2004b). Consequently, Hou et al. (2004b) concluded that the ortho-dihydroxyphenyl structure on the B-ring of anthocyanidin was the critical structure to suppress this cell transformation and AP-1 activity. The ortho-dihydroxyphenyl structure at the B-ring also appears essential for apoptosis actions through an oxidative stress-involved JNK signaling pathway (Hou et al., 2003). Anthocyanidins with ortho-dihydroxyphenyl structure (cyanidin and delphinidin) may have anti-inflammatory properties through the inhibition of MAPK-mediated COX-2 expression (Hou et al., 2005). In our experimental data, pelargonidin derivatives, which do not possess the ortho-dihydroxyphenyl structure on B-ring, showed relatively low inhibition on HT29 cells in vitro (Jing et al., 2008).

In some studies, malvidin bearing two methoxy substituents in the 3′- and 5′-positions on the B-ring, showed the highest inhibitive effect among the common six anthocyanidins. Zhang et al. (2005) found that malvidin exerted the greatest inhibition among cyanidin, delphinidin, pelargonidin and petunidin, closely followed by pelargonidin at 200 μg/mL on AGS, HCT116, NCIH460, MCF7 and SF268 cancer cell growth (Zhang et al., 2005). Of five anthocyanidins (cyanidin, delphinidin, malvidin, pelargonidin, and peonidin) and four glycosylated anthocyanins (cyanidin 3-glucoside, malvidin 3-glucoside, pelargonidin 3-glucoside and peonidin 3-glucoside), malvidin showed the most potent antiproliferation effect on AGS cells with cell cycle arrest of AGS cells at the G0/G1 phase and induced apoptosis (Shih et al., 2005). In this study, malvidin increased Bax/Bcl-2 ratio for 1.6-fold of control at 100 μM and significantly induced up-regulation of p38 kinase expression and down-regulation of the ERK activity. Malvidin most effectively inhibited cAMP-specific phosphodiesterases (PDEs), which is required to achieve a shut-down of MAPK pathway, a signaling cascade crucial for the regulation of cell growth (Doris et al., 2004). Doris et al. (2004) found that the absence of methoxy groups and/or replacement by hydroxyl substitutes was found to diminish PDE-inhibitory property. Delphinidin/cyanidin and malvidin bearing different substitution pattern at the B-ring might interfere with different signaling cascades involved in the regulation of cell growth and apoptosis.

In addition, a few studies have been conducted regarding the relationship of structure/function in glycosylated anthocyanins with/without acylation groups. The glycosidic pattern also affected the anthocyanin's biological activities (Koide et al., 1997; Jing et al., 2008). Koide et al. (1997) found that an extract containing mostly cyanidin-glucoside and cyanidin-rhamnoside was more effective in suppressing the HCT15 cell growth in vitro than the extract rich in cyanidin-rhamnoside, suggesting that cyanidin-3-glucoside resulted in greater cell growth inhibition than the corresponding cyanidin-3-rhamnoside. We studied the relationship between chemical characteristics of anthocyanins and their biological activity, determined as the GI_{50}, through multiple regression analyses. The statistical analyses demonstrated that anthocyanins with structure properties of mono-glycoside were more potent inhibitors of the proliferation of HT29 carcinoma cells than their tri-glycosylated counterparts (Jing et al., 2008). We also found that cyanidin was more effective than pelargonidin, regardless of the glycosylation pattern. The effect of anthocyanin acylation on the antiproliferation activity of the pigments was related to the type of aglycone (Jing et al., 2008).

Yoshimoto et al. (2001) found that cyanidin 3-sophoroside-5-glucoside with or without acylation with cinnamic acids showed greater antimutagenic activity than did peonidin-type anthocyanins with similar structure patterns by using *Salmonella typhimurium* TA 98 (Yoshimoto et al., 2001). Yoshimoto et al. (2001) also found that deacylation of the cyanidin-type pigment increased antimutagenicity, while the antimutagenicity of peonidin-type pigment markedly decreased after deacylation.

6 Interaction Effects of Anthocyanins with Other Phytochemicals in Berries

Anthocyanin-rich berry fruits contain multiple bioactive phytochemicals, including polyphenols (flavonoids, phenolic acids, etc), stilbenoids, lignans, and triterpenoids. The anticancer potential of berries can be attributed to the combined performance of those bioactive compounds, either in an additive, synergistic or inhibitory manner. The interaction of anthocyanins with other bioactive phytochemicals has been discussed in a few studies. Liu (2004) reported that the major part of total antioxidant activity is from the combination of phytochemicals of fruits and vegetables, which is related to reduce the risk of developing cancer. Therefore, he proposed that the additive and synergistic effects of phytochemicals in fruits and vegetables are responsible for these potent antioxidant and anticancer activities (Liu, 2004). In another study, an additive or synergistic interaction of anthocyanins, proanthocyanidins, and flavonol glycosides from cranberries have been suggested for the growth inhibition of HT29 and HCT116 cells (Seeram et al., 2004). We studied the interaction of anthocyanins with other phenolics from chokeberry on the HT-29 cell system by using the combination index (CI) reported by Chou and Talalay (1984). The combination indexes obtained with our fractions indicated an additive interaction between chokeberry anthocyanins and other phenolics, suggesting that anthocyanins and other phenolics in chokeberry might exert chemoprotective effects by a similar mechanism on the growth inhibition of HT29 cells (Jing et al., 2008).

7 Bioavailability

Based on recent scientific reports, the bioavailability of anthocyanins is generally described as low, with very low absorption of anthocyanins into the plasma and low levels detected in the urine after large dietary intake of anthocyanin-rich extracts or berries.

McGhie et al. (2003) studied the bioabsorption of anthocyanins with structures containing different aglycons and conjugated sugars extracted from blueberry, boysenberry, black raspberry, and black currant. The bioavailability of anthocyanins with diverse molecular structure was confirmed by detection of intact and unmetabolized anthocyanins in urine of rats and humans. The total amount of anthocyanins excreted as a percentage of the amount consumed was less than 0.1% for all anthocyanins (McGhie et al., 2003). The urinary excretion of anthocyanins from strawberries corresponded to 1.8% of pelargonidin 3-glucoside consumed by humans (Felgines et al., 2003), while total urinary excretion of blackberry anthocyanin was

0.16% of the amount of anthocyanins ingested (Felgines et al., 2005). Average concentrations of anthocyanins and their metabolites in human urine reached to 17.9 μmol/L within 5 h and detected in the serum were observed at 5,917 nmol/within 2 h after consumption of 20 g chokeberry extracts (1.3 g of cyanidin 3-glycosides) (Kay et al., 2004). Anthocyanins were detected in glycosylated form in plasma and urine after a consumption of 720 mg anthocyanins by elderly women, the concentration can reach up to 168 nmol/L in plasma (Cao et al., 2001). Delphinidin 3-glucoside rapidly appeared in the blood plasma within 15 min of oral administration (100 mg/kg body wt) to rats and maintained at approximately 30 nmol/L even after 4 h (Ichiyanagi et al., 2004). Rechner et al. (2002) detected four major native anthocyanins (delphinidin 3-glucoside, delphinidin 3-rutinoside, cyanidin 3-glucoside and cyanidin 3-rutinoside) of black currant juice in human plasma and urine post-ingestion in all volunteers. The total excreted anthocyanins were less than 0.133% of total anthocyanins ingested (Rechner et al., 2002). Matsumoto et al. (2006) found that intact forms of black currant anthocyanins were detected in the plasma and whole eye after oral and intraperitoneal (i.p.) administration in rats. Four anthocyanins were identified in the plasma and several ocular tissues after intravenous (i.v.) administration in rabbits. This study indicates that intact forms of anthocyanins could pass through the blood–aqueous barrier and blood–retinal barrier in both rats and rabbits (Matsumoto et al., 2006). Cyanidin 3-glucoside and cyanidin 3-rutinoside, the major anthocyanins in wild mulberry, showed maximum concentration in plasma and kidney in rats at 15 min after oral administration of mulberry anthocyanin-rich extract (Hassimotto et al., 2008). Felgines et al. (2009) evaluated distribution of anthocyanins to various organs (bladder, prostate, testes, heart and adipose tissue) in rats after a blackberry anthocyanin-enriched diet for 12 days. As a result, anthocyanin derivatives were widely distributed to all tested organs, among which the bladder contained the highest levels of anthocyanins followed by the prostate (Felgines et al., 2009). He also found that profile of anthocyanin derivatives differed according to the organ.

Anthocyanin metabolism has been reported to occur via methylation, glucuronidation, and sulfoconjugation after absorption in weanling pigs that had a single meal with a freeze-dried powder of chokeberry, black currant, or elderberry. Anthocyanins with different aglycons were found to be metabolized differently in vivo. Metabolites of delphinidin anthocyanins were not detected, whereas anthocyanins of cyanidin were metabolized by methylation, glucuronidation or both (Wu et al., 2005). In a human study, metabolites were identified as glucuronide conjugates, as well as methylated and oxidised derivatives of cyanidin 3-galactoside and cyanidin glucuronide in urine after consumption of chokeberry extracts (Kay et al., 2004).

In a human study involving dietary intake of strawberries, five metabolites were found in urine samples, including three monoglucuronides of pelargonidin, one sulfoconjugate of pelargonidin and pelargonidin, among which monoglucuronide was more than 80%. These metabolites were found in addition to pelargonidin-3-glucoside, the intact pigment present in the strawberry fruit itself (Felgines et al., 2003). Besides native cyanidin 3-glucoside, several other anthocyanin metabolites were detected in the human urine: methylated glycosides, glucuronides of anthocyanidins and anthocyanins, a sulfoconjugate of cyanidin, and anthocyanidins after consumption of blackberries, among which monoglucuronides of anthocyanidins were major metabolites in urine (>60% of excretion) (Felgines et al., 2005). Malvidin-3-glucoside was detected in plasma and urine after ingestion of red wine, dealcoholized red wine, and red grape juice while its metabolites including the aglycon, sulfate or glucuronate conjugates were not detected in plasma and urine (Bub et al., 2001). The metabolism of delphinidin 3- glucoside was investigated in rats. Two peaks appeared at 15 and 60 min in blood plasma after ingestion. Besides the delphinidin 3- glucoside peak, a single major metabolite peak was identified as methylation of the 4′-OH on the delphinidin B-ring by means of MS and NMR spectroscopy (Ichiyanagi et al., 2004). Ichiyanagi et al. (2007) found that neither protocatechuic acid as the major intestinal metabolite of cyanidin 3- glucoside was absorbed after oral administration nor formed as the metabolite in liver after intravenous administration (Ichiyanagi et al., 2007).

McGhie et al. (2003) found that individual anthocyanin concentration in urine appeared to be different in berry extracts, suggesting that absorption and excretion of anthocyanins were influenced by structure of the conjugated sugar, especially for single glucose moiety. Anthocyanins with either a di- or trisaccharide moiety were excreted in the urine primarily as the intact form in higher percentage of ingested doses than intact forms of monoglycoside (Wu et al., 2005), which can be partially explained by a larger proportion of the anthocyanin rutinosides than of the glucosides absorbed into blood stream (Nielsen et al., 2003).

Metabolism by intestinal microflora and transformation of pure anthocyanins and anthocyanin-rich extracts has been evaluated. Anthocyanins extracts from radish, and the assumed degradation products, were evaluated in models to mimic in vivo conditions (Fleschhut et al., 2006). Glycosylated and acylated anthocyanins were rapidly degraded by the intestinal microflora after anaerobic incubation with a human fecal suspension with an increase of degradation product protocatechuic acid. Anthocyanins were glucuronidated, but no hydroxylation and demethylation, by cytochrome P450 enzymes from rat liver microsomes in the presence of the cofactor NADPH (Fleschhut et al., 2006). In another study, in vitro fermentation showed that cyanidin glycosides were totally metabolized by the rat colonic microflora, whereas cyanidin and protocatechuic acid as the products of their fermentation degradation were not detected in plasma (Hassimotto et al., 2008).

The reasons that anthocyanins have such poor absorption are not yet clear. A possible reason is that many anthocyanin chemical structures are not efficiently hydrolyzed by β-glucosidase in the GI tract, resulting in a low absorption into the blood stream (Nemeth et al., 2003). The degradation of anthocyanins due to neutral and mild alkaline condition in intestines could be one possible reason. However, it has been reported that after a 14-day dietary intake of anthocyanin-rich extracts from chokeberries, bilberries or grapes, the anthocyanins were abundant in rat feces (0.7/1.8/2.0 g/kg wet feces for chokeberry/bilberry/grape, respectively) (He et al., 2005). Food matrix may exert a protective effect on anthocyanin stability after ingestion. In humans, the absorption and urinary excretion of anthocyanins from blackcurrant juice were found to be proportional with dose and not influenced by the ingestion of a rice cake (Nielsen et al., 2003), suggesting that food ingredients such as protein may enhance anthocyanin stability in vivo. In another study, a formulated mucoadhesive gel containing freeze-dried black raspberries for oral cancer prevention was proven to improve absorption and penetration of anthocyanins into the target oral mucosal tissue site (Mallery et al., 2007). Hassimotto et al. (2008) proposed fund by the everted sac model that anthocyanins were transported across the enterocyte by the sodium-dependent glucose transporter. Dreiseitel et al. (2009) reported that berry anthocyanins and anthocyanidins showed distinct affinities for the efflux transporters breast cancer resistance protein (BCRP) and multidrug resistance protein 1 (MDR1). That indicated that they may be actively transported out of intestinal tissues and endothelia, resulting in the low bioavailability in plasma and brain (Dreiseitel et al., 2009).

Evidence is compounding that indicate anthocyanins in berries play a very important role on the protective effects of fruits and vegetables against chronic diseases, cancer in particular. Their contribution is likely to be additive or synergistic in combination with the many other phytochemicals present in berries. However, because of their color characteristics, anthocyanins are a group of compounds whose concentration can be easily assessed by consumers. Increased consumption of fruits and vegetables has been long recommended. Consumption of darkly colored berries will increase dietary intake of anthocyanins, increasing their potential for impacting health.

References

Afaq F, Syed DN, Malik A et al (2006) Delphinidin, an anthocyanidin in pigmented fruits and vegetables, protects human hacat keratinocytes and mouse skin against UVB-mediated oxidative stress and apoptosis. J Invest Dermatol 127:222–232

Andersen ØM (1985) Chromatographic separation of anthocyanins in cowberry (lingonberry) *Vaccinium vites-idaea* L. J Food Sci 50:1230–1232

Andersen ØM (1987) Anthocyanins in fruits of *Vaccinium uliginosum* L. (bog whortleberry). J Food Sci 52:665–666, 680

Andersen ØM (1989) Anthocyanins in fruits of *Vaccinium oxycoccus* L. (small cranberry). J Food Sci 54:383–384, 387

Andersen ØM, Fossen T, Torskangerpoll K et al (2004) Anthocyanin from strawberry (*Fragaria x ananassa*) with the novel aglycone, 5-carboxypyranopelargonidin. Phytochemistry 65:405–410

Andersen ØM, Jordheim M (2005) The anthocyanins. In: Andersen ØM, Markham KR (eds) Flavonoids: chemistry, biochemistry and applications, 1st edn. CRC press, Boca Raton, FL

Angel P, Karin M (1991) The role of Jun, fos and the AP-1 complex in cell-proliferation and transformation. Biochim Biophys Acta 1072:129–157

Aziz RM, Nines R, Rodrigo K et al (2002) The effect of freeze-dried blueberries on N-nitrosomethylbenzylamine tumorigenesis in the rat esophagus. Pharm Biol 40(Suppl):43–49

Bakowska-Barczak AM, Kolodziejczyk P (2008) Evaluation of Saskatoon berry (Amelanchier alnifolia Nutt.) cultivars for their polyphenol content, antioxidant properties, and storage stability. J Agric Food Chem 56:9933–9940

Balkwill F, Mantovani A (2001) Inflammation and cancer: back to Virchow? Lancet 357:539–545

Benvenuti S, Pellati F, Melegari M et al (2004) Polyphenols, anthocyanins, ascorbic acid, and radical scavenging activity of *Rubus, Ribes*, and *Aronia*. J Food Sci 69:FCT164–FCT169
Boateng J, Verghese M, Shackelford L et al (2007) Selected fruits reduce azoxymethane (AOM)-induced aberrant crypt foci (ACF) in Fisher 344 male rats. Food Chem Toxicol 45:725–732
Bomser J, Madhavi DL, Singletary K et al (1996) In vitro anticancer activity of fruit extracts from *Vaccinium* species. Planta Med 62:212–216
Bovin D, Blanchette M, Barrette S et al (2007) Inhibition of cancer cell proliferation and suppression of TNF-induced activation of NFκB by edible berry juice. Anticancer Res 27:937–948
Bub A, Watzl B, Heeb D et al (2001) Malvidin-3-glucoside bioavailability in humans after ingestion of red wine, dealcoholized red wine and red grape juice. Eur J Nutr 40:113–120
Burrows C, Moore PP (2002) Genotype x environment effects on raspberry fruit quality. Acta Hortic 585:467–473
Cao G, Muccitelli HU, Sanchez-Moreno C et al (2001) Anthocyanins are absorbed in glycated forms in elderly women: a pharmacokinetic study. Am J Clin Nutr 73:920–926
Carlton PS, Kresty LA, Siglin JC et al (2001) Inhibition of N-nitrosomethylbenzylamine-induced tumorigenesis in the rat esophagus by dietary freeze-dried strawberries. Carcinogenesis 22:441–446
Casto BC, Kresty LA, Kraly CL et al (2002) Chemoprevention of oral cancer by black raspberries. Anticancer Res 22:4005–4015
Chen PN, Chu SC, Chiou HL et al (2005) Cyanidin 3-glucoside and peonidin 3-glucoside inhibit tumor cell growth and induce apoptosis in vitro and suppress tumor growth in vivo. Nutr Cancer 53:232–243
Chen PN, Chu SC, Chiou HL et al (2006a) Mulberry anthocyanins, cyanidin 3-rutinoside and cyanidin 3-glucoside, exhibited an inhibitory effect on the migration and invasion of a human lung cancer cell line. Cancer Lett 235:248–259
Chen PN, Kuo WH, Chiang CL et al (2006b) Black rice anthocyanins inhibit cancer cells invasion via repressions of MMPs and u-PA expression. Chem Biol Interact 163:218–229
Cho MJ, Howard LR, Prior RL et al (2004) Flavonoid glycosides and antioxidant capacity of various blackberry, blueberry and red grape genotypes determined by high-performance liquid chromatography/mass spectrometry. J Sci Food Agric 84:1771–1782
Chou TC, Talalay P (1984) Quantitative analysis of dose-effect relationships: the combined effects of multiple drugs or enzyme inhibitors. Adv Enzyme Regul 22:27–55
Clark JR, Howard L, Talcott S (2002) Antioxidant activity of blackberry genotypes. Acta Hortic 585:475–480
Clifford MN (2000) Anthocyanins – nature, occurrence and dietary burden. J Sci Food Agric 80:1063–1072
Coates E, Popa G, Gill C et al (2007) Colon-available raspberry polyphenols exhibit anti-cancer effects on in vitro models of colon cancer. J Carcinog 6:4
Connor AM, Luby JJ, Hancock JF et al (2002) Changes in fruit antioxidant activity among blueberry cultivars during cold-temperature storage. J Agric Food Chem 50:893–898
Cooke D, Schwarz M, Boocock D et al (2006) Effect of cyanidin-3-glucoside and an anthocyanin mixture from bilberry on adenoma development in the Apc^{Min} mouse model of intestinal carcinogenesis-relationship with tissue anthocyanin levels. Int J Cancer 119: 2213–2220
Cordenunsi BR, Oliveira do Nascimento JR, Genovese MI et al (2002) Influence of cultivar on quality parameters and chemical composition of strawberry fruits grown in Brazil. J Agric Food Chem 50:2581–2586
Dai J, Gupte A, Gates L et al (2009) A comprehensive study of anthocyanin-containing extracts from selected blackberry cultivars: extraction methods, stability, anticancer properties and mechanisms. Food Chem Toxicol 47:837–847
Deighton N, Brennan R, Finn C et al (2000) Antioxidant properties of domesticated and wild *Rubus* species. J Sci Food Agric 80:1307–1313

Ding M, Feng R, Wang SY et al (2006) Cyanidin-3-glucoside, a natural product derived from blackberry, exhibits chemopreventive and chemotherapeutic activity. J Biol Chem 281: 17359–17368
Doris M, Nicole P, Zeina T et al (2004) The substitution pattern of anthocyanidins affects different cellular signaling cascades regulating cell proliferation. Mol Nutr Food Res 48:318–325
Dreiseitel A, Oosterhuis B, Vukman KV, et al (2009) Berry anthocyanins and anthocyanidins exhibit distinct affinities for the efflux transporters BCRP and MDR1. Br J Clin Pharmacol 158:1942–1950
Dreiseitel A, Schreier P, Oehme A et al (2008) Inhibition of proteasome activity by anthocyanins and anthocyanidins. Biochem Biophys Res Commun 372:57–61
Dugo P, Mondello L, Errante G et al (2001) Identification of anthocyanins in berries by narrow-bore high-performance liquid chromatography with electrospray ionization detection. J Agric Food Chem 49:3987–3992
Elisia I, Hu C, Popovich DG et al (2007) Antioxidant assessment of an anthocyanin-enriched blackberry extract. Food Chem 101:1052–1058
Escribano-Bailón MT, Alcalde-Eon C, Muñoz O et al (2006) Anthocyanins in berries of Maqui (*Aristotelia chilensis* (Mol.) Stuntz). Phytochem Anal 17:8–14
Evan GI, Vousden KH (2001) Proliferation, cell cycle and apoptosis in cancer. Nature 411:342–348
Felgines C, Talavera S, Gonthier MP et al (2003) Strawberry anthocyanins are recovered in urine as glucuro- and sulfoconjugates in humans. J Nutr 133:1296–1301
Felgines C, Talavera S, Texier O et al (2005) Blackberry anthocyanins are mainly recovered from urine as methylated and gucuronidated conjugates in humans. J Agric Food Chem 53: 7721–7727
Felgines C, Texier O, Garcin P et al (2009) Tissue distribution of anthocyanins in rats fed a blackberry anthocyanin-enriched diet. Mol Nutr Food Res 53:1098
Feng R, Ni H-M, Wang SY et al (2007) Cyanidin-3-rutinoside, a natural polyphenol antioxidant, selectively kills leukemic cells by induction of oxidative stress. J Biol Chem 282: 13468–13476
Fimognari C, Berti F, Nüsse M et al (2004) Induction of apoptosis in two human leukemia cell lines as well as differentiation in human promyelocytic cells by cyanidin-3-O-[beta]-glucopyranoside. Biochem Pharmacol 67:2047–2056
Fiorini M (1995) Preparative high-performance liquid chromatography for the purification of natural anthocyanins. J Chromatogr A 692:213–219
Fleschhut J, Kratzer F, Rechkemmer G et al (2006) Stability and biotransformation of various dietary anthocyanins in vitro. Eur J Nutr 45:7–18
Fox SB (2006) Quantitative angiogenesis in breast cancer. Methods Mol Med 120:161–187
Garzón GA, Riedl KM, Schwartz SJ (2009) Determination of anthocyanins, total phenolic content, and antioxidant activity in Andes berry (*Rubus glaucus* Benth). J Food Sci 74:C227–C232
Giusti MM, Jing P (2007) Natural pigments of berry fruits: functionality and application. In: Zhao Y (ed) Berry fruit: value-added products for health promotion, 1st edn. Taylor & Francis, Boca Raton, FL
Giusti MM, Wrolstad RE (2003) Acylated anthocyanins from edible sources and their applications in food systems. Biochem Eng J 14:217–225
Goiffon JP, Brun M, Bourrier MJ (1991) High-performance liquid chromatography of red fruit anthocyanins. J Chromatogr 537:101–121
Hafeez BB, Siddiqui IA, Asim M, Malik A et al (2008) A dietary anthocyanidin delphinidin induces apoptosis of human prostate cancer PC3 cells in vitro and in vivo: involvement of nuclear factor-{kappa}B signaling. Cancer Res 68:8564–8572
Haffner K, Rosenfeld HJ, Skrede G et al (2002) Quality of red raspberry *Rubus idaeus* L cultivars after storage in controlled and normal atmospheres. Postharvest Biol Technol 24:279–289
Hakimuddin F, Paliyath G, Meckling K (2004) Selective cytotoxicity of a red grape wine flavonoid fraction against MCF-7 cells. Breast Cancer Res Treat 85:65–79
Han C, Ding H, Casto B et al (2005) Inhibition of the growth of premalignant and malignant human oral cell lines by extracts and components of black raspberries. Nutr Cancer 51:207–217

Harborne JB (1979) Correlations between flavonoid chemistry, anatomy and geography in the restionaceae from Australasia and South Africa. Phytochemistry 18:1323–1327

Harris GK, Gupta A, Nines RG et al (2001) Effects of lyophilized black raspberries on azoxymethane-induced colon cancer and 8-hydroxy-2′-deoxyguanosine levels in the Fischer 344 rat. Nutr Cancer 40:125–133

Hassimotto NMA, Genovese MI, Lajolo FM (2008) Absorption and metabolism of cyanidin-3-glucoside and cyanidin-3-rutinoside extracted from wild mulberry (*Morus nigra* L.) in rats. Nutr Res 28:198–207

He J, Magnuson BA, Giusti MM (2005) Analysis of anthocyanins in rat intestinal contents – impact of anthocyanin chemical structure on fecal excretion. J Agric Food Chem 53:2859–2866

Hogan S, Chung H, Zhang L et al (2010) Antiproliferative and antioxidant properties of anthocyanin-rich extract from açai. Food Chem 118:208–214

Hosseinian FS, Beta T (2007) Saskatoon and wild blueberries have higher anthocyanin contents than other Manitoba berries. J Agric Food Chem 55:10832–10838

Hou DX, Fujii M, Terahara N et al (2004a) Molecular mechanisms behind the chemopreventive effects of anthocyanidins. J Biomed Biotechnol 5:321–325

Hou DX, Kai K, Li JJ et al (2004b) Anthocyanidins inhibit activator protein 1 activity and cell transformation: structure-activity relationship and molecular mechanisms. Carcinogenesis 25:29–36

Hou DX, Ose T, Lin S et al (2003) Anthocyanidins induce apoptosis in human promyelocytic leukemia cells: structure-activity relationship and mechanisms involved. Int J Oncol 23: 705–712

Hou DX, Tong X, Terahara N et al (2005a) Delphinidin 3-sambubioside, a Hibiscus anthocyanin, induces apoptosis in human leukemia cells through reactive oxygen species-mediated mitochondrial pathway. Arch Biochem Biophys 440:101–109

Hou DX, Yanagita T, Uto T et al (2005b) Anthocyanidins inhibit cyclooxygenase-2 expression in LPS-evoked macrophages: structure-activity relationship and molecular mechanisms involved. Biochem Pharmacol 70:417–425

Huang C, Huang Y, Li J et al (2002) Inhibition of Benzo(a)Pyrene diol-epoxide-induced transactivation of activated protein 1 and nuclear factor B by black raspberry extracts. Cancer Res 62:6857–6863

Huang C, Li J, Song L et al (2006) Black raspberry extracts inhibit Benzo(a)Pyrene diol-epoxide-induced activator protein 1 activation and VEGF transcription by targeting the phosphotidylinositol 3-kinase/Akt pathway. Cancer Res 66:581–587

Huopalahti R, Järvenpää E, Katina K (2000) A novel solid-phase extraction-HPLC method for the analysis of anthocyanin and organic acid composition of Finnish cranberry. J Liq Chromatogr Relat Technol 23:2695–2701

Ichiyanagi T, Rahman MM, Hatano Y et al (2007) Protocatechuic acid is not the major metabolite in rat blood plasma after oral administration of cyanidin 3-O-β-d-glucopyranoside. Food Chem 105:1032–1039

Ichiyanagi T, Rahman MM, Kashiwada Y et al (2004) Absorption and metabolism of delphinidin 3-O-β-d-glucopyranoside in rats. Free Radic Biol Med 36:930–937

Inami O, Tamura I, Kikuzaki H et al (1996) Stability of anthocyanins of *Sambucus canadensis* and *Sambucus nigra*. J Agric Food Chem 44:3090–3096

Jing P, Bomser JA, Schwartz SJ et al (2008) Structure-function relationships of anthocyanins from various anthocyanin-rich extracts on the inhibition of colon cancer cell growth. J Agric Food Chem 56:9391–9398

Jung KJ, Wallig MA, Singletary KW (2006) Purple grape juice inhibits 7,12-dimethylbenz[a]anthracene (DMBA)-induced rat mammary tumorigenesis and in vivo DMBA-DNA adduct formation. Cancer Lett 233:279–288

Kaack K, Kuhn BF (1992) Black chokeberry (*Aronia melanocarpa*) for manufacture of a food colorant. Tidsskrift Planteavl 96:183–196

Kähkönen MP, Heinamaki J, Ollilainen V et al (2003) Berry anthocyanins: isolation, identification and antioxidant properties. J Sci Food Agric 83:1403–1411
Kalt W, Forney CF, Martin A et al (1999) Antioxidant capacity, vitamin C, phenolics, and anthocyanins after fresh storage of small fruits. J Agric Food Chem 47:4638–4644
Kamei H, Hashimoto Y, Koide T et al (1998) Antitumor effect of methanol extracts from red and white wines. Cancer Biother Radiopharm 13:447–452
Kampuse S, Kampuss K, Pizika L (2002) Stability of anthocyanins and ascorbic acid in raspberry and blackcurrant cultivars during frozen storage. Acta Hortic 585:507–510
Katsube N, Iwashita K, Tsushida T et al (2003) Induction of apoptosis in cancer cells by bilberry (*Vaccinium myrtillus*) and the anthocyanins. J Agric Food Chem 51:68–75
Kay CD, Mazza G, Holub BJ et al (2004) Anthocyanin metabolites in human urine and serum. Br J Nutr 91:933–942
Klopotek Y, Otto K, Bohm V (2005) Processing strawberries to different products alters contents of vitamin C, total phenolics, total anthocyanins, and antioxidant capacity. J Agric Food Chem 53:5640–5646
Koide T, Hashimoto Y, Kamei H et al (1997) Antitumor effect of anthocyanin fractions extracted from red soybeans and red beans in vitro and in vivo. Cancer Biother Radiopharm 12:277–280
Kong JM, Chia LS, Goh NK et al (2003) Analysis and biological activities of anthocyanins. Phytochemistry 64:923–933
Kresty LA, Frankel WL, Hammond CD et al (2006) Transitioning from preclinical to clinical chemopreventive assessments of lyophilized black raspberries: interim results show berries modulate markers of oxidative stress in Barrett's esophagus patients. Nutr Cancer 54(1):148–156
Kresty LA, Morse MA, Morgan C et al (2001) Chemoprevention of esophageal tumorigenesis by dietary administration of lyophilized black raspberries. Cancer Res 61:6112–6119
Kuskoski EM, Vega JM, Rios JJ et al (2003) Characterization of anthocyanins from the fruits of baguaçu (*Eugenia umbelliflora* Berg). J Agric Food Chem 51:5450–5454
Lala G, Malik M, Zhao C et al (2006) Anthocyanin-rich extracts inhibit multiple biomarkers of colonic cancer in rats. Nutr Cancer 54:84–93
Lazze MC, Savio M, Pizzala R et al (2004) Anthocyanins induce cell cycle perturbations and apoptosis in different human cell lines. Carcinogenesis 25:1427–1433
Lee J, Finn CE, Wrolstad RE (2004) Comparison of anthocyanin pigment and other phenolic compounds of *Vaccinium membranaceum* and *Vaccinium ovatum* native to the Pacific Northwest of North America. J Agric Food Chem 52:7039–7044
Lister CE, Wilson PE, Sutton KH et al (2002) Understanding the health benefits of blackcurrants. Acta Hortic 585:443–449
Liu RH (2004) Potential synergy of phytochemicals in cancer prevention: mechanism of action. J Nutr 134:3479S–3485S
Liu M, Li XQ, Weber C et al (2002) Antioxidant and antiproliferative activities of raspberries. J Agric Food Chem 50:2926–2930
Longo L, Vasapollo G (2005) Anthocyanins from Bay (*Laurus nobilis* L.) berries. J Agric Food Chem 53:8063–8067
Longo L, Vasapollo G, Rescio L (2005) Identification of anthocyanins in *Rhamnus alaternus* L. Berries. J Agric Food Chem 53:1723–1727
Lopes-da-Silva F, de Pascual-Teresa S, Rivas-Gonzalo J et al (2002) Identification of anthocyanin pigments in strawberry (cv Camarosa) by LC using DAD and ESI-MS detection. Eur Food Res Technol 214:248–253
Maatta KR, Kamal-Eldin A, Torronen AR (2003) High-performance liquid chromatography (HPLC) analysis of phenolic compounds in berries with diode array and electrospray ionization mass spectrometric (MS) detection: ribes species. J Agric Food Chem 51:6736–6744
Maatta-Riihinen KR, Kamal-Eldin A, Mattila PH et al (2004) Distribution and contents of phenolic compounds in eighteen Scandinavian berry species. J Agric Food Chem 52:4477–4486
Malik M, Zhao C, Schoene N et al (2003) Anthocyanin-rich extract from *Aronia meloncarpa* E induces a cell cycle block in colon cancer but not normal colonic cells. Nutr Cancer 46:186–196

Mallery SR, Stoner GD, Larsen PE et al (2007) Formulation and in-vitro and in-vivo evaluation of a mucoadhesive gel containing freeze dried black raspberries: implications for oral cancer chemoprevention. Pharm Res 24:728

Martin S, Favot L, Matz R et al (2003) Delphinidin inhibits endothelial cell proliferation and cell cycle progression through a transient activation of ERK-1/-2. Biochem Pharmacol 65:669–675

Matsumoto H, Nakamura Y, Iida H et al (2006) Comparative assessment of distribution of blackcurrant anthocyanins in rabbit and rat ocular tissues. Exp Eye Res 83:348–356

McGhie TK, Ainge GD, Barnett LE et al (2003) Anthocyanin glycosides from berry fruit are absorbed and excreted unmetabolized by both humans and rats. J Agric Food Chem 51: 4539–4548

McGhie TK, Hall HK, Ainge GD et al (2002) Breeding *Rubus* cultivars for high anthocyanin content and high antioxidant capacity. Acta Hortic 585:495–500

Meiers S, Kemeny M, Weyand U et al (2001) The anthocyanidins cyanidin and delphinidin are potent inhibitors of the epidermal growth-factor receptor. J Agric Food Chem 49:958–962

Meyers KJ, Watkins CB, Pritts MP et al (2003) Antioxidant and antiproliferative activities of strawberries. J Agric Food Chem 51:6887–6892

Moyer RA, Hummer KE, Finn CE et al (2002) Anthocyanins, phenolics, and antioxidant capacity in diverse small fruits: *Vaccinium, Rubus*, and *Ribes*. J Agric Food Chem 50:519–525

Mullen W, Lean ME, Crozier A (2002) Rapid characterization of anthocyanins in red raspberry fruit by high-performance liquid chromatography coupled to single quadrupole mass spectrometry. J Chromatogr A 966:63–70

Nemeth K, Plumb GW, Berrin JG et al (2003) Deglycosylation by small intestinal epithelial cell beta-glucosidases is a critical step in the absorption and metabolism of dietary flavonoid glycosides in humans. Eur J Nutr 42:29–42

Nickavar B, Amin G (2004) Anthocyanins from *Vaccinium arctostaphylos* berries. Pharm Biol 42:289–291

Nielsen IL, Dragsted LO, Ravn-Haren G et al (2003) Absorption and excretion of black currant anthocyanins in humans and watanabe heritable hyperlipidemic rabbits. J Agric Food Chem 51:2813–2820

Olsson ME, Gustavsson KE, Andersson S et al (2004) Inhibition of cancer cell proliferation in vitro by fruit and berry extracts and correlations with antioxidant levels. J Agric Food Chem 52:7264–7271

Oszmianski J, Sapis JC (1988) Anthocyanins in fruits of *Aronia melanocarpa* (chokeberry). J Food Sci 53:1241–1242

Padhani AR, Harvey CJ, Cosgrove DO (2005) Angiogenesis imaging in the management of prostate cancer. Nat Clin Pract Urol 2:596–607

Perkins-Veazie P, Kalt W (2002) Postharvest storage of blackberry fruit does not increase antioxidant levels. Acta Hortic 585:521–524

Poulsen HE, Prieme H, Loft S (1998) Role of oxidative DNA damage in cancer initiation and promotion. Eur J Cancer Prev 7:9–16

Prior RL, Cao G, Martin A et al (1998) Antioxidant capacity as influenced by total phenolic and anthocyanin content, maturity, and variety of *Vaccinium* species. J Agric Food Chem 46: 2686–2693

Prior RL, Lazarus SA, Cao G et al (2001) Identification of procyanidins and anthocyanins in blueberries and cranberries (*Vaccinium Spp*.) Using high-performance liquid chromatography/mass spectrometry. J Agric Food Chem 49:1270–1276

Rechner AR, Kuhnle G, Hu H et al (2002) The metabolism of dietary polyphenols and the relevance to circulating levels of conjugated metabolites. Free Radic Res 36:1229–1241

Reddy MK, Alexander-Lindo RL, Nair MG (2005) Relative inhibition of lipid peroxidation, cyclooxygenase enzymes, and human tumor cell proliferation by natural food colors. J Agric Food Chem 53:9268–9273

Renis M, Calandra L, Scifo C et al (2008) Response of cell cycle/stress-related protein expression and DNA damage upon treatment of CaCo2 cells with anthocyanins. Br J Nutr 100: 27–35

Rodrigo KA, Rawal Y, Renner RJ et al (2006) Suppression of the tumorigenic phenotype in human oral squamous cell carcinoma cells by an ethanol extract derived from freeze-dried black raspberries. Nutr Cancer 54:58–68

Roy S, Khanna S, Alessio HM et al (2002) Anti-angiogenic property of edible berries. Free Radic Res 36:1023–1031

Saario M (2000) Fresh lingonberry quality as affected by storage conditions and packaging. J Food Qual 23:453–463

Sandler AB (2005) Targeting angiogenesis in lung cancer. Semin Oncol 32:S16–S22

Sarma AD, Sharma R (1999) Anthocyanin-DNA copigmentation complex: mutual protection against oxidative damage. Phytochemistry 52:1313–1318

Seeram NP, Adams LS, Hardy ML et al (2004) Total cranberry extract versus its phytochemical constituents: antiproliferative and synergistic effects against human tumor cell lines. J Agric Food Chem 52:2512–2517

Seeram NP, Adams LS, Zhang Y et al (2006) Blackberry, black raspberry, blueberry, cranberry, red raspberry, and strawberry extracts inhibit growth and stimulate apoptosis of human cancer cells in vitro. J Agric Food Chem 54:9329–9339

Seeram NP, Momin RA, Nair MG et al (2001) Cyclooxygenase inhibitory and antioxidant cyanidin glycosides in cherries and berries. Phytomedicine 8:362–369

Shih PH, Yeh CT, Yen GC (2005) Effects of anthocyanidin on the inhibition of proliferation and induction of apoptosis in human gastric adenocarcinoma cells. Food Chem Toxicol 43: 1557–1566

Shih P-H, Yeh C-T, Yen G-C (2007) Anthocyanins induce the activation of phase II enzymes through the antioxidant response element pathway against oxidative stress-induced apoptosis. J Agric Food Chem 55:9427

Singletary KW, Jung KJ, Giusti MM (2007) Anthocyanin-rich grape extract blocks breast cell DNA damage. J Med Food 10:244–251

Slimestad R, Torskangerpoll K, Nateland HS et al (2005) Flavonoids from black chokeberries, *Aronia melanocarpa*. J Food Compost Anal 18:61–68

Stoner GD, Wang L-S, Casto BC (2008) Laboratory and clinical studies of cancer chemoprevention by antioxidants in berries. Carcinogenesis 29:1665–1674

Stoner GD, Wang L-S, Zikri N et al (2007) Cancer prevention with freeze-dried berries and berry components. Semin Cancer Biol 17:403–410

Strigl AW, Leitner E, Pfannhauser W (1995) Chokeberries as natural food colorant source. Dtsch Lebensmitt Rundsch 91:177–180

Strik BC (2007) Berry crops: worldwide area and production systems. In: Zhao Y (ed) Berry fruit: value-added products for health promotion, 1st edn. Taylor & Francis, Boca Raton, FL

Strik BC, Finn C, Wrolstad R (2003) Performance of chokeberry (*Aronia melanocarpa*) in Oregon, USA. Paper presented at the Berry Crop Breeding, Production and Utilization for a New Century (ISHS), 626, pp 439–443

Sun J, Chu YF, Wu X et al (2002) Antioxidant and antiproliferative activities of common fruits. J Agric Food Chem 50:7449–7454

Thomasset S, Berry DP, Cai H et al (2009) Pilot study of oral anthocyanins for colorectal cancer chemoprevention. Cancer Prev Res 2:625–633

Tian Q, Giusti MM, Stoner GD et al (2006) Characterization of a new anthocyanin in black raspberries (*Rubus occidentalis*) by liquid chromatography electrospray ionization tandem mass spectrometry. Food Chem 94:465–468

Wada L, Ou B (2002) Antioxidant activity and phenolic content of oregon caneberries. J Agric Food Chem 50:3495–3500

Wang SY, Feng R, Bowman L et al (2005) Antioxidant activity in lingonberries (*Vaccinium vitis-idaea* L.) And its inhibitory effect on activator protein-1, nuclear factor-kappab, and mitogen-activated protein kinases activation. J Agric Food Chem 53:3156–3166

Wang SY, Lin HS (2000) Antioxidant activity in fruits and leaves of blackberry, raspberry, and strawberry varies with cultivar and developmental stage. J Agric Food Chem 48:140–146

Wang LS, Stoner GD (2008) Anthocyanins and their role in cancer prevention. Cancer Lett 269:281–290

Wang SY, Stretch AW (2001) Antioxidant capacity in cranberry is influenced by cultivar and storage temperature. J Agric Food Chem 49:969–974

Weisel T, Baum M, Eisenbrand G et al (2006) An anthocyanin/polyphenolic-rich fruit juice reduces oxidative DNA damage and increases glutathione level in healthy probands. Biotechnol J 1:388–397

Wu X, Gu L, Prior RL et al (2004) Characterization of anthocyanins and proanthocyanidins in some cultivars of *Ribes, Aronia*, and *Sambucus* and their antioxidant capacity. J Agric Food Chem 52:7846–7856

Wu X, Pittman HE, McKay S et al (2005) Aglycones and sugar moieties alter anthocyanin absorption and metabolism after berry consumption in weanling pigs. J Nutr 135: 2417–2424

Wu X, Prior RL (2005) Systematic identification and characterization of anthocyanins by HPLC-ESI-MS/MS in common foods in the United States: fruits and berries. J Agric Food Chem 53:2589–2599

Yance DR Jr, Sagar SM (2006) Targeting angiogenesis with integrative cancer therapies. Integr Cancer Ther 5:9–29

Yi W, Akoh CC, Fischer J et al (2006) Effects of phenolic compounds in blueberries and muscadine grapes on HepG2 cell viability and apoptosis. Food Res Int 39:628–638

Yi W, Fischer J, Krewer G et al (2005) Phenolic compounds from blueberries can inhibit colon cancer cell proliferation and induce apoptosis. J Agric Food Chem 53:7320–7329

Yoshimoto M, Okuno S, Yamaguchi M et al (2001) Antimutagenicity of deacylated anthocyanins in purple-fleshed sweetpotato. Biosci Biotechnol Biochem 65:1652–1655

Youdim KA, Martin A, Joseph JA (2000) Incorporation of the elderberry anthocyanins by endothelial cells increases protection against oxidative stress. Free Radic Biol Med 29:51–60

Zhang Y, Vareed SK, Nair MG (2005) Human tumor cell growth inhibition by nontoxic anthocyanidins, the pigments in fruits and vegetables. Life Sci 76:1465–1472

Zhao C, Giusti MM, Malik M et al (2004) Effects of commercial anthocyanin-rich extracts on colonic cancer and nontumorigenic colonic cell growth. J Agric Food Chem 52:6122–6128

Zheng W, Wang SY (2003) Oxygen radical absorbing capacity of phenolics in blueberries, cranberries, chokeberries, and lingonberries. J Agric Food Chem 51:502–509

Chapter 2
Ursolic Acid and Other Pentacyclic Triterpenoids: Anticancer Activities and Occurrence in Berries

Catherine C. Neto

Abstract Ursolic acid and related pentacyclic triterpenoids have been isolated and identified as constituents of various berries, particularly cranberries (*Vaccinium macrocarpon*) and other *Vaccinium* species. In vitro studies have shown that these compounds possess anti-inflammatory and anti-cancer activities. These compounds reportedly inhibit the growth of numerous tumor cell lines including colon, breast, liver, prostate and leukemia and inhibit the expression and activity of cyclooxygenases. Among the berry triterpenoids, ursolic acid is the most studied. Ursolic acid has been found to induce apoptosis in tumor cells by activation of caspases and modulation of other pathways involved in cell proliferation and migration. These compounds may therefore play a complementary or synergistic role together with other berry constituents in chemoprevention. Further studies of bioavailability and in vivo activities are needed.

Keywords Ursolic acid · Triterpenoids · Anti-cancer · Cranberry · Blueberry · Vaccinium · Anti-inflammatory · Tumor · Apoptosis

1 Introduction

Ursolic acid (3β-hydroxyurs-12-en-28-oic acid) is a pentacyclic triterpenoid that occurs in numerous plants and is a constituent of several herbal medicines marketed in Asia and worldwide for inflammatory conditions (Kim et al., 2004). As a potential functional food phytochemical, ursolic acid (UA) has received relatively scant attention, perhaps because little is known about its general distribution among edible plants or its oral bioavailability. Numerous reports of UA's in vitro activities against tumor cell lines have appeared in the literature (Novotny et al., 2001) and the possible mechanisms of action have been reviewed recently (Neto, 2007).

C.C. Neto (✉)
Department of Chemistry and Biochemistry, University of Massachusetts Dartmouth, North Dartmouth, MA 02747, USA
e-mail: cneto@umassd.edu

G.D. Stoner, N.P. Seeram (eds.), *Berries and Cancer Prevention*,
DOI 10.1007/978-1-4419-7554-6_2,

The pentacyclic triterpenoids are a class of C_{30} isoprenoid compounds occurring widely in plants. Folding and cyclization of squalene leads to the dammarenyl ring system, which has a slightly different stereochemistry and ring structure from that of the major sterols (Dewick, 2001). Ring expansion and additional cyclization forms the characteristic fifth ring found in the lupeol, α-amyrin and β-amyrin skeletons (Fig. 2.1). Ursolic acid contains the β-amyrin skeleton; its C30 isomer α-amyrin is found in oleanolic acid. The 3-OH may be esterified with a phenolic acid. As these compounds are relatively nonpolar, they can be found in the waxy outer coating of fruits and other plant parts. Their role in the plant is not well understood.

2 Occurrence of Ursolic Acid and Other Triterpenoids in *Vaccinium* Berries

Among berries, North American cranberry fruit (*Vaccinium macrocarpon*), in particular, contains a significant quantity of ursolic acid (Fig. 2.1a) in its peel. It is found in the aglycone form and as the *cis* and *trans* p-hydroxycinnamate esters (Murphy et al., 2003) shown in Fig. 2.1b, c. Quantitative analysis of cranberry fruit and products by liquid chromatography-mass spectrometry (LC-MS) found the ursolic acid content of whole cranberry fruit of different cultivars to range between 60 and 110 mg per 100 g of fresh fruit (Kondo, 2006). A similar content is found in sweetened, dried fruit. Considerably less ursolic acid is detected in jellied cranberry sauce or commercial cranberry juice due presumably to its low solubility in water.

A bioassay-guided fractionation approach was used to examine in vitro antitumor activities of whole cranberry fruit and juice, extracts and fractions, and finally, individual compounds or subfractions within structural classes. Initially, it was determined that an ethyl-acetate extract of whole cranberry fruit inhibited growth of human tumor cell lines in vitro (Yan et al., 2002). From ethyl-acetate soluble extracts we isolated and identified two hydroxycinnamate esters of ursolic acid that inhibited the growth of several types of tumor cells in vitro, including MCF-7 breast, HT-29 colon, DU-145 prostate, H460 lung, ME180 cervical epidermoid, and K562 leukemia cell lines (Murphy et al., 2003). The concentration at which 50% growth inhibition occurred (GI_{50}) ranged from 11 to 28 μg/mL for these esters depending on cell line. LC-MS analysis of various cranberry cultivars found that in addition to the parent ursolic acid, the hydroxycinnamate esters are present in whole cranberry fruit in quantities averaging about 15–20 mg per 100 g of fresh fruit (Kondo, 2006). Ursolic acid isolated from cranberry fruit was also reported to inhibit the proliferation of HepG2 human liver cancer cells (He and Liu, 2006).

Other members of the genus *Vaccinium* have been found to contain ursolic acid. Highbush blueberries (*Vaccinium corymbosum*) also contain some ursolic acid in the peel. In a systematic study identifying the ethyl-acetate soluble constituents of highbush blueberry fruit, several sterols and triterpenoids, as well as phenolic acids, were isolated (Wang et al., 2000). Ursolic acid and its 19-hydroxy derivative,

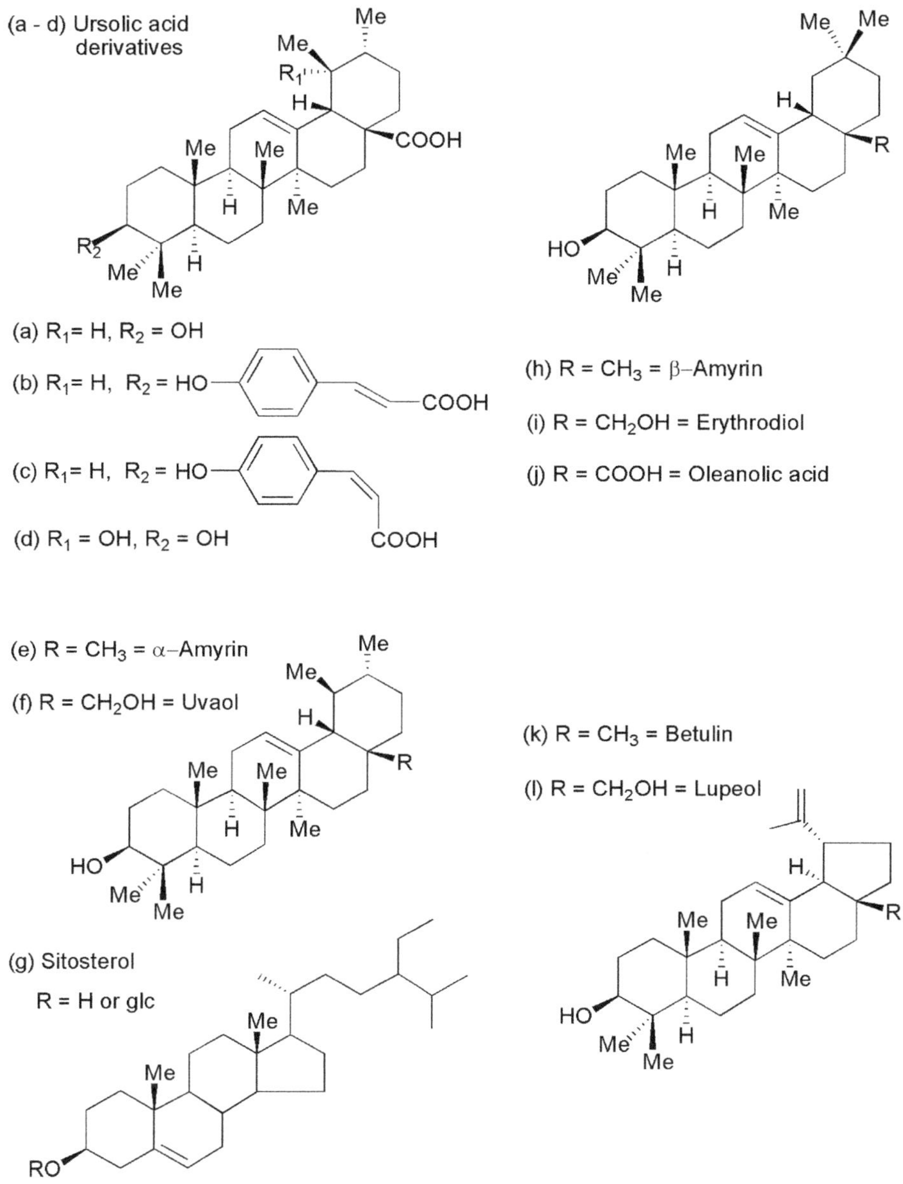

Fig. 2.1 Triterpenoids (C_{30}) identified in berry fruit include (*a–f*): ursolic acid and others derived from α-amyrin skeleton; (*h–j*) oleanolic acid and others derived from the β-amyrin skeleton; (*k–l*) betulins, and (*g*) the common plant sterol β-sitosterol

pomolic acid (Fig. 2.1d), both isolated from blueberry fruit, were reported to inhibit proliferation and DNA synthesis in the HL-60 leukemia cell line at μM concentrations (Wang et al., 2000). A study of triterpenes and sterols isolated from the fruit of "rabbiteye" blueberry (*Vaccinium ashei*) also found that ursolic acid, β-amyrin and a glucoside of the common sterol β-sitosterol (Fig. 2.1g) inhibited the growth of HCT 116 human colon cancer cells and PC-12 adrenal pheochromocytoma cells at micromolar concentrations (Ono et al., 2004). Other triterpenes identified in the fruit with lesser activity were α-amyrin (Fig. 2.1e), uvaol (Fig. 2.1f), erythrodiol (Fig. 2.1i), lupeol and betulin (Fig. 2.1k, l).

Vaccinium vitis-idaea, known variously as cowberry, lingonberry and partridge berry, was reported to contain ursolic acid in fruits and leaves, with somewhat lesser amounts in the stems and rhizomes (Szakiel and Mroczek, 2007). Oleanolic acid (Fig. 2.1h), an isomer of ursolic acid differing only in the position of the C-29 methyl group, was also found in the plant. Both ursolic and oleanolic acid have been recognized as having anti-inflammatory properties (Safayhi and Sailer, 1997).

3 Triterpenoids in Other Berries

Sea buckthorn (*Hippophae rhamnoides* L.) is cultivated in the Baltic Sea region of northern Europe for use in food, fodder, pharmaceuticals and cosmetics, and has been investigated for its antiproliferative effects. A recent study examined the comparative activities of sea buckthorn berry extracts having varying compositions against cell proliferation in the Caco-2 (colon) and Hep G2 (liver) cancer cell lines (Grey et al., 2010). Among the extracts, the ethyl-acetate soluble extract showed the strongest antiproliferative effects on Caco-2 cells. Phytochemical analysis showed that ursolic acid was much higher in this extract than the others. Apoptosis was also detected based on an assay for histone-associated DNA fragments in the cytoplasm. The antiproliferative activity of the ursolic-acid containing fraction was somewhat weaker in the HepG2 cell line, with polyphenolics-rich ethanol-soluble extract showing greater activity. The authors suggest that synergistic effects between the constituents are possible (Grey et al., 2010).

Red berries of the decorative shrub winterberry (*Ilex verticillata*) were investigated for cytotoxic principles using a brine shrimp lethality assay (Fang and McLaughlin, 1989). Solvent partitioning resulted in a bioactive fraction from which ursolic acid was isolated as the active compound. However, winterberry is not recommended for human consumption (USDA/NRCS plant fact sheet at http://plants.usda.gov/factsheet/pdf/fs_ilve.pdf).

Derivatives of ursolic and oleanolic acid have recently been reported as constituents of non-berry fruits including apples (*Malus pumila*), where the aglycones and several cinnamoyl and hydroxycinnamoyl esters were isolated from the peels (He and Liu, 2007). Anti-proliferative activities were measured in three tumor cell lines: HepG2 liver, MCF-7 breast and Caco-2 colon. Most of the triterpenoids exhibited EC_{50} values between 10 and 100 μM. The most effective inhibitors were 2α-hydroxyursolic acid and the coumaroyl esters of maslinic acid (2α-hydroxyoleanolic acid).

4 Anti-cancer and Anti-inflammatory Activities of Ursolic Acid and Its Esters

The anti-proliferative activity of ursolic acid has been reported in a wide variety of cancer cell lines (Neto, 2007). Ursolic acid hydroxycinnamate esters isolated by us from cranberry fruit were evaluated for anti-tumor activity in a 60 tumor cell line panel through the National Cancer Institute's Developmental Therapeutics program (http://dtp.nci.nih.gov/about.html). The esters inhibited the growth of several lung, colon, breast and renal cancers, melanoma and leukemia cell lines with GI_{50} values based on sulforhodamine B (SRB) assay of between 1.2 and 11 μM (Kondo 2006).

Ursolic acid may also affect migration and colony formation by cancer cells. We used clonogenic assays to assess effects of cranberry constituents on tumor colony formation over a 2 week period, showing that ursolic acid and cranberry proanthocyanidins separately inhibited tumor colony formation in a dose-dependent manner in HT-29 and HCT116 colon tumor models (Liberty et al., 2009). In this study, the ursolic acid and cranberry proanthocyanidins both induced apoptosis, as detected by DNA fragmentation, but the effect varied with cell line. Both compounds caused a dose-dependent induction of apoptosis in HT-29 cells, whereas in the HCT116 cells, ursolic acid effectively induced apoptosis, but the proanthocyanidins had a weaker effect. Complementary effects of these compounds are likely to play a role in decreased tumor cell proliferation (Liberty et al., 2009).

Most of the existing bioactivity studies on ursolic acid examine the activity of purified ursolic acid, either isolated from a plant or commercially obtained. The anti-inflammatory actions of pentacyclic triterpenoids are well known and structure-activity relationships have been reviewed (Safayhi and Sailer, 1997). For ursolic acid, several studies report anti-inflammatory activities in vivo, primarily observing reduced inflammation in mouse-ear edema models (Recio et al., 1995; Baricevic et al., 2001). The effects of ursolic acid on proinflammatory pathways observed in vitro include inhibition of COX-2 catalyzed prostaglandin biosynthesis (Ringbom et al., 1998). Ursolic acid inhibited COX-2 transcription in a human mammary oncogenic epithelial cell line (184B5/HER) and the observed suppression of gene expression involved the protein kinase C signal transduction pathway (Subbaramaiah et al., 2000).

Recently, cranberry extracts were evaluated for their anti-inflammatory activity, and a methanol-soluble extract was found to inhibit the activity of COX-2 at 50 μg/mL based on measuring conversion of arachidonic acid to prostaglandin E2 (Huang et al., 2009). The most active subfraction in this study, which inhibited COX-2 activity by 85% at a concentration of 10 μg/mL, was analyzed by LC-MS and found to contain ursolic acid and its hydroxycinnamate esters. The methanol fraction and active subfractions also inhibited the TNF-induced activation of NF-κB in Jurkat cells as well as NF-κB transcription in human T lymphocytes.

Other possible anti-inflammatory mechanisms for ursolic acid include induction of NF-κB mediated expression of inducible nitric oxide synthase (iNOS) and TNF-α in macrophages, implying a possible anti-carcinogenic mechanism involving enhanced NO production (You et al., 2001). In the same cranberry anti-inflammation study described above, cranberry extracts were also evaluated for iNOS activity in RAW 264.7 mouse macrophages. However, the extracts had no effect on iNOS activity at concentrations of 100 μg/mL or less (Huang et al., 2009).

Despite its being recognized as an anti-inflammatory (Kim et al., 2004), ursolic acid has received relatively little attention as a functional food factor. Data on in vivo anti-cancer effects are quite scarce and most involve mouse paw edema models. One of the few in vivo anticancer studies of ursolic acid appeared in 2001. This mouse model study reported that a dose of 100 mg/kg inhibited murine fibrosarcoma FSaII growth (Lee et al., 2001).

5 Mechanisms of Action

The in vitro anti-tumor activity of ursolic acid was reviewed in 2001 (Novotny et al., 2001). In addition to its anti-inflammatory activity, ursolic acid reduces the proliferation of many tumor cell lines and many possible mechanisms of action have been addressed. Studies in B16 cells and MCF-7 breast carcinoma cells showed an early G1 cytostatic effect for ursolic acid (Es-saady et al., 1996a, b). Enhancement of intracellular Ca^{2+} signaling is thought to play a role in reducing proliferation (Novotny et al., 2001).

Ursolic acid's ability to induce apoptosis in many different cell types is likely to play a major role in its anti-proliferative activity. In HT-29 colon cells, ursolic acid decreased proliferation by induction of apoptosis accompanied by activation of caspases-3, 8 and 9 (Andersson et al., 2003). Ursolic acid-induced apoptosis in HL-60 leukemia cells was observed to be mediated by intracellular Ca^{2+} release (Baek et al., 1997). In human prostate cells, apoptosis was accompanied by enhanced release of cytochrome c, caspase activation, and down-regulation of inhibitor of apoptosis proteins (c-IAPs) (Choi et al., 2000). Increased expression of $p21^{WAF1}$, a gene regulated by p53 and thought to induce tumor suppression through inhibition of cyclin-dependent kinases (CDKs), has also been reported (Kim et al., 2000). In B16F-10 melanoma cells, ursolic acid at non-cytotoxic concentrations (10–50 μM) resulted in apoptosis accompanied by upregulation of the tumor suppressor gene p53 and caspase-3 and down-regulation of anti-apoptotic gene Bcl-2 (Manu and Kuttan, 2008). This decrease in NF-κB-mediated activation of Bcl-2 occurred with the inhibition of several transcription factors in the NF-κB pathway. A reduction was seen in the expression of pro-inflammatory cytokines IL-1β and IL-6, and TNF-α and GM-CSF. Caspase-3 activation by ursolic acid through the mitochondrial pathway with upregulation of pro-apototic Bax and a decrease in Bcl-2 was reported in M4Beu human melanoma cells (Duval et al., 2008). Further, studies in an endometrial cancer cell line SNG-II showed that treatment with 50 μM ursolic acid decreased activation of the phosphatidylinositol-3-kinase-Akt (PI3K-Akt) pathway and the mitogen activated protein kinase (MAPK) pathways, which are associated with the high level of Akt phosphorylation often seen in endometrial tumors (Achiwa et al., 2007)

Ursolic acid has been shown to decrease the expression of matrix metalloproteinase-9 (MMP-9) (Cha et al., 1996) 31. Matrix metalloproteinase activities are involved in the remodeling of the extracellular matrix, part of the tumor micro-environment, and are thus linked to tumor invasion and increased risk of metastasis (Björklund and Koivunen, 2005). Ursolic acid has been shown to decrease cell viabililty and induce apoptosis in prostate cancer cells (Kassi et al., 2007). Since prostate cancers often metastasize, we have studied the effects of cranberry constituents on matrix metalloproteinase expression in DU-145 prostate tumor cells. The hydroxycinnamoyl esters of ursolic acid were evaluated by us in a DU-145 prostate tumor model and were found to strongly inhibit expression of both MMP-2 and MMP-9 at micromolar concentrations (Kondo et al., unpublished results). While polyphenolics from cranberry fruit also inhibited MMP expression (Neto et al., 2006), the triterpenoids were observed to do so at much lower concentrations.

6 Future Research Directions

Considering the anti-proliferative activities of triterpenoids such as ursolic acid in cancer cells, the various molecular pathways affected, and the occurrence of these compounds in cranberries and other fruit, there is a clear need for further research on these compounds as potential functional food factors. Studies on their bioavailability and the nature of metabolites formed in vivo would be helpful in determining the role triterpenoids may play in preventing cancers and inflammatory diseases. The oral bioavailability of these compounds is not well-known and should be evaluated. Complementary or synergistic effects with other berry constituents such as flavonoids and carotenoids should be considered, as well as the effect of processing on the triterpenoid content in products derived from fruits.

References

Achiwa Y, Hasegawa K, Udagawa Y (2007) Regulation of the phosphatidylinositol 3-kinase-Akt and the mitogen-activated protein kinase pathways by ursolic acid in human endometrial cancer cells. Biosci Biotechnol Biochem 71:31–37

Andersson D, Liu JJ, Nilsson A, Duan RD (2003) Ursolic acid inhibits proliferation and stimulates apoptosis in HT29 cells following activation of alkaline sphingomyelinase. Anticancer Res 23:3317–3322

Baek JH, Lue YS, Kang CM, Kim JA, Kwon KS, Son HC, Kim KW (1997) Intracellular Ca^{2+} release mediates ursolic acid-induced apoptosis in human leukemic HL-60 cells. Int J Cancer 73:725–728

Baricevic D, Sosa S, Della Loggia R, Tubaro A, Simonovska B, Krasna A, Zupancic A (2001) Topical anti-inflammatory activity of *Salvia officianalis* L. leaves: the relevance of ursolic acid. J Ethnopharmacol 75:125–132

Björklund M, Koivunen E (2005). Gelatinase-mediated migration and invasion of cancer cells. Biochim Biophys Acta 1755:37–69

Cha HJ, Bae SK, Lee HY, Lee O.H, Sato H, Setki M, Park BC, Kim KW (1996) Anti-invasive activity of ursolic acid correlates with the reduced expression of matrix metalloproteinase-9 (MMP-9) in HT1080 human fibrosarcoma cells. Cancer Res 56:2281–2284

Choi YH, Baek JH, Yoo MA, Chung HY, Kim ND, Kim KW (2000) Induction of apoptosis by ursolic acid through activation of caspases and down-regulation of c-IAPs in human prostate epithelial cells. Int J Oncol 17:565–571

Dewick PM (2001) Medicinal natural products, a biosynthetic approach, 2nd edn. Wiley, Chichester, pp 212–219

Duval RE, Harmand PO, Jayat-Vignoles C, Cook-Moreau J, Pinon A, Delage C, Simon A (2008) Differential involvement of mitochondria during ursolic-acid induced apoptotic process in HaCaT and M4Beu cells. Oncol Rep 19:145–149

Es-saady D, Simon A, Jayat-Vignoles C, Chulia AJ, Delage C (1996a) MCF-7 cell cycle arrested at G_1 through ursolic acid and increased reduction of tetrazolium salts. Anticancer Res 16: 481–486

Es-saady D, Simon A, Ollier M, Maurizis JC, Chulia AJ, Delage C (1996b) Inhibitory effect of ursolic acid on B16 proliferation through cell cycle arrest. Cancer Lett 106:193–197

Fang XP, McLaughlin JL (1989) Ursolic acid, a cytotoxic component of the berries of Ilex verticillata. Fitoterapia 61:176–177

Grey C, Widen C, Adlercreutz P, Rumpunen K, Duan RD (2010) Antiproliferative effects of sea buckthorn (Hippophae rhamnoides L.) extracts on human colon and liver cancer cell lines. Food Chem 120:1004–1010

He X, Liu RH (2006) Cranberry phytochemicals: isolation, structure elucidation and their anti-proliferative and antioxidant activities. J Agric Food Chem 54:7069–7074

He X, Liu RH (2007) Triterpenoids isolated from apple peels have potent anti-proliferative activity and may be partially responsible for apple's anticancer activity. J Agric Food Chem 55: 4366–4370

Huang Y, Nikolic D, Pendland S, Doyle BJ, Locklear TJ, Mahady GB (2009) Effects of cranberry extracts and ursolic acid derivatives on P-fimbriated Escherichia coli, COX-2 activity, pro-inflammatory cytokine release and the NF-κB transcriptional response in vitro. Pharm Biol 47:18–25

Kassi E, Papoutsi Z, Pratsinis H, Aligiannis N, Manoussakis M, Moutsatsou P (2007) Ursolic acid, a naturally occurring triterpenoid, demonstrates anticancer activity on human prostate cancer cells. J Cancer Res Clin Oncol 133:493–500

Kim DK, Baek JH, Kang CM, Yoo MA, Sung JW, Kim DK, Chung HY, Kim ND, Choi YH et al (2000) Apoptotic activity of ursolic acid may correlated with the inhibition of initiation of DNA replication. Int J Cancer 87:629–636

Kim KA, Lee JS, Park HJ, Kim JW, Kim CJ, Shim IS, Kim NJ, Han SM Lim S (2004) Inhibition of cytochrome P450 activities by oleanolic acid and ursolic acid in human liver microsomes. Life Sci 74:2769–2779

Kondo M (2006) Phytochemical studies of extracts from cranberry (*Vaccinium macrocarpon*) with anti-cancer, anti-fungal and cardioprotective properties. M.S. Thesis, University of Massachusetts Dartmouth

Lee I, Lee J, Lee YH, Leonard J (2001) Ursolic-acid induced changes in tumor growth, O_2 consumption, and tumor interstitial fluid pressure. Anticancer Res 21(4A): 2827–2833

Liberty AM, Amoroso JW, Hart PE, Neto CC (2009) Cranberry PACs and triterpenoids: anti-cancer activities in colon tumor cell lines. Proceedings of the second international symposium on human health effects of fruits and vegetables. Acta Hortic 841:61–66

Manu KA, Kuttan G (2008) Ursolic acid induces apoptosis by activating p53 and caspase-3 gene expressions and suppressing NF-kB mediated activation of bcl-2 in B16F-10 melanoma cells. Int Immunopharmacol 8:974–981

Murphy BT, MacKinnon SL, Yan X, Hammond GB, Vaisberg AJ, Neto CC (2003) Identification of triterpene hydroxycinnamates with in vitro anti-tumor activity from whole cranberry fruit *(Vaccinium macrocarpon)*. J Agric Food Chem 51:3541–3545

Neto CC (2007) Cranberry and its phytochemicals: a review of in vitro anticancer studies. J Nutr 137:186S–193S

Neto CC, Krueger CG, Lamoureaux TL, Kondo M, Vaisberg AJ, Hurta RAR, Curtis S, Matchett MD, Yeung H, Sweeney-Nixon MI, Reed JD (2006) MALDI-TOF MS characterization of proanthocyanidins from cranberry fruit (*Vaccinium macrocarpon*) that inhibit tumor cell growth and matrix metalloproteinase expression *in vitro*. J Sci Food Agric 86:18–25

Novotny L, Vachalkova A, Biggs D (2001) Ursolic acid: an anti-tumorigenic and chemopreventive activity minireview. Neoplasma 48:241–246

Ono M, Koto M, Komatsu H, Igoshi K, Kobayashi H, Ito Y, Nohara T (2004) Cytotoxic triterpenes and sterol from the fruit of rabbiteye blueberry (*Vaccinium ashei*). Food Sci Technol Res 10: 56–59

Recio MC, Giner RM, Manez S, Gueho J, Julien HR, Hostettmann K, Rios JL (1995) Investigations on the steroidal anti-inflammatory activity of triterpenoids from *Diospyros leucomelas*. Planta Med 61:9–12

Ringbom T, Segura L, Noreen Y, Perera P, Bohlin L (1998) Ursolic acid from *Plantago major*, a selective inhibitor of cyclooxygenase-2 catalyzed prostaglandin biosynthesis. J Nat Prod 61:1212–1215

Safayhi H, Sailer E-R (1997) Anti-Inflammatory actions of pentacyclic triterpenes. Planta Med 63:487–493

Subbaramaiah K, Michaluart P, Sporn MB, Dannenberg AJ (2000) Ursolic acid inhibits cyclooxygenase-2 transcription in human mammary epithelial cells. Cancer Res 60:2399–2404

Szakiel A, Mroczek A (2007) Distribution of triterpene acids and their derivatives in organs of cowberry (*Vaccinium vits-idaea*, L.) plant. Acta Biochim 54:733–740

Wang M, Li J, Shao Y, Huang T, Huang C, Chin C, Rosen RT, Ho CT (2000) Anti-oxidative and cytotoxic components of highbush blueberry (*Vaccinium corymbosum* L.), In: Phytochemicals and phytopharmaceuticals. AOCS Press, Champaign, IL, pp 271–277

Yan X, Murphy BT, Hammond GB, Vinson JA, Neto CC (2002) Antioxidant activities and anti-tumor screening of extracts from cranberry fruit (*Vaccinium macrocarpon*). J Agric Food Chem 20:5844–5849

You HJ, Choi CY, Kim JY, Park SJ, Hahm KS, Jeong HG (2001) Ursolic acid enhances nitric oxide and tumor necrosis factor-a production via nuclear factor-kB activation in the resting macrophages. FEBS Lett 509:156–160

Chapter 3
The Effects of Berry Extracts on Cell Signaling Pathways: Leading to Cellular Transformation

Tongjian Cai and Chuanshu Huang

Abstract Cell signaling pathways play fundamental roles in modulating various biological processes such as cell cycle, cell proliferation, differentiation, and survival. The abnormal activation of several signaling pathways has been linked to the development of various cancers, whereas the inhibition of these pathways has also been considered as a strategy for cancer prevention and therapy. A series of in vitro studies have shown that berry extracts may exert their chemopreventive effects through targeting different cellular signaling pathways, including transcription factors (NFκB, AP-1), their upstream kinases (RTKs, PI3K/Akt, MAPKs), and their downstream target genes (COX-2, VEGF). This chapter outlined the current progresses in this research area. It should be noted that more efforts are needed to address the direct targets of berry extracts and their active compounds, as well as the crosstalk among the various pathways that are inhibited for chemopreventive effects by the berries and berry components because of the complexity and diversity of cancers, cell signaling pathways, and extracts themselves.

Keywords Berry extracts · Signaling pathways · Cellular transformation

Abbreviations

AML	Acute myeloid leukemia
AP-1	Activator protein-1
AR	Androgen receptor
B[a]P	Benzo(a)pyrene
B[a]PDE	Benzo(a)pyrene diol-epoxide
C3G	Cyanidin-3-glucoside
CLA	Conjugated linoleic acid
COX	Cyclooxygenase

C. Huang (✉)
Nelson Institute of Environmental Medicine, New York University School of Medicine, Tuxedo, NY 10987, USA
e-mail: chuanshu.huang@nyumc.org; huangc05@med.nyu.edu

G.D. Stoner, N.P. Seeram (eds.), *Berries and Cancer Prevention*,
DOI 10.1007/978-1-4419-7554-6_3,

CyR	Cyanidin-3-rutinoside
DEN	Diethylnitrosamine
EGF	Epidermal growth factor
EGFR	Epidermal growth factor receptor
ERK	Extracellular signal-regulated kinase
FGF	Fibroblast growth factor
FGFR	Fibroblast growth factor receptor
GSK3β	Glycogen synthase kinase 3β
HCC	Human hepatocellular carcinoma
HIF	Hypoxia-induced factor
HNSCC	Head and neck squamous cell carcinoma
IGF	Insulin-like growth factor
IGFR	Insulin-like growth factor receptor
IL-6	Interleukin-6
JNK	c-jun amino-terminal kinase
MAPK	Mitogen-activated protein kinase
ME	Methanol extract
MKP	Mitogen-activated protein kinase phosphatase
MMP	Matrix metalloproteinase
mTOR	Mammalian target of rapamycin
mTORC1	Mammalian target of rapamycin complex-1
NFAT	Nuclear factor of activated T cells
NFκB	Nuclear factor κB
NSAID	Non-steroidal anti-inflammatory drug
p70S6K	70 kDa ribosomal S6 kinase
PDGF	Platelet-derived growth factor
PDGFR	Platelet-derived growth factor receptor
PG	Prostaglandin
PI3K/Akt	Phosphatidylinositol-3-kinase/Akt
PIP3	Phosphatidylinositol (3, 4, 5)-triphosphate
PTEN	Phosphatase and tensin homolog
RTK	Receptor tyrosine kinase
SCC	Squamous cell carcinoma
SMC	Smooth muscle cell
TGF	Transforming growth factor
TNF	Tumor necrosis factor
TPA	Tetradecanoylphorbol-13-acetate
TSC2	Tuberous sclerosis complex 2
UV	Ultraviolet
UVB	Ultraviolet-B
UVC	Ultraviolet-C
VEGF	Vascular endothelial growth factor
VEGFR	Vascular endothelial growth factor receptor

1 Introduction

In recent years, both in vivo and in vitro studies have shown that extracts and compounds isolated from berries show anti-cancer activities in several types of tumors, such as esophageal tumors (Chen et al., 2006; Wang et al., 2009), colon cancer (Harris et al., 2001), prostate cancer (Goldmann et al., 2001; Scholtysek et al., 2009), and breast cancer (Lu et al., 2006). However, the molecular mechanisms responsible for such anti-cancer activities remain ambiguous. Cell signaling is a complex net system that governs basic cellular activities and coordinates cell actions. After activated, cell signaling pathway components regulate their target proteins such as transcription factors, which further modulate the expression of different target genes. Thus, these pathways play fundamental roles in modulating various biological processes, including cell cycle, cell proliferation, differentiation, and survival. The abnormal activation of several signaling pathways has been linked to the development of various cancers and the inhibition of these pathways has also been considered as a strategy for cancer prevention and therapy. Up to present, a series of in vitro studies have been carried out to elucidate the inhibition of cellular signaling pathways leading to anti-cancer effects of berry extracts. Several pathways, such as receptor tyrosine kinases (RTKs), phosphatidylinositol-3-kinase/Akt (PI3K/Akt), and mitogen-activated protein kinases (MAPKs), have been reported to participate in the chemopreventive effects of berry extracts. As a result, several transcription factors and their downstream target genes, such as nuclear factor κB (NFκB), activator protein-1 (AP-1), cyclooxygenase-2 (COX-2), and vascular endothelial growth factor (VEGF), have also been connected to the chemopreventive effects of berry extracts. In the present chapter, we summarize the studies in this specific field.

2 Receptor Tyrosine Kinases (RTKs)

2.1 RTK Signaling Pathways and Cancers

Various growth factors, such as epidermal growth factor (EGF), platelet-derived growth factor (PDGF), insulin-like growth factor (IGF), fibroblast growth factor (FGF), and vascular endothelial growth factor (VEGF), transduce their mitogenic signals through the activation of receptor tyrosine kinases (RTKs) (Gouni-Berthold and Sachinidis, 2004). RTKs are transmembrane proteins that have multiple functional domains, including an extracellular ligand-binding domain, a transmembrane segment, and intracellular domains, which contain the juxtamembrane segment, the tyrosine kinase catalytic domain, and a carboxy-terminal tail (Castellone et al., 2008). Upon growth factor binding to its specific receptor, mutual transphosphorylation of tyrosine residues within active RTK dimers recruits intracellular proteins endowed with phosphotyrosine-binding domains. Proximal targets of RTKs invoke PI3K/AKT and MAPKs pathways, which leads to further diverse biological responses (Castellone et al., 2008).

RTKs have been shown to be involved in malignant transformation and tumor proliferation (Porter and Vaillancourt, 1998). It is well known that the aberrant signaling by RTKs is critically involved in human cancers and other hyper-proliferative diseases. Constitutive activation of RTKs, which has been shown to be important for malignant transformation and tumor proliferation, can occur by several mechanisms. In most cases, gene amplification, overexpression, and mutations, are responsible for the acquired transforming potential of oncogenic RTKs (Zwick et al., 2001). Oncogenic mutations disrupt normal regulatory mechanisms and lead to the constitutive activation of the kinases. Point mutations or rearrangements in the extracellular domain mimic ligand-binding, thereby causing constitutive dimerization (Castellone et al., 2008). Vascular endothelial growth factor receptor (VEGFR) is a key modulator of angiogenesis (Teller et al., 2009). Highly expressed in a variety of human malignancies, epidermal growth factor receptor (EGFR) is correlated with poor tumor differentiation, fast tumor growth, and high metastatic rate (Bellezza et al., 2006). EGFR binding with its ligand activates multiple signaling pathways, including the PI3K/AKT pathway. Approximately 10–15% of patients with non-small cell lung cancer have tumors that depend on the activation of EGFR (Riely, 2008). Abnormal expression and function of human EGFR have also been found to be responsible for the development and progression of prostate cancer (Gross et al., 2004). Deregulation of fibroblast growth factor receptor (FGFR) signaling, another important member of RTKs, by either mutations or ligand/receptor overexpression could make it constitutively active, leading to cancer development (Acevedo et al., 2009). Overexpression of other growth factor receptors, including insulin-like growth factor receptor (IGFR), platelet-derived growth factor receptor (PDGFR), and EGFR, has also been considered to be associated with poor prognosis in breast cancer.

The inhibition of RTKs has been considered as a strategy for chemoprevention of cancers. Targeted agents inhibit receptor tyrosine kinase signaling by binding the extracellular component of a growth receptor, the soluble ligand that triggers the receptor, or intracellular sites that interfere with downstream signaling events (Zureikat and McKee, 2008). Due to its universal expression in head and neck squamous cell carcinoma (HNSCC), EGFR has long been a target for the treatment of HNSCC (Cooper and Cohen, 2009). Gefitinib is an orally-active EGFR inhibitor that blocks EGFR signaling in vitro. It thereby inhibits the growth, proliferation, and survival of many solid tumors (Von Pawel, 2004). Clinical trial data show that gefitinib mono-therapy is generally well tolerated in patients with a wide range of tumor types (Ranson, 2002; Von Pawel, 2004). Targeted therapies against ErbB family have shown some promise in the treatment of hormone-refractory prostate cancer (Chen et al., 2008). RTK inhibitors against the receptors for different growth factors manifest significant antiangiogenic activities. These compounds can also enhance tumor radiation response by attacking tumor microvasculature (Lu et al., 2005).

2.2 The Effects of Berry Extracts on RTK Pathways and Their Chemoprevention

Although large numbers of studies have reported that RTKs are important in carcinogenesis, the research on the potential of targeting RTKs by berry extracts is still in its early stages. Mirtocyan is a standardized anthocyanin-rich extract of bilberries. A recent report has shown that both mirtocyan and oenocyanin E163, an extract of red grape pomace, can inhibit the kinase activity of recombinant kinase domains of each RTK at concentrations $\leq$12.9 μg/ml, with preferential inhibition of VEGFR-2 and EGFR ($\leq$3.4 μg/ml) (Teller et al., 2009). Similarly, ligand-induced autophosphorylation of these RTKs in human vulva carcinoma or porcine aortic endothelial cells is suppressed by the mixtures. Such anthocyanin-rich extracts completely abrogate VEGFR-3 phosphorylation at concentrations of $\geq$50 μg/ml. Further results indicate that these mixtures can inhibit RTKs with low specificity (Teller et al., 2009). As we have mentioned above, different VEGFRs are key modulators of angiogenesis. After binding to VEGF, VEGFRs further activate intracellular signaling pathways, eliciting angiogenesis by inducing the migration and proliferation of endothelial cells (Lu et al., 2006). Anthocyanidins are a major series of flavonoid constituents present in berries (Taruscio et al., 2004; Cooke et al., 2005). Lamy et al. have investigated the antiangiogenic effects of six kinds of anthocyanidins, including cyanidin, delphinidin, malvidin, pelargonidin, peonidin, and petunidin. Among six contents, delphinidin is the most effective in inhibiting the differentiation of endothelial cells (Lamy et al., 2006). Delphinidin can also potently inhibit VEGF-induced capillary-like structure formation and endothelial cell migration in vitro (Lamy et al., 2006). Lamy et al's work further shows that delphinidin inhibits VEGF-induced phosphorylation of VEGFR-2 and ERK1/2, a substrate of VEGFR-2, which may be involved in VEGF-induced endothelial cell migration and capillary-like structure formation (Lamy et al., 2006). Although the mechanism by which delphinidin elicits its inhibitory effect on VEGFR-2 is not yet known, structure–function analysis suggests that the inhibitory effects of delphinidin can be enhanced by the presence of three hydroxyl groups at the B-ring, as compared to other anthocyanidins. Such a free hydroxyl group at Position 3 seems to be essential for its potent inhibitory effects (Lamy et al., 2006). Delphinidin can be not only a potent inhibitor of VEGF-induced capillary-like structure formation and endothelial cells migration, but also an inhibitor of smooth muscle cells (SMCs) migration, which is important for the mature and normal function of vasculature (Lamy et al., 2008). In another research from the same group, delphinidin is shown to inhibit PDGF-induced migration of SMCs, as well as the differentiation and stabilization of endothelial cells (ECs) and SMCs into capillary-like tubular structures. Such effects of delphinidin may be related to its inhibitory effects on PDGFR-β, which in turn leads to the inhibition of ERK1/2 activation and the chemotactic motility of SMCs (Lamy et al., 2008). Similarly, delphinidin is an effective inhibitor of EGFR signaling, which mediates the suppression of PI3K, AKT, and MAPK. This inhibition is thought to be responsible for its inhibitory effects on the invasion, growth, and induction of apoptosis in breast cancer cells (Afaq et al., 2008).

3 PI3K/Akt Signaling Pathway

3.1 PI3K/Akt Signaling Pathway and Cancer

PI3K consists of a regulatory subunit (p85) and a catalytic subunit (p110) (Dhand et al., 1994), which is well-known as being involved in the regulation of multiple cellular events, including cell survival, growth, and transformation (Huang et al., 1996, 1997b; Rahmani et al., 2009). Activated PI3K preferentially phosphorylates the membrane phospholipid, phosphatidylinositol (4, 5)-biphosphate, to produce phosphatidylinositol(3, 4, 5)-triphosphate (PIP3). PIP3 functions as a second messenger to recruit pleckstrin homology domain-containing proteins, such as Akt and phosphoinositide-dependent kinases (Xiao et al., 2009). PI3K signaling is inhibited by phosphatase and tensin homolog (PTEN) through the dephosphorylation of PIP3 (Yap et al., 2008). Akt is one of the major downstream targets of PI3K (Du et al., 2009). As a serine/threonine kinase, Akt activity is tightly regulated by PI3K. Phosphorylation of Akt at Thr^{308} and Ser^{473} is necessary for its full activation, which subsequently regulates many biological responses by targeting downstream effectors (Wang et al., 2010). One of the well-known Akt substrates, glycogen synthase kinase 3β (GSK3β), is involved in numerous cellular functions such as metabolism, survival, gene expression, and cytoskeletal dynamics, while its activity is inhibited by the phosphorylation at its Ser^{9} residue (Uranga et al., 2009). The accumulation of GSK3β in the nucleus mediates cyclin D1 phosphorylation, nuclear export, and subsequent ubiquitin-dependent degradation of cyclin D1, thereby linking PI3K/Akt pathway to cell proliferation (Gu et al., 2009). Another key effector downstream of Akt is mammalian target of rapamycin (mTOR). PI3K/Akt/mTOR is an important pathway for cellular growth, survival, and energy homeostasis. The mammalian target of rapamycin complex-1 (mTORC1) mediates numerous intracellular processes, including protein synthesis and survival, through its actions on target molecules including the 70 kDa ribosomal S6 kinase (p70S6K) (Patel and Mohan, 2005; Matheny and Adamo, 2009).

The activation of Akt generally promotes cell survival due to the inactivation of proapoptotic effectors such as Bad and Bim (Rahmani et al., 2009; Zhou et al., 2009b). Activated Akt phosphorylates BAD, which prevents its binding with Bcl-xL (Zhou et al., 2009a). Akt can also promote cell survival through the activation of NFκB and the upregulation of anti-apoptotic protein Bcl-2, by which growth factors mediate cell survival (Dai et al., 2009). The activation of Akt results in IκB degradation and allows NFκB to enter the nucleus and up-regulate the anti-apoptotic genes (Zhou et al., 2009b). PI3K/Akt signaling has also been reported to suppress $p27^{Kip1}$ and thus precede cell cycle (Li et al., 2010). In addition to promoting cell proliferation and survival, the PI3K/Akt pathway can also influence apoptotic cell death machinery through its interaction with other pathways such as MAPKs (Xie et al., 2009).

The role of PI3K/Akt pathway in the development of cell transformation has been extensively investigated (Huang et al., 1996, 1997b; Agarwal et al., 2009). Altered expression or mutation of many components in this pathway have been implicated in human cancers (Garcia-Echeverria and Sellers, 2008; Xie et al., 2009). The mutations in PI3K pathway components account for up to 30% of all human cancers (Cakir and Grossman, 2009). A high level of phosphorylated Akt correlates with a poor prognosis in cases of prostate cancer, whereas in normal prostate tissue, phosphorylated Akt is undetectable (Assinder et al., 2009). The PI3K/Akt/mTOR pathway is constitutively activated in many types of cancers. Once activated, this pathway confers resistance to many types of cancer therapy (LoPiccolo et al., 2008; Assinder et al., 2009). Activated Akt inhibits GSK3β, which normally prevents up-regulation of cell proliferation due to increased cyclin D1 degradation (Assinder et al., 2009). Also, the inhibition of GSK3β has been shown to spare free β-catenin from degradation in prostate-cancer cells (Assinder et al., 2009). As a bridge between cytoskeleton and cadherin motifs in cell-to-cell junctions, increased β-catenin can bind and stabilize cyclin D1 mRNA, which leads to the enhanced cyclin D1 protein expression. Such overexpression may further promote G1-phase/S-phase progression (Assinder et al., 2009). The upregulation of PI3K/PTEN/Akt/mTOR and Ras/Raf/MEK/ERK pathways and the phosphorylation of the downstream target Bad are observed frequently in acute myeloid leukemia (AML) patient specimens and are associated with the poorer prognosis than patients lacking these changes (McCubrey et al., 2008). p53 is a well-known tumor suppressor. Our work has demonstrated that the knockout of p53 also results in PI3k/Akt activation (Wang et al., 2005).

PI3k/Akt plays a key role in chemically-induced carcinogenesis. Our results have demonstrated that PI3K/Akt-mediated cyclin D1 expression is a key event implicated in arsenite-induced human keratinocyte transformation. Repeated exposure of HaCat cells, an immortalized human keratinocytes cell line, to arsenite causes malignant transformation (Ouyang et al., 2008). The arsenite exposure also increases in PI3K/Akt activation and the inhibition of PI3K/Akt activation blocks such cell transformation in HaCat cells (Ouyang et al., 2008). Further studies show that this effect of the PI3K/Akt-dependent pathway is through the upregulation of cyclin D1 expression (Ouyang et al., 2008). Our work also shows that arsenite can induce cyclin D1 expression through PI3K/Akt/JNK/c-Jun signaling in human bronchial epithelial Beas-2B cells (Ding et al., 2009b) or through the PI3K/Akt/IKKβ/NFκB signal cascade in mouse epidermal Cl41 cells (Ouyang et al., 2006). In addition to arsenite, our work also shows that the activation of PI3K/Akt may be responsible for various biological effects due to exposure to other carcinogens, such as benzo(a)pyrene diol-epoxide (B[a]PDE) (Ding et al., 2006a), 5-MCDE (Ding et al., 2006a), nickel (Li et al., 2004b; Ouyang et al., 2005), and ultraviolet (UV) (Huang et al., 2001).

Constitutive activation of PI3K/Akt may also be due to the aberrant expression of its natural antagonist PTEN. The loss of heterozygosity at the PTEN locus has been observed in 27–32% of the hepatocellular cancers (HCC) (Michl and Downward, 2005). The PTEN gene is commonly inactivated by mutation and deletion. Such aberrations have been implicated in the development of glioblastoma, endometrial, prostate, and other cancers (Yap et al., 2008). The loss of PTEN appears to be the most common mechanism responsible for PI3K activation in human cancers (Cakir and Grossman, 2009).

Moreover, the inhibition of PI3K/Akt pathway is a major molecular mechanism implicated in anti-cancer effects of several natural products. Inositol hexaphosphate (InsP6) is an abundant inositol phosphate found in plants. In our early study, we found that InsP6 could direct interact with PI3K, by which InsP6 markedly blocks EGF-induced PI3K activity in a dose-dependent manner in C141 cells. Such interaction profoundly impairs EGF- or phorbol ester-induced cell transformation and ERK1/2 MAPK-regulated protein kinases activation, as well as AP-1 activation in C141 cells (Huang et al., 1997a). Conjugated linoleic acid (CLA) is an important naturally occurring fatty acid. A recent study has shown that CLA could reduce the growth and invasion of breast cancer through the inhibition of PI3K/AKT pathway (Bocca et al., 2010). Fisetin (3,3′,4′,7-tetrahydroxyflavone) is a naturally occurring flavonoid that has been reported to possess anti-cancer and anti-inflammation capabilities. Recently, it has been found to exhibit its inhibitory effects on the adhesion, migration, and invasion ability of a highly metastatic PC-3 cells under non-cytotoxic concentrations through the inhibition of PI3K/AKT and JNK pathways, which further reduce the protein expression of MMP-2 and MMP-9 (Chien et al., 2010).

3.2 The Effects of Berry Extracts on PI3K/Akt Pathway and Their Chemoprevention

Our studies have demonstrated that the PI3K/Akt pathway is critical for B[a]PDE-induced AP-1 activation in mouse epidermal C141 cells (Huang et al., 2006), and overexpression of the dominant negative PI3K mutant p85 (Δp85) has been found to reduce the VEGF induction due to B[a]PDE exposure (Huang et al., 2006). Our published studies further demonstrate that two black raspberry fractions, RO-FOO3 and RO-ME, show their inhibitory effect on AP-1 activation and AP-1-mediated VEGF induction due to B[a]PDE exposure (Huang et al., 2006). Consistent with the inhibition of AP-1 activation, the RO-ME fraction also markedly inhibits the activation of PI3K, Akt, and p70S6K in C141 cells under same experimental conditions (Huang et al., 2006), revealing that the inhibitory effects of RO-FOO3 and RO-ME on B[a]PDE-induced VEGF expression is mediated by targeting PI3K/Akt/AP-1 pathway. In view of the important roles of AP-1 and VEGF in tumor development, we anticipate that the inhibition of PI3K/Akt/AP-1/VEGF pathway is at least one of the mechanisms responsible for the chemopreventive activity of black raspberries (Huang et al., 2006), and that RO-ME is the major fraction for the inhibition of both AP-1 activation and VEGF production due to B[a]PDE exposure (Huang et al., 2006). In contrast, our further work shows that the extract fraction FA-ME from strawberries does not show such effect on the AP-1 activation and VEGF expression under the same experimental condition (Li et al., 2008). Akt and p70S6K are two major PI3K downstream targets responsible for mediation of chemical carcinogen-induced AP-1 activation (Li et al., 2004a; Ding et al., 2006a). In our studies, FA-ME failed to inhibit Akt activation, while RO-ME blocked B[a]PDE-induced Akt phosphorylation at Thr^{308} and Ser^{473}. The effects of RO-ME and FA-ME on p70S6K are similar to those on Akt activation. Finally, we have shown that RO-ME and FA-ME have different effects on MAPKs activation (Li et al., 2008). FA-ME does not affect MAPK activation, while RO-ME does show an inhibitory effect (Li et al., 2008). Our studies strongly indicate that RO-ME inhibits the carcinogenic PI3K/Akt-p70S6K/MAPKs-AP-1/NFkB signaling pathway triggering by B[a]PDE, whereas FA-ME does not show any inhibition on such pathway (Li et al., 2008). Although we do not know what specific compound(s) in the RO-ME fraction is responsible for such inhibition, the fraction is abundant in anthocyanins, which exhibit a marked ability to down-regulate B[a]PDE-induced NFκB activity in C141 cells (Huang et al., 2002). Anthocyanins also exist richly in mulberry plants and have been well characterized as having various bioactive properties. In addition, mulberry anthocyanins can inhibit the metastasis of B16-F1 cells, a murine melanoma cell line, which is mediated by inhibiting MMP-2 and MMP-9 activities through the suppression of Ras/PI3K signaling pathway (Huang et al., 2008). Further investigation show that mulberry anthocyanins can significantly suppress the activation of Akt by decreasing the expression of p85 regulatory subunit (Huang et al., 2008). Taken together, berry extract fractions, especially black raspberry extract fractions, show significant inhibition of PI3K/Akt pathway and its related downstream gene expression as well as cellular function.

4 Mitogen-Activated Protein Kinases (MAPKs)

4.1 MAPK Signaling Pathways and Cancers

Mitogen-activated protein kinases (MAPKs) are a family of highly conserved proline-directed protein kinases found in all organisms from yeast to human (Widmann et al., 1999). As a superfamily of serine/threonine protein kinases involved in the regulation of large numbers of intracellular signaling, mammalian MAPKs are grouped into at least six major subfamilies: extracellular signal-regulated kinases ERK1 and 2 (ERK1/2, also known as p44 and p42 MAPK), c-Jun-N-terminal kinases (JNKs), p38, ERK-3, ERK-5 (also called big MAP kinase 1), and ERK-6 (Robinson and Cobb, 1997; Zhang et al., 2007). ERK1/2 primarily regulate cellular growth and differentiation, whereas JNKs and p38 mainly function as mediators of cellular stresses such as inflammation and apoptosis (Zheng et al., 2008). MAP kinase families are composed of MAPKs, MAPK kinases (MAPKKs), and MAPKK kinases (MAPKKKs). MAPKKKs can be activated by small GTPases such as Rho and Rac. Activated MAPKKKs subsequently activate MAPKKs, which include MKK1/2, MKK3/6, and MKK4/7. MAPKKs in turn phosphorylate individual MAPKs (Sweeney and Firestein, 2006; Wu, 2007). Activated MAPKs phosphorylate their downstream targets, such as transcription factors, enzymes, and other kinases (Roux and Blenis, 2004). Since phosphorylation is required for the activation of MAPKs, several mitogen-activated protein kinase phosphatases (MKPs) are important negative regulators for MAPKs by mediating their dephosphorylation (Wu, 2007). The MAPKs, implicated in the regulation of cell growth and survival, have been reported to be aberrantly activated in a broad spectrum of human tumors (Kuno et al., 1998; Hoshino et al., 1999).

The Ras/Raf/MEK/ERK signaling pathway regulates cell proliferation, differentiation, and survival (Song et al., 2009). Aberrant activation of this pathway plays a critical role in the development of human cancers (Liu et al., 2007). ERK1/2 have been reported to link to the invasive and migratory behavior of a number of malignancies, such as colon cancer, melanoma, breast cancer, and prostate cancer (Zhou et al., 2007a). The key components of the Ras/Raf/MEK/ERK signal module are frequently altered in human cancers (Whyte et al., 2009). As an ERK1/2 downstream transcription factor, c-Myc is involved in carcinogenesis and is overexpressed in several human tumors (Sun et al., 2008). Downregulation of c-Myc following MEK/ERK inhibition has been found to halt the proliferation of carcinoma cells (Sun et al., 2008). Matrix metalloproteinases (MMPs) play a pivotal role in matrix degradation during tumor growth and invasion, and tumor-induced angiogenesis (Johansson et al., 2000; Nabeshima et al., 2002). It is well known that MMP-9 mRNA expression is modulated by MAPK pathways. Both ERK1/2 and p38 pathways have been found to regulate MMP-9 expression in cancer cells (Gao et al., 2008). In our published studies, we have found that ERK1/2 can be the upstream kinases of AP-1 responsible for tumor necrosis factor-α (TNF-α) induction in cellular response to nickel exposure, which might play a role in nickel-induced lung chronic inflammation and carcinogenicity (Ding et al., 2009a). We have also found that ERK1/2 activation is critical for tetradecanoylphorbol-13-acetate (TPA)-, EGF-, and arsenite-induced cell transformation (Huang et al., 1998, 1999c). At present, pharmacological inhibitors of the Raf/MEK/ERK pathway have been proposed as anti-cancer drugs, which represent a promising anti-cancer strategy. Several agents have been designed to target this pathway and are in various stages of clinical trials (Zhou et al., 2007a; Daouti et al., 2009).

A series of studies have shown that p38 MAPK is involved in several types of cancer development. Androgen receptor (AR) signaling is involved in the development and progression of prostate cancer (Khandrika et al., 2009). As an early response to hypoxia, the inhibition of p38 MAPK pathway activation can abolish hypoxia-reoxygenation-induced AR activity and survival increase, clonogenicity, and invasiveness of prostate cancer cells (Khandrika et al., 2009). p38 MAPK has been demonstrated to be an important mediator of H-Ras-stimulated motility in human breast epithelial cells (Zhou et al., 2007a). Highly activated p38 has been regarded as a marker of poor prognosis for breast cancers (Chen et al., 2009). It has been found to be implicated in breast cancer progression by up-regulating uPA expression. Thus p38 MAPK might be important in the invasion and metastasis of breast cancer (Han et al., 2007). Furthermore, the activation of the p38 MAPK pathway can not only contribute to the loss of cell-cell contact and the round cell shape characteristic of poorly differentiated gastric cancer (Atsumi et al., 2007), it could also be responsible for the chemotherapy resistance in human gastric cancer cells (Guo et al., 2008).

The c-Jun N-terminal kinase (JNK) pathway is an evolutionarily conserved kinase cascade that regulates the apoptotic machinery. There are three jnk genes, jnk1, jnk2, and jnk3, which result in at least 10 different JNK proteins varying in size from 46 to 55 kDa. Both JNK1 and JNK2 proteins are widely expressed, whereas JNK3 expression is largely restricted to neurons in the central nervous system, cardiac smooth muscle, and testis (Sun et al., 2007). In mammal cells, JNK signaling has been implicated in stress-induced apoptosis (Igaki, 2009). JNKs activate apoptotic signaling by upregulating pro-apoptotic genes through the transactivation of specific transcription factors or by directly modulating the activities of pro- and antiapoptotic proteins through distinctly different phosphorylation events (Dhanasekaran and Reddy, 2008). Following activation, JNKs further phosphorylate more than 20 nuclear substrates, many of which are transcription factors. These substrates provide a link to a wide range of cellular functions, such as cell death and cell migration (Bogoyevitch and Kobe, 2006). One of main JNK targets is the transcription factor AP-1, which is composed of Jun and Fos family members. In many human cancers, JNKs can exert dual functions, that can be either oncogenic or tumor suppressive. The oncogenic functions of JNKs are mostly associated with their ability to phosphorylate c-Jun and activate AP-1, whereas their tumor-suppressive function is related to their pro-apoptotic activity (Wagner and Nebreda, 2009). For example, transforming growth factor-β (TGF-β) is involved in actin cytoskeleton reorganization and tumor progression. It promotes the invasion and metastasis of gastric cancer cells by increasing the expression of fascin1, an actin-binding protein involved in cell invasiveness and motility in various transformed cells, via the ERK and JNK signal pathways (Fu et al., 2009). Hepatocyte growth factor enhances proteolysis and invasiveness of human nasopharyngeal cancer cells through the activation of PI3K and JNKs (Zhou et al., 2008). Human hepatocellular carcinoma (HCC) is the third most common cause of death from cancers worldwide. The deficiency of JNK1 (but not JNK2 deficiency) has been shown to significantly decrease susceptibility to diethylnitrosamine (DEN)-induced HCC formation (Wagner and Nebreda, 2009). Our early studies have shown that JNK activation is required for TNF-α-induced cell transformation (Huang et al., 1999a). Recently, we have also demonstrated that JNK1 is implicated in HIF-1α stabilization in nickel-mimicked hypoxia conditions through regulation of Hsp90/Hsp70 expression as well as HDAC6-mediated Hsp90 acetylating modification, which may play an important role in nickel-related carcinogenesis (Zhang et al., 2010). Several chemotherapeutic agents have been shown to exert their effects via the activation of JNK pathway, such as gonadotropin-releasing hormone-II antagonists (Fister et al., 2009), surfactin (Cao et al., 2010), NSC-741909 (Wei et al., 2009), statins (Liu et al., 2009), pseudolaric acid B (Yu et al., 2008), simvastatin (Koyuturk et al., 2007), sphingoid (Ahn and Schroeder, 2006), and isothiocyanates (Xu et al., 2006). We have found that arsenite may induce the apoptosis of Cl41 cells through the activation of JNKs (Huang et al., 1999b). Other studies by our group further show that IκB kinase β (IKKβ)-NF-κB p50 acts as the activator of the MKK4/JNK pathway through the induction of GADD45α in response to arsenite (Song et al., 2006).

4.2 The Effects of Berry Extracts on MAPK Pathways and Their Role in Chemoprevention

Several kinds of berry extracts have been shown to exert their chemopreventive effects through the inhibition of MAPKs. Black raspberry extracts have been shown to inhibit benzo(a)pyrene (B[a]P)-induced cell transformation in vitro (Xue et al., 2001). Our work further shows that the biological effects of black raspberry extracts appear to be mediated via the inhibition of MAPKs activation (Huang et al., 2002). Our data show that RO-ME, a methanol extract (ME) fraction from black raspberries, can inhibit the activation of AP-1 induced by B[a]PDE through its inhibitory effect on the activation of MAPK family, including ERK1/2, JNKs, and p38, suggesting that all these three MAPK family members are involved in the inhibitory effect of RO-ME on AP-1 activation (Huang et al., 2002). Deerberry fruit extracts have been proven to inhibit phosphorylation of ERKs and MEK1/2 due to TPA or UVB exposure in HL-60 cancer cells (Wang et al., 2007).

5 Transcription Factors and Their Downstream Target Genes

5.1 The Role of NFκB, AP-1, COX-2, and VEGF in Cancers

NFκB is implicated in multiple physiological and pathological processes, including cell proliferation and differentiation, cell survival and apoptosis, as well as tumorigenesis (Liu and Lin, 2007; Yu et al., 2009). NFκB family consists of five members: p50/p105, p52/p100, c-Rel, RelA (p65), and RelB, forming several homo- and hetero-dimers (Verstrepen et al., 2009). Under nonstimulated conditions, NFκB complex, formed mainly by a p50/p65 heterodimer, binds to a member of NFκB inhibitors (the IκB family). The nuclear localization signal of NFκB is effectively inhibited due to its noncovalent binding with IκB (Ahmed and Li, 2008). Upon stimulation, IκB is phosphorylated at specific residues, which tags it for ubiquitination and degradation by the proteasome. The degradation of IκB allows NFκB to translocate into the nucleus where it acts as a transcription factor (D'Acquisto et al., 2002). In addition to shuttling in and out of the nucleus, NFκB proteins are post-translationally modified by phosphorylation, acetylation, or ubiquitination. These modifications can alter its binding specificity to different promoters (Bai et al., 2009). Misregulation of NFκB signaling has severe health consequences, which have a broad biomedical impact on understanding pathology of the diseases and devising therapeutic strategies (Kearns and Hoffmann, 2009). As a ubiquitous transcriptional activator, AP-1 is composed of members of Jun and Fos families that form homodimers or heterodimers and bind to a distinct DNA response element. Elevated AP-1 activities and its upstream regulators, such as MAPKs, are found to be involved in neoplastic transformation, tumor progression, metastasis, and angiogenesis (Feng et al., 2004). Many studies have shown that both NFκB and AP-1 play important roles, not only in carcinogenesis, but also in the anti-apoptosis and chemotherapy drug resistance of tumor cells (He et al., 2009). TGF-β suppresses PTEN in pancreatic cancer cells through NFκB activation, which enhances cell motility and invasiveness (Chow et al., 2010). Interleukin-6 (IL-6) is involved in cancer-related inflammation, promotes transformation, proliferation, invasion, angiogenesis, and metastasis (Aggarwal and Gehlot, 2009). The results of a recent research show that hyperactivated NFκB and AP-1 promote highly accessible chromatin and constitutive transcription across the IL-6 gene promoter in metastatic breast cancer cells (Ndlovu et al., 2009). Our previous work shows that the transactivation of NFκB and AP-1 are activated in response to some environmental carcinogens, such as B[a]PDE and UV radiation (Huang et al., 2002, 2007). Some anti-cancer agents have been shown to exert chemopreventive effects through their inhibition of NFκB and AP-1, thereby inhibiting promotion and progression (Zhou et al., 2007b; Gopalakrishnan and Kong, 2008).

Cyclooxygenase-2 (COX) is a major downstream target gene that is regulated by both AP-1 and NFκB, while vascular endothelial growth factor (VEGF) could also be regulated by AP-1 (Lu et al., 2006). COX-1 is expressed constitutively in most tissues, whereas COX-2 is induced by a wide variety of stimuli and was initially identified as an immediate-early growth response gene (Williams et al., 1999). COX-2 is known to produce PGs that regulate tumor-associated angiogenesis, modulate immune system, regulate cell migration and invasion, and inhibit apoptosis, all of which promote cancer progression (Cha and DuBois, 2007). The main product of COX-2, prostaglandin E2 (PGE2), has been found to be at high levels in tumor cells (Mazhar et al., 2006). Other byproducts of the COX-2 pathway, such as malondialdehyde, directly interact with DNA and form DNA adducts that may initiate carcinogenesis (Cha and DuBois, 2007). A significant reversal association between COX-2 overexpression and survival of patients with various cancers has been reported in retrospective studies (Mazhar et al., 2005). For example, the overexpression of COX-2 is an independent predictor of an unfavorable outcome for node-negative breast cancer (Schmitz et al., 2006). As inhibitors of COX activity and PG formation, non-steroidal anti-inflammatory drugs (NSAIDs) are assumed to be effective in the prevention of cancers (Baek and Eling, 2006). Preclinical and clinical studies have clearly shown a benefit of utilization of NSAIDs in reducing cancer risk (Cha and DuBois, 2007).

VEGF, another AP-1-regulated gene, has long been found to be involved in the regulation of vascularization and growth of primary tumors as well as cancer metastases (Martiny-Baron and Marme, 1995). In 1989, Ferrara et al. reported the isolation of VEGF from medium conditioned by bovine pituitary follicular cells (Ferrara and Henzel, 1989). At least five members of VEGF family, including VEGF-A, -B, -C, -D, and -E, have been described in previous studies (Carmeliet, 2005; Bremnes et al., 2006). VEGF-A is of prime importance for angiogenesis (Carmeliet, 2005; Bremnes et al., 2006). A well-established action of VEGF is to promote the growth of vascular endothelial cells derived from arteries, veins, and lymphomatics (Ferrara et al., 2004). In vivo, VEGF induces a potent angiogenic response, which is essential for normal embryonic vasculogenesis and angiogenesis. The inactivation of a single VEGF allele in mice results in embryonic lethality. VEGF can induce the expression of anti-apoptotic protein Bcl-2 in endothelial cells (Ferrara et al., 2005). The most significant regulator of VEGF expression is hypoxia. As a tumor increases in mass, it becomes hypoxic, which leads to VEGF induction and in turn stimulates growth of new vessels. The transcription of VEGF mRNA is up-regulated in hypoxia through hypoxia-induced factors (HIFs) that bind to the VEGF promoter (Ferrara, 2005). VEGF-mediated angiogenesis is thought to play a critical role in tumor growth and metastasis (Cardones and Banez, 2006). As a major regulator of normal and pathological angiogenesis, VEGF is enabled to be a significant target for the effective treatment of cancers, and several VEGF inhibitors have been approved by the US Food and Drug Administration for the treatment of cancers (Ferrara et al., 2007).

5.2 *The Effects of Berry Extracts on Activation of NFκB and AP-1, and Expression of COX-2 and VEGF*

Several studies concerning the effects of berry extracts on transcription factor AP-1 and NFκB have been published. We have reported that pretreatment of C141 cells with various black raspberry extracts results in the inhibition of B[a]PDE-induced AP-1 and NFκB activities and that RO-ME fraction is the most potent inhibitor among the fractions tested (Huang et al., 2002). We have also shown that the inhibitory effects of RO-ME on B[a]PDE-induced activation of AP-1 and NFκB are mediated via inhibition of MAPK activation and inhibitory subunit IκB phosphorylation, respectively (Huang et al., 2002).

While berry extracts show their inhibitory effects on AP-1 and NFκB, they also have inhibitory effects on their target gene expression, such as VEGF and COX-2. In our previous studies, we have shown that pretreatment of C141 cells with RO-ME, a methanol extract (ME) fraction from black raspberries, can result in a significant inhibition of B[a]PDE-induced expression of VEGF and COX-2 (Lu et al., 2006). The ability of black raspberries to down-regulate VEGF and COX-2 expression may be due to their inhibition of the signal transduction pathways that lead to the activation of AP-1 and NFκB (Lu et al., 2006). Using cell lines isolated from human oral squamous cell carcinoma (SCC), Rodrigo et al. have found that a freeze-dried black raspberry ethanol extract, RO-ET, suppresses cell proliferation, VEGF expression, and nitric oxide synthase activity, and induces both apoptosis and terminal differentiation (Rodrigo et al., 2006). Bagchi et al. have evaluated various combinations of edible berry extracts and have developed a synergistic formula, OptiBerry

IH141, which inhibits both H_2O_2- and TNF-α-induced VEGF expression in human keratinocytes (Bagchi et al., 2004).

Our published studies indicate that the fractions from various berries show differential effects on transcription factor activation and gene expression. For example, black raspberry fractions inhibit the activation of AP-1, NFκB, and NFAT as well as their upstream PI3K/Akt/p70S6K and MAPK pathways in C141 cells following B[a]PDE exposure, while strawberry fractions only inhibit NFAT activation, but do not have any inhibitory effect on AP-1, NFκB, PI3K/Akt/p70S6K, or MAPK pathways (Li et al., 2008). Consistent with the effects on NFAT activation, TNF-α induction by B[a]PDE was blocked by extract fractions of both black raspberries and strawberries, whereas VEGF expression, which is mediated by AP-1 activation, is only suppressed by black raspberry fractions, but not strawberry fractions (Li et al., 2008). In another research, we compared the effects of methanol fractions from black raspberries, strawberries, and blueberries on UV-induced activation of NFκB and AP-1 in C141 cells. In this study, only the fractions from black raspberries inhibited UVB-induced NFκB activation in a time- and dose-dependent manner; whereas the methanol fractions from strawberries and blueberries did not show such inhibitory effect. Interestingly, none of the fractions from all three berry types inhibited UVB- or UVC-induced AP-1 activation, suggesting that NFκB is specifically targeted by black raspberries (Huang et al., 2007). This notion is supported by the studies performed by Boivin et al., in which the chemopreventive effects of the extracts from 13 berries have been tested. In terms of cell growth inhibition, only the juice of 6 berries can significantly inhibit TNF-induced COX-2 expression and NFκB activation in various cancer cells, including those of stomach, prostate, intestine, and breast (Boivin et al., 2007). It has also been noted that even the same extract may have different effects on the same pathway that has been activated by different carcinogens. For example, our work has shown that black raspberry fraction RO-ME inhibits the activation of AP-1, NFκB, and NFAT in C141 cells following B[a]PDE exposure (Li et al., 2008), whereas the same fraction only inhibits NFκB activation, but not AP-1 activation in same cells exposed to UVB radiation (Huang et al., 2007). Thus, the biological effects of berries and their extract fractions are dependent on berry types, berry fractions, and carcinogen types.

Anthocyanins are one of the most abundant types of phenolics in nature and are responsible for the red, purple, and blue colors of most fruits and vegetables (Cooke et al., 2005). The anticarcinogenic activities of anthocyanins and anthocyanin-rich extracts have been confirmed in cell culture models and in animal tumor models (Wang and Stoner, 2008). In collaboration with Dr. Hecht's and Stoner's group, we have identified that cyanidin-3-rutinoside (CyR) is the most abundant anthocyanin in freeze-dried black raspberries (Tian et al., 2006). CyR is the most abundant anthocyanin in alcohol extracts of black raspberries (Huang et al., 2007). In both freeze-dried black raspberries and methanol fraction, CyR represents about 60% of the total anthocyanins, while cyanidin-3-glucoside (C3G), cyanidin-2G-xylosylrutinoside, and cyanidin-3- sambubioside represent about 16, 20, and 4%, respectively (Huang et al., 2007). Thus, we anticipate that the differential inhibitory effects of extracts from different berries may be related to the differences in their chemical compounds, such as profiles of anthocyanins.

The potential roles of different constituents from berries in anti-carcinogenic effects have drawn considerable attention in recent years. It has been shown that 40 μM anthocyanidins decreased COX-1 and -2 activities by 52 and 74%, respectively (Cooke et al., 2005). In a research performed by Seeram et al., anthocyanins from raspberries and sweet cherries demonstrated 45 and 47% COX-1 and COX-2 inhibitory activities, respectively, at dose of 125 μg/ml (Seeram et al., 2001). Delphinidin is an important anthocyanidin that presents in berries. The treatment of human colon cancer HCT116 cells with delphinidin has been found to result in G2/M phase arrest and apoptosis with the NFκB inhibition (Yun et al., 2009). CyR, an abundant anthocyanin found in black raspberries but not in strawberries or highbush blueberries, has been found to contribute to the inhibition of UVB-induced NFκB activation (Huang et al., 2007). Cyanidin-3-glucoside (C3G) is a compound found in blackberry and other food products (Ding et al., 2006b). While showing its chemopreventive and chemotherapeutic activities, C3G can inhibit TPA-induced transactivation of NFκB and AP-1 and the expression of COX-2 and TNF-α in C141 cells (Ding et al., 2006b). These inhibitory effects appear to be mediated through the inhibition of MAPK activity (Ding et al., 2006b). C3G can also block TPA-induced neoplastic transformation in C141 cells (Ding et al., 2006b). C3G and cyanidin chloride, both from freeze-dried black raspberries, have been reported to be good inhibitors of B[a]PDE-induced NFκB activity in C141 cells, which may be account for the anti-cancer effects of freeze-dried black raspberries (Hecht et al., 2006).

6 Conclusion

In summary, a series of in vitro studies have shown that berry extracts may exert their chemopreventive effects through targeting different cellular signaling pathways, including transcription factors, their upstream kinases (RTKs, PI3K/Akt, MAPKs), and their downstream target genes. Because of the complexity and diversity of cancers, cell signaling pathways, and extracts themselves, it is difficult to draw a simple conclusion with respect to the effects of berry extracts on cell signaling pathways related to carcinogenesis. We summarized current knowledge regarding multi-functional cell signaling pathways that have been demonstrated to be associated with the anti-carcinogenic effects of berry extracts and their active compound, as illustrated in Fig. 3.1. It is important to be aware that more efforts are needed to address the direct targets of berry extracts and their active compounds, as well as the crosstalk among the various pathways that are inhibited for chemopreventive effects of berries and berry components. In addition, we need to pay more attention to the design and synthesis of new chemical compounds for chemoprevention and therapy based on the information that we have obtained from studies of active anti-cancer compounds that we identified from berry extracts.

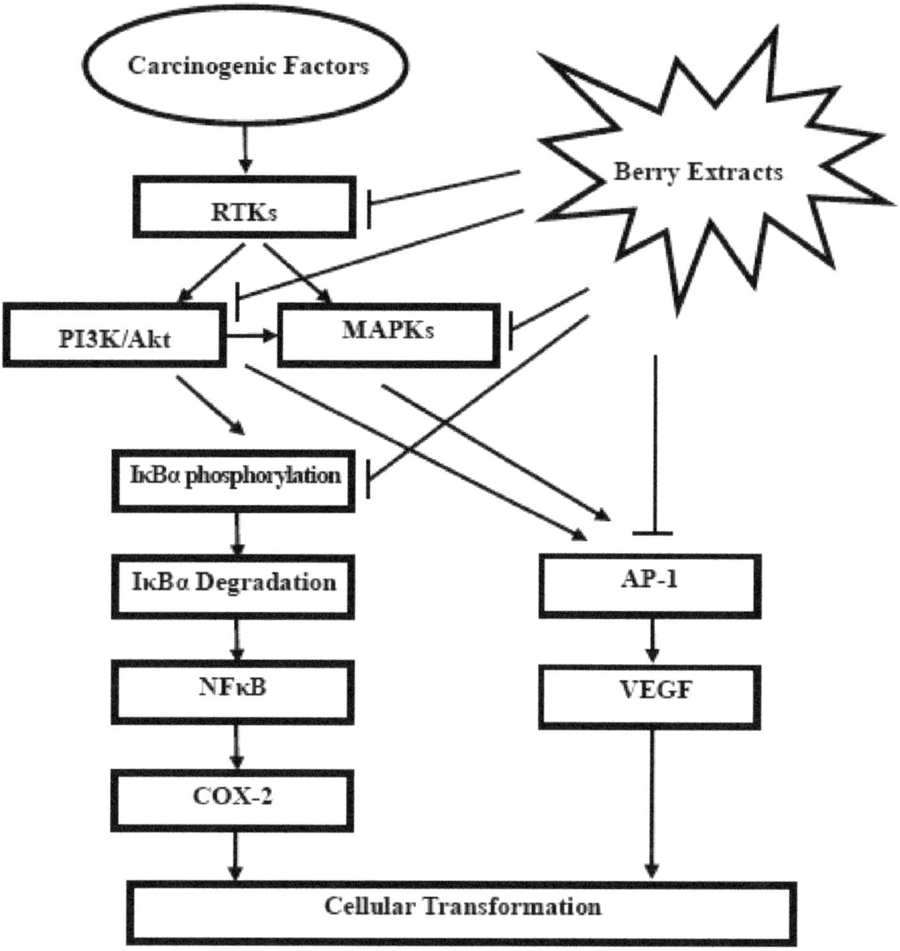

Fig. 3.1 Schematic illustration of cell signaling pathways targeted by berry extracts

References

Acevedo VD, Ittmann M, Spencer DM (2009) Paths of FGFR-driven tumorigenesis. Cell Cycle 8:580–588

Afaq F, Zaman N, Khan N, Syed DN, Sarfaraz S, Zaid MA, Mukhtar H (2008) Inhibition of epidermal growth factor receptor signaling pathway by delphinidin, an anthocyanidin in pigmented fruits and vegetables. Int J Cancer 123:1508–1515

Agarwal S, Achari C, Praveen D, Roy KR, Reddy GV, Reddanna P (2009) Inhibition of 12-LOX and COX-2 reduces the proliferation of human epidermoid carcinoma cells (A431) by modulating the ERK and PI3K-Akt signalling pathways. Exp Dermatol 18:939–946

Aggarwal BB, Gehlot P (2009) Inflammation and cancer: how friendly is the relationship for cancer patients? Curr Opin Pharmacol 9:351–369

Ahmed KM, Li JJ (2008) NF-kappa B-mediated adaptive resistance to ionizing radiation. Free Radic Biol Med 44:1–13

Ahn EH, Schroeder JJ (2006) Sphinganine causes early activation of JNK and p38 MAPK and inhibition of AKT activation in HT-29 human colon cancer cells. Anticancer Res 26:121–127

Assinder SJ, Dong Q, Kovacevic Z, Richardson DR (2009) The TGF-beta, PI3K/Akt and PTEN pathways: established and proposed biochemical integration in prostate cancer. Biochem J 417:411–421

Atsumi T, Kato K, Uno K, Iijima K, Koike T, Imatani A, Ohara S, Shimosegawa T (2007) Pathophysiological role of the activation of p38 mitogen-activated protein kinases in poorly differentiated gastric cancer. Pathol Int 57:635–644

Baek SJ, Eling TE (2006) Changes in gene expression contribute to cancer prevention by COX inhibitors. Prog Lipid Res 45:1–16

Bagchi D, Sen CK, Bagchi M, Atalay M (2004) Anti-angiogenic, antioxidant, and anti-carcinogenic properties of a novel anthocyanin-rich berry extract formula. Biochemistry 69:75–80, 71 p preceding 75

Bai D, Ueno L, Vogt PK (2009) Akt-mediated regulation of NFkappaB and the essentialness of NFkappaB for the oncogenicity of PI3K and Akt. Int J Cancer 125:2863–2870

Bellezza I, Bracarda S, Caserta C, Minelli A (2006) Targeting of EGFR tyrosine kinase by ZD1839 ("Iressa") in androgen-responsive prostate cancer in vitro. Mol Genet Metab 88:114–122

Bocca C, Bozzo F, Cannito S, Colombatto S, Miglietta A (2010) CLA reduces breast cancer cell growth and invasion through ERalpha and PI3K/Akt pathways. Chem Biol Interact 183:187–193

Bogoyevitch MA, Kobe B (2006) Uses for JNK: the many and varied substrates of the c-Jun N-terminal kinases. Microbiol Mol Biol Rev 70:1061–1095

Boivin D, Blanchette M, Barrette S, Moghrabi A, Beliveau R (2007) Inhibition of cancer cell proliferation and suppression of TNF-induced activation of NFkappaB by edible berry juice. Anticancer Res 27:937–948

Bremnes RM, Camps C, Sirera R (2006) Angiogenesis in non-small cell lung cancer: the prognostic impact of neoangiogenesis and the cytokines VEGF and bFGF in tumours and blood. Lung Cancer 51:143–158

Cakir M, Grossman AB (2009) Targeting MAPK (Ras/ERK) and PI3K/Akt pathways in pituitary tumorigenesis. Expert Opin Ther Targets 13:1121–1134

Cao XH, Wang AH, Wang CL, Mao DZ, Lu MF, Cui YQ, Jiao RZ (2010) Surfactin induces apoptosis in human breast cancer MCF-7 cells through a ROS/JNK-mediated mitochondrial/caspase pathway. Chem Biol Interact 183:357–362

Cardones AR, Banez LL (2006) VEGF inhibitors in cancer therapy. Curr Pharm Des 12:387–394

Carmeliet P (2005) VEGF as a key mediator of angiogenesis in cancer. Oncology 69(Suppl 3):4–10

Castellone MD, Carlomagno F, Salvatore G, Santoro M (2008) Receptor tyrosine kinase inhibitors in thyroid cancer. Best Pract Res 22:1023–1038

Cha YI, DuBois RN (2007) NSAIDs and cancer prevention: targets downstream of COX-2. Annu Rev Med 58:239–252

Chen FL, Armstrong AJ, George DJ (2008) Cell signaling modifiers in prostate cancer. Cancer J 14:40–45

Chen L, Mayer JA, Krisko TI, Speers CW, Wang T, Hilsenbeck SG, Brown PH (2009) Inhibition of the p38 kinase suppresses the proliferation of human ER-negative breast cancer cells. Cancer Res 69:8853–8861

Chen T, Rose ME, Hwang H, Nines RG, Stoner GD (2006) Black raspberries inhibit N-nitrosomethylbenzylamine (NMBA)-induced angiogenesis in rat esophagus parallel to the suppression of COX-2 and iNOS. Carcinogenesis 27:2301–2307

Chien CS, Shen KH, Huang JS, Ko SC, Shih YW (2010) Antimetastatic potential of fisetin involves inactivation of the PI3K/Akt and JNK signaling pathways with downregulation of MMP-2/9 expressions in prostate cancer PC-3 cells. Mol Cell Biochem 333:169–180

Chow JY, Ban M, Wu HL, Nguyen F, Huang M, Chung H, Dong H, Carethers JM (2010) TGF-beta downregulates PTEN via activation of NF-kappaB in pancreatic cancer cells. Am J Physiol 298:G275–G282

Cooke D, Steward WP, Gescher AJ, Marczylo T (2005) Anthocyans from fruits and vegetables–does bright colour signal cancer chemopreventive activity? Eur J Cancer 41:1931–1940

Cooper JB, Cohen EE (2009) Mechanisms of resistance to EGFR inhibitors in head and neck cancer. Head & Neck 31:1086–1094

Dai J, Peng L, Fan K, Wang H, Wei R, Ji G, Cai J, Lu B, Li B, Zhang D, Kang Y, Tan M, Qian W, Guo Y (2009) Osteopontin induces angiogenesis through activation of PI3K/AKT and ERK1/2 in endothelial cells. Oncogene 28:3412–3422

Daouti S, Wang H, Li WH, Higgins B, Kolinsky K, Packman K, Specian A Jr, Kong N, Huby N, Wen Y, Xiang Q, Podlaski FJ, He Y, Fotouhi N, Heimbrook D, Niu H (2009) Characterization of a novel mitogen-activated protein kinase kinase 1/2 inhibitor with a unique mechanism of action for cancer therapy. Cancer Res 69:1924–1932

Dhanasekaran DN, Reddy EP (2008) JNK signaling in apoptosis. Oncogene 27:6245–6251

Dhand R, Hiles I, Panayotou G, Roche S, Fry MJ, Gout I, Totty NF, Truong O, Vicendo P, Yonezawa K et al. (1994) PI 3-kinase is a dual specificity enzyme: autoregulation by an intrinsic protein-serine kinase activity. EMBO J 13:522–533

Ding M, Feng R, Wang SY, Bowman L, Lu Y, Qian Y, Castranova V, Jiang BH, Shi X (2006b) Cyanidin-3-glucoside, a natural product derived from blackberry, exhibits chemopreventive and chemotherapeutic activity. J Biol Chem 281:17359–17368

Ding J, Huang Y, Ning B, Gong W, Li J, Wang H, Chen CY, Huang C (2009a) TNF-alpha induction by nickel compounds is specific through ERKs/AP-1-dependent pathway in human bronchial epithelial cells. Curr Cancer Drug Targets 9:81–90

Ding J, Li J, Chen J, Chen H, Ouyang W, Zhang R, Xue C, Zhang D, Amin S, Desai D, Huang C (2006a) Effects of polycyclic aromatic hydrocarbons (PAHs) on vascular endothelial growth factor induction through phosphatidylinositol 3-kinase/AP-1-dependent, HIF-1alpha-independent pathway. J Biol Chem 281:9093–9100

Ding J, Ning B, Huang Y, Zhang D, Li J, Chen CY, Huang C (2009b) PI3K/Akt/JNK/c-Jun signaling pathway is a mediator for arsenite-induced cyclin D1 expression and cell growth in human bronchial epithelial cells. Curr Cancer Drug Targets 9:500–509

Du F, Wang L, Qian W, Liu S (2009) Loss of enteric neurons accompanied by decreased expression of GDNF and PI3K/Akt pathway in diabetic rats. Neurogastroenterol Motil 21: 1229–e1114

D'Acquisto F, May MJ, Ghosh S (2002) Inhibition of nuclear factor kappa B (NF-B): an emerging theme in anti-inflammatory therapies. Mol Interv 2:22–35

Feng R, Bowman LL, Lu Y, Leonard SS, Shi X, Jiang BH, Castranova V, Vallyathan V, Ding M (2004) Blackberry extracts inhibit activating protein 1 activation and cell transformation by perturbing the mitogenic signaling pathway. Nutr Cancer 50:80–89

Ferrara N (2005) VEGF as a therapeutic target in cancer. Oncology 69(Suppl 3):11–16

Ferrara N, Henzel WJ (1989) Pituitary follicular cells secrete a novel heparin-binding growth factor specific for vascular endothelial cells. Biochem Biophys Res Commun 161:851–858

Ferrara N, Hillan KJ, Gerber HP, Novotny W (2004) Discovery and development of bevacizumab, an anti-VEGF antibody for treating cancer. Nat Rev Drug Discov 3:391–400

Ferrara N, Hillan KJ, Novotny W (2005) Bevacizumab (avastin), a humanized anti-VEGF monoclonal antibody for cancer therapy. Biochem Biophys Res Commun 333:328–335

Ferrara N, Mass RD, Campa C, Kim R (2007) Targeting VEGF-A to treat cancer and age-related macular degeneration. Annu Rev Med 58:491–504

Fister S, Gunthert AR, Aicher B, Paulini KW, Emons G, Grundker C (2009) GnRH-I antagonists induce apoptosis in human endometrial, ovarian, and breast cancer cells via activation of stress-induced MAPKs p38 and JNK and proapoptotic protein bax. Cancer Res 69:6473–6481

Fu H, Hu Z, Wen J, Wang K, Liu Y (2009) TGF-beta promotes invasion and metastasis of gastric cancer cells by increasing fascin1 expression via ERK and JNK signal pathways. Acta Biochim Biophys Sin 41:648–656

Gao JL, Shi JM, He K, Zhang QW, Li SP, Lee SM, Wang YT (2008) Yanhusuo extract inhibits metastasis of breast cancer cells by modulating mitogen-activated protein kinase signaling pathways. Oncol Rep 20:819–824

Garcia-Echeverria C, Sellers WR (2008) Drug discovery approaches targeting the PI3K/Akt pathway in cancer. Oncogene 27:5511–5526

Goldmann WH, Sharma AL, Currier SJ, Johnston PD, Rana A, Sharma CP (2001) Saw palmetto berry extract inhibits cell growth and Cox-2 expression in prostatic cancer cells. Cell Biol Int 25:1117–1124

Gopalakrishnan A, Tony Kong AN (2008) Anticarcinogenesis by dietary phytochemicals: cytoprotection by nrf2 in normal cells and cytotoxicity by modulation of transcription factors NF-kappa B and AP-1 in abnormal cancer cells. Food Chem Toxicol 46:1257–1270

Gouni-Berthold I, Sachinidis A (2004) Molecular mechanisms explaining the preventive effects of catechins on the development of proliferative diseases. Curr Pharm Des 10:1261–1271

Gross ME, Jo S, Agus DB (2004) Update on HER-kinase-directed therapy in prostate cancer. Clin Adv Hematol Oncol 2:53–56

Gu M, Roy S, Raina K, Agarwal C, Agarwal R (2009) Inositol hexaphosphate suppresses growth and induces apoptosis in prostate carcinoma cells in culture and nude mouse xenograft: PI3K-Akt pathway as potential target. Cancer Res 69:9465–9472

Guo X, Ma N, Wang J, Song J, Bu X, Cheng Y, Sun K, Xiong H, Jiang G, Zhang B, Wu M, Wei L (2008) Increased p38-MAPK is responsible for chemotherapy resistance in human gastric cancer cells. BMC Cancer 8:375

Han YC, Zeng XX, Wang R, Zhao Y, Li BL, Song M (2007) Correlation of p38 mitogen-activated protein kinase signal transduction pathway to uPA expression in breast cancer. Chin J Cancer 26:48–53

Harris GK, Gupta A, Nines RG, Kresty LA, Habib SG, Frankel WL, LaPerle K, Gallaher DD, Schwartz SJ, Stoner GD (2001) Effects of lyophilized black raspberries on azoxymethane-induced colon cancer and 8-hydroxy-2′-deoxyguanosine levels in the Fischer 344 rat. Nutr Cancer 40:125–133

He D, Xu Q, Yan M, Zhang P, Zhou X, Zhang Z, Duan W, Zhong L, Ye D, Chen W (2009) The NF-kappa B inhibitor, celastrol, could enhance the anti-cancer effect of gambogic acid on oral squamous cell carcinoma. BMC Cancer 9:343

Hecht SS, Huang C, Stoner GD, Li J, Kenney PM, Sturla SJ, Carmella SG (2006) Identification of cyanidin glycosides as constituents of freeze-dried black raspberries which inhibit anti-benzo[a]pyrene-7,8-diol-9,10-epoxide induced NFkappaB and AP-1 activity. Carcinogenesis 27:1617–1626

Hoshino R, Chatani Y, Yamori T, Tsuruo T, Oka H, Yoshida O, Shimada Y, Ari-i S, Wada H, Fujimoto J, Kohno M (1999) Constitutive activation of the 41-/43-kDa mitogen-activated protein kinase signaling pathway in human tumors. Oncogene 18:813–822

Huang C, Huang Y, Li J, Hu W, Aziz R, Tang MS, Sun N, Cassady J, Stoner GD (2002) Inhibition of benzo(a)pyrene diol-epoxide-induced transactivation of activated protein 1 and nuclear factor kappaB by black raspberry extracts. Cancer Res 62:6857–6863

Huang C, Li J, Ding M, Leonard SS, Wang L, Castranova V, Vallyathan V, Shi X (2001) UV induces phosphorylation of protein kinase B (Akt) at Ser-473 and Thr-308 in mouse epidermal Cl 41 cells through hydrogen peroxide. J Biol Chem 276:40234–40240

Huang C, Li J, Ma WY, Dong Z (1999a) JNK activation is required for JB6 cell transformation induced by tumor necrosis factor-alpha but not by 12-O-tetradecanoylphorbol-13-acetate. J Biol Chem 274:29672–29676

Huang C, Li J, Song L, Zhang D, Tong Q, Ding M, Bowman L, Aziz R, Stoner GD (2006) Black raspberry extracts inhibit benzo(a)pyrene diol-epoxide-induced activator protein 1 activation and VEGF transcription by targeting the phosphatidylinositol 3-kinase/Akt pathway. Cancer Res 66:581–587

Huang C, Ma WY, Dong Z (1996) Requirement for phosphatidylinositol 3-kinase in epidermal growth factor-induced AP-1 transactivation and transformation in JB6 P+ cells. Mol Cell Biol 16:6427–6435

Huang C, Ma WY, Hecht SS, Dong Z (1997a) Inositol hexaphosphate inhibits cell transformation and activator protein 1 activation by targeting phosphatidylinositol-3′ kinase. Cancer Res 57:2873–2878

Huang C, Ma WY, Li J, Dong Z (1999b) Arsenic induces apoptosis through a c-Jun NH2-terminal kinase-dependent, p53-independent pathway. Cancer Res 59:3053–3058

Huang C, Ma WY, Li J, Goranson A, Dong Z (1999c) Requirement of erk, but not JNK, for arsenite-induced cell transformation. J Biol Chem 274:14595–14601

Huang C, Ma WY, Young MR, Colburn N, Dong Z (1998) Shortage of mitogen-activated protein kinase is responsible for resistance to AP-1 transactivation and transformation in mouse JB6 cells. Proc Natl Acad Sci USA 95:156–161

Huang C, Schmid PC, Ma WY, Schmid HH, Dong Z (1997b) Phosphatidylinositol-3 kinase is necessary for 12-O-tetradecanoylphorbol-13-acetate-induced cell transformation and activated protein 1 activation. J Biol Chem 272:4187–4194

Huang HP, Shih YW, Chang YC, Hung CN, Wang CJ (2008) Chemoinhibitory effect of mulberry anthocyanins on melanoma metastasis involved in the ras/PI3K pathway. J Agric Food Chem 56:9286–9293

Huang C, Zhang D, Li J, Tong Q, Stoner GD (2007) Differential inhibition of UV-induced activation of NF kappa B and AP-1 by extracts from black raspberries, strawberries, and blueberries. Nutr Cancer 58:205–212

Igaki T (2009) Correcting developmental errors by apoptosis: lessons from drosophila JNK signaling. Apoptosis 14:1021–1028

Johansson N, Ahonen M, Kahari VM (2000) Matrix metalloproteinases in tumor invasion. Cell Mol Life Sci 57:5–15

Kearns JD, Hoffmann A (2009) Integrating computational and biochemical studies to explore mechanisms in NF-{kappa}B signaling. J Biol Chem 284:5439–5443

Khandrika L, Lieberman R, Koul S, Kumar B, Maroni P, Chandhoke R, Meacham RB, Koul HK (2009) Hypoxia-associated p38 mitogen-activated protein kinase-mediated androgen receptor activation and increased HIF-1alpha levels contribute to emergence of an aggressive phenotype in prostate cancer. Oncogene 28:1248–1260

Koyuturk M, Ersoz M, Altiok N (2007) Simvastatin induces apoptosis in human breast cancer cells: p53 and estrogen receptor independent pathway requiring signalling through JNK. Cancer Lett 250:220–228

Kuno Y, Kondo K, Iwata H, Senga T, Akiyama S, Ito K, Takagi H, Hamaguchi M (1998) Tumor-specific activation of mitogen-activated protein kinase in human colorectal and gastric carcinoma tissues. Jpn J Cancer Res 89:903–909

Lamy S, Beaulieu E, Labbe D, Bedard V, Moghrabi A, Barrette S, Gingras D, Beliveau R (2008) Delphinidin, a dietary anthocyanidin, inhibits platelet-derived growth factor ligand/receptor (PDGF/PDGFR) signaling. Carcinogenesis 29:1033–1041

Lamy S, Blanchette M, Michaud-Levesque J, Lafleur R, Durocher Y, Moghrabi A, Barrette S, Gingras D, Beliveau R (2006) Delphinidin, a dietary anthocyanidin, inhibits vascular endothelial growth factor receptor-2 phosphorylation. Carcinogenesis 27:989–996

Li CJ, Chang JK, Chou CH, Wang GJ, Ho ML (2010) The PI3K/Akt/FOXO3a/p27Kip1 signaling contributes to anti-inflammatory drug-suppressed proliferation of human osteoblasts. Biochem Pharmacol 79:926–937

Li J, Chen H, Tang MS, Shi X, Amin S, Desai D, Costa M, Huang CPI (2004a) PI-3 K and Akt are mediators of AP-1 induction by 5-MCDE in mouse epidermal cl41 cells. J Cell Biol 165: 77–86

Li J, Davidson G, Huang Y, Jiang BH, Shi X, Costa M, Huang C (2004b) Nickel compounds act through phosphatidylinositol-3-kinase/Akt-dependent, p70(S6k)-independent pathway to induce hypoxia inducible factor transactivation and Cap43 expression in mouse epidermal Cl41 cells. Cancer Res 64:94–101

Li J, Zhang D, Stoner GD, Huang C (2008) Differential effects of black raspberry and strawberry extracts on BaPDE-induced activation of transcription factors and their target genes. Mol Carcinog 47:286–294

Liu H, Liang SL, Kumar S, Weyman CM, Liu W, Zhou A (2009) Statins induce apoptosis in ovarian cancer cells through activation of JNK and enhancement of bim expression. Cancer Chemother Pharmacol 63:997–1005

Liu J, Lin A (2007) Wiring the cell signaling circuitry by the NF-kappa B and JNK1 crosstalk and its applications in human diseases. Oncogene 26:3267–3278

Liu D, Liu Z, Jiang D, Dackiw AP, Xing M (2007) Inhibitory effects of the mitogen-activated protein kinase kinase inhibitor CI-1040 on the proliferation and tumor growth of thyroid cancer cells with BRAF or RAS mutations. J Clin Endocrinol Metab 92:4686–4695

LoPiccolo J, Blumenthal GM, Bernstein WB, Dennis PA (2008) Targeting the PI3K/Akt/mTOR pathway: effective combinations and clinical considerations. Drug Resist Updat 11: 32–50

Lu H, Li J, Zhang D, Stoner GD, Huang C (2006) Molecular mechanisms involved in chemoprevention of black raspberry extracts: from transcription factors to their target genes. Nutr Cancer 54:69–78

Lu B, Shinohara ET, Edwards E, Geng L, Tan J, Hallahan DE (2005) The use of tyrosine kinase inhibitors in modifying the response of tumor microvasculature to radiotherapy. Technol Cancer Res Treat 4:691–698

Martiny-Baron G, Marme D (1995) VEGF-mediated tumour angiogenesis: a new target for cancer therapy. Curr Opin Biotechnol 6:675–680

Matheny RW Jr, Adamo ML (2009) Effects of PI3K catalytic subunit and Akt isoform deficiency on mTOR and p70S6K activation in myoblasts. Biochem Biophys Res Commun 390: 252–257

Mazhar D, Ang R, Waxman J (2006) COX inhibitors and breast cancer. Br J Cancer 94:346–350

Mazhar D, Gillmore R, Waxman J (2005) COX and cancer. Q J Med 98:711–718

McCubrey JA, Steelman LS, Abrams SL, Bertrand FE, Ludwig DE, Basecke J, Libra M, Stivala F, Milella M, Tafuri A, Lunghi P, Bonati A, Martelli AM (2008) Targeting survival cascades induced by activation of Ras/Raf/MEK/ERK, PI3K/PTEN/Akt/mTOR and Jak/STAT pathways for effective leukemia therapy. Leukemia 22:708–722

Michl P, Downward J (2005) Mechanisms of disease: PI3K/AKT signaling in gastrointestinal cancers. Z Gastroenterol 43:1133–1139

Nabeshima K, Inoue T, Shimao Y, Sameshima T (2002) Matrix metalloproteinases in tumor invasion: role for cell migration. Pathol Int 52:255–264

Ndlovu N, Van Lint C, Van Wesemael K, Callebert P, Chalbos D, Haegeman G, Vanden Berghe W (2009) Hyperactivated NF-{Kappa}B and AP-1 transcription factors promote highly accessible chromatin and constitutive transcription across the interleukin-6 gene promoter in metastatic breast cancer cells. Mol Cell Biol 29:5488–5504

Ouyang W, Li J, Ma Q, Huang C (2006) Essential roles of PI-3 k/Akt/IKKbeta/NFkappaB pathway in cyclin D1 induction by arsenite in JB6 Cl41 cells. Carcinogenesis 27:864–873

Ouyang W, Li J, Shi X, Costa M, Huang C (2005) Essential role of PI-3 K, ERKs and calcium signal pathways in nickel-induced VEGF expression. Mol Cell Biochem 279:35–43

Ouyang W, Luo W, Zhang D, Jian J, Ma Q, Li J, Shi X, Chen J, Gao J, Huang C (2008) PI-3 K/Akt pathway-dependent cyclin D1 expression is responsible for arsenite-induced human keratinocyte transformation. Environ Health Perspect 116:1–6

Patel RK, Mohan C (2005) PI3K/AKT signaling and systemic autoimmunity. Immunol Res 31: 47–55

Porter AC, Vaillancourt RR (1998) Tyrosine kinase receptor-activated signal transduction pathways which lead to oncogenesis. Oncogene 17:1343–1352

Rahmani M, Anderson A, Habibi JR, Crabtree TR, Mayo M, Harada H, Ferreira-Gonzalez A, Dent P, Grant S (2009) The BH3-only protein bim plays a critical role in leukemia cell death triggered by concomitant inhibition of the PI3K/Akt and MEK/ERK1/2 pathways. Blood 114:4507–4516

Ranson M (2002) ZD1839 (Iressa): for more than just non-small cell lung cancer. Oncologist 7(Suppl 4):16–24

Riely GJ (2008) Second-generation epidermal growth factor receptor tyrosine kinase inhibitors in non-small cell lung cancer. J Thorac Oncol 3:S146–S149

Robinson MJ, Cobb MH (1997) Mitogen-activated protein kinase pathways. Curr Opin Cell Biol 9:180–186

Rodrigo KA, Rawal Y, Renner RJ, Schwartz SJ, Tian Q, Larsen PE, Mallery SR (2006) Suppression of the tumorigenic phenotype in human oral squamous cell carcinoma cells by an ethanol extract derived from freeze-dried black raspberries. Nutr Cancer 54:58–68

Roux PP, Blenis J (2004) ERK and p38 MAPK-activated protein kinases: a family of protein kinases with diverse biological functions. Microbiol Mol Biol Rev 68:320–344

Schmitz KJ, Callies R, Wohlschlaeger J, Kimmig R, Otterbach F, Bohr J, Lee HS, Takeda A, Schmid KW, Baba HA (2006) Overexpression of cyclo-oxygenase-2 is an independent predictor of unfavourable outcome in node-negative breast cancer, but is not associated with protein kinase B (Akt) and mitogen-activated protein kinase (ERK1/2, p38) activation or with her-2/neu signalling pathways. J Clin Pathol 59:685–691

Scholtysek C, Krukiewicz AA, Alonso JL, Sharma KP, Sharma PC, Goldmann WH (2009) Characterizing components of the saw palmetto berry extract (SPBE) on prostate cancer cell growth and traction. Biochem Biophys Res Commun 379:795–798

Seeram NP, Momin RA, Nair MG, Bourquin LD (2001) Cyclooxygenase inhibitory and antioxidant cyanidin glycosides in cherries and berries. Phytomedicine 8:362–369

Song L, Li J, Zhang D, Liu ZG, Ye J, Zhan Q, Shen HM, Whiteman M, Huang C (2006) IKKbeta programs to turn on the GADD45alpha-MKK4-JNK apoptotic cascade specifically via p50 NF-kappaB in arsenite response. J Cell Biol 175:607–617

Song C, Wang W, Li M, Liu Y, Zheng D (2009) Tax1 enhances cancer cell proliferation via ras-raf-MEK-ERK signaling pathway. IUBMB Life 61:685–692

Sun W, Wang Q, Chen B, Liu J, Liu H, Xu W (2008) Gamma-tocotrienol-induced apoptosis in human gastric cancer SGC-7901 cells is associated with a suppression in mitogen-activated protein kinase signalling. Br J Nutr 99:1247–1254

Sun Y, Yang T, Xu Z (2007) The JNK pathway and neuronal migration. J Genet Genomics 34: 957–965

Sweeney SE, Firestein GS (2006) Mitogen activated protein kinase inhibitors: where are we now and where are we going? Ann the Rheum Dis 65(Suppl 3):iii83–88

Taruscio TG, Barney DL, Exon J (2004) Content and profile of flavanoid and phenolic acid compounds in conjunction with the antioxidant capacity for a variety of northwest vaccinium berries. J Agric Food Chem 52:3169–3176

Teller N, Thiele W, Marczylo TH, Gescher AJ, Boettler U, Sleeman J, Marko D (2009) Suppression of the kinase activity of receptor tyrosine kinases by anthocyanin-rich mixtures extracted from bilberries and grapes. J Agric Food Chem 57:3094–3101

Tian Q, Giusti MM, Stoner GD, Schwartz SJ (2006) Urinary excretion of black raspberry (rubus occidentalis) anthocyanins and their metabolites. J Agric Food Chem 54: 1467–1472

Uranga RM, Giusto NM, Salvador GA (2009) Iron-induced oxidative injury differentially regulates PI3K/Akt/GSK3beta pathway in synaptic endings from adult and aged rats. Toxicol Sci 111:331–344

Verstrepen L, Carpentier I, Verhelst K, Beyaert R (2009) ABINs: A20 binding inhibitors of NF-kappa B and apoptosis signaling. Biochem Pharmacol 78:105–114

Von Pawel J (2004) Gefitinib (Iressa, ZD1839): a novel targeted approach for the treatment of solid tumors. Bull Cancer 91:E70–E76

Wagner EF, Nebreda AR (2009) Signal integration by JNK and p38 MAPK pathways in cancer development. Nat Rev 9:537–549

Wang SY, Feng R, Bowman L, Lu Y, Ballington JR, Ding M (2007) Antioxidant activity of vaccinium stamineum: exhibition of anticancer capability in human lung and leukemia cells. Planta Med 73:451–460

Wang LS, Hecht SS, Carmella SG, Yu N, Larue B, Henry C, McIntyre C, Rocha C, Lechner JF, Stoner GD (2009) Anthocyanins in black raspberries prevent esophageal tumors in rats. Cancer Prev Res 2:84–93

Wang J, Ouyang W, Li J, Wei L, Ma Q, Zhang Z, Tong Q, He J, Huang C (2005) Loss of tumor suppressor p53 decreases PTEN expression and enhances signaling pathways leading

to activation of activator protein 1 and nuclear factor kappaB induced by UV radiation. Cancer Res 65:6601–6611
Wang LS, Stoner GD (2008) Anthocyanins and their role in cancer prevention. Cancer Lett 269:281–290
Wang X, Zhang X, Cheng Y, Li C, Zhang W, Liu L, Ding Z (2010) Alpha-lipoic acid prevents bupivacaine-induced neuron injury in vitro through a PI3K/Akt-dependent mechanism. Neurotoxicology 31:101–112
Wei X, Guo W, Wu S, Wang L, Lu Y, Xu B, Liu J, Fang B (2009) Inhibiting JNK dephosphorylation and induction of apoptosis by novel anticancer agent NSC-741909 in cancer cells. J Biol Chem 284:16948–16955
Whyte J, Bergin O, Bianchi A, McNally S, Martin F (2009) Key signalling nodes in mammary gland development and cancer. Mitogen-Activated protein kinase signalling in experimental models of breast cancer progression and in mammary gland development. Breast Cancer Res 11:209
Widmann C, Gibson S, Jarpe MB, Johnson GL (1999) Mitogen-activated protein kinase: conservation of a three-kinase module from yeast to human. Physiol Rev 79:143–180
Williams C, Shattuck-Brandt RL, DuBois RN (1999) The role of COX-2 in intestinal cancer. Ann N Y Acad Sci 889:72–83
Wu GS (2007) Role of mitogen-activated protein kinase phosphatases (MKPs) in cancer. Cancer Metastasis Rev 26:579–585
Xiao W, Yang Y, Weng Q, Lin T, Yuan M, Yang K, Pang Y (2009) The role of the PI3K-Akt signal transduction pathway in autographa californica multiple nucleopolyhedrovirus infection of spodoptera frugiperda cells. Virology 391:83–89
Xie D, Gore C, Zhou J, Pong RC, Zhang H, Yu L, Vessella RL, Min W, Hsieh JT (2009) DAB2IP coordinates both PI3K-Akt and ASK1 pathways for cell survival and apoptosis. Proc Natl Acad Sci USA 106:19878–19883
Xu C, Shen G, Yuan X, Kim JH, Gopalkrishnan A, Keum YS (2006) Kong AN ERK and JNK signaling pathways are involved in the regulation of activator protein 1 and cell death elicited by three isothiocyanates in human prostate cancer PC-3 cells. Carcinogenesis 27:437–445
Xue H, Aziz RM, Sun N, Cassady JM, Kamendulis LM, Xu Y, Stoner GD, Klaunig JE (2001) Inhibition of cellular transformation by berry extracts. Carcinogenesis 22:351–356
Yap TA, Garrett MD, Walton MI, Raynaud F, de Bono JS, Workman P (2008) Targeting the PI3K-AKT-mTOR pathway: progress, pitfalls, and promises. Curr Opin Pharmacol 8:393–412
Yu Y, Wan Y, Huang C (2009) The biological functions of NF-kappaB1 (p50) and its potential as an anti-cancer target. Curr Cancer Drug Targets 9:566–571
Yu JH, Wang HJ, Li XR, Tashiro S, Onodera S, Ikejima T (2008) Protein tyrosine kinase, JNK, and ERK involvement in pseudolaric acid B-induced apoptosis of human breast cancer MCF-7 cells. Acta Pharmacol Sin 29:1069–1076
Yun JM, Afaq F, Khan N, Mukhtar H (2009) Delphinidin, an anthocyanidin in pigmented fruits and vegetables, induces apoptosis and cell cycle arrest in human colon cancer HCT116 cells. Mol Carcinog 48:260–270
Zhang D, Li J, Costa M, Gao J, Huang C (2010) JNK1 mediates degradation HIF-1alpha by a VHL-independent mechanism that involves the chaperones hsp90/hsp70. Cancer Res 70: 813–823
Zhang GX, Lu XM, Kimura S, Nishiyama A (2007) Role of mitochondria in angiotensin II-induced reactive oxygen species and mitogen-activated protein kinase activation. Cardiovasc Res 76:204–212
Zheng G, Chen Y, Zhang X, Cai T, Liu M, Zhao F, Luo W, Chen J (2008) Acute cold exposure and rewarming enhanced spatial memory and activated the MAPK cascades in the rat brain. Brain Res 1239:171–180
Zhou HY, Pon YL, Wong AS (2007a) Synergistic effects of epidermal growth factor and hepatocyte growth factor on human ovarian cancer cell invasion and migration: role of extracellular signal-regulated kinase 1/2 and p38 mitogen-activated protein kinase. Endocrinology 148:5195–5208

Zhou HY, Wan KF, Ip CK, Wong CK, Mak NK, Lo KW, Wong AS (2008) Hepatocyte growth factor enhances proteolysis and invasiveness of human nasopharyngeal cancer cells through activation of PI3K and JNK. FEBS Lett 582:3415–3422

Zhou YJ, Yang HW, Wang XG, Zhang H (2009b) Hepatocyte growth factor prevents advanced glycation end products-induced injury and oxidative stress through a PI3K/Akt-dependent pathway in human endothelial cells. Life Sci 85:670–677

Zhou Y, Yau C, Gray JW, Chew K, Dairkee SH, Moore DH, Eppenberger U, Eppenberger-Castori S, Benz CC (2007b) Enhanced NF kappa B and AP-1 transcriptional activity associated with antiestrogen resistant breast cancer. BMC Cancer 7:59

Zhou Y, Zhen H, Mei Y, Wang Y, Feng J, Xu S, Fu X (2009a) PI3K/AKT mediated p53 down-regulation participates in CpG DNA inhibition of spontaneous B cell apoptosis. Cell Mol Immunol 6:175–180

Zureikat AH, McKee MD (2008) Targeted therapy for solid tumors: current status. Surg Oncol Clin N Am 17:279–301

Zwick E, Bange J, Ullrich A (2001) Receptor tyrosine kinase signalling as a target for cancer intervention strategies. Endocr Relat Cancer 8:161–173

Part II
Antioxidant Capacity of Berry Components

Chapter 4
Correlation of Antioxidants and Antioxidant Enzymes to Oxygen Radical Scavenging Activities in Berries

Shiow Y. Wang

Abstract Berry fruits contain high levels of antioxidant compounds. In addition to the usual nutrients such as vitamins and minerals, berry fruits are also rich in flavonols, anthocyanidins, proanthocyanidins, catechins, flavones, and glycosides. These antioxidants are capable of performing a number of functions including free radical scavenging, peroxide decomposition, singlet and triplet oxygen quenching, enzyme inhibition, and synergism. Some antioxidants exhibit additive and synergistic effects; therefore, a single phytochemical alone usually is not a good index to reflect antioxidant activity. A positive correlation was found between antioxidant activity and antioxidant enzyme activity, and phenolic content and anthocyanin content. In general, antioxidant values are highly correlated with total phenol content, whereas a smaller linear correlation exists between antioxidant capacity and total anthocyanin content. Genotype variation, the degree of maturity at harvest, different parts of fruit tissues, preharvest conditions, and postharvest handling techniques could all affect the antioxidant profiles. This chapter discusses the factors affecting antioxidants, antioxidant enzymes, oxygen radical scavenging activities and their correlations in berry fruits.

Keywords Correlation · Antioxidants · Antioxidant enzymes · Oxygen radical scavenging activity · Species and genotypes · Maturation · Preharvest conditions · Postharvest techniques

1 Introduction

In recent years, increasing attention has been paid by consumers to the health and nutritional aspects of horticultural products (Scalzo et al., 2005). Fruits and vegetables contain significant levels of biologically active components that

S.Y. Wang (✉)
Genetic Improvement of Fruits and Vegetables Lab, US Department of Agriculture, ARS, Beltsville, MD 20705, USA
e-mail: shiow.wang@ars.usda.gov

G.D. Stoner, N.P. Seeram (eds.), *Berries and Cancer Prevention*,
DOI 10.1007/978-1-4419-7554-6_4,

positively impact health beyond basic nutrients (Velioglu et al., 1998). High consumption of fruits and vegetables has been associated with decreasing the risk of several chronic diseases caused by oxidative stress (Ames et al., 1993). Berry fruits are a good source of natural antioxidant substances such as anthocyanins, flavonoids, and phenolic acids and have high antioxidant enzymes and oxygen radical scavenging activities which could act effectively as free radical inhibitors and provide protection against harmful damage (Heinonen et al., 1998).

Many phenolic compounds important to our diets, such as hydroxybenzolic and hydroxycinnamic acid derivatives, anthocyanins, flavonol glycosides, flavan-3-ols, and proanthocyanidins are abundant in berry fruits (Macheix et al., 1990). Positive correlations have also been found between oxygen radical absorbance capacity (ORAC) and anthocyanin or phenolic content in various berries (Prior et al., 1998; Wang and Lin, 2000; Wang and Jiao, 2000; Zheng and Wang, 2003). Some phytochemicals have exhibited additive and synergistic effects on antioxidant activity when they were combined in different concentrations. This ability of antioxidant compounds to reinforce each other can have a significant effect on the antioxidant responses and their correlations. Research also indicates better health functionality of whole foods compared to single active compounds suggesting a synergistic interaction of phenolic phytochemicals in the diet (Lila and Raskin, 2005).

Antioxidant activities are positively correlated to antioxidant enzyme activities. Antioxidant enzymes include superoxide dismutatse (SOD), peroxidase (POD), catalase (CAT), and glutathione peroxidase (GSH-POD) among others. The main function of these antioxidant enzymes is to neutralize free radicals. Antioxidant enzymes may stop free radical formation in the first place or interrupt an oxidizing chain reaction to minimize the damage caused by free radicals. The risk of free radical-related health problems could be reduced by decreasing exposure to free radicals and increasing the intake of antioxidants and antioxidant enzyme rich foods.

It has been demonstrated that there is a wide diversity of phytochemical levels and antioxidant capacities within and across genera of small fruits (Moyer et al., 2002). Increasing evidence suggests that genotype has a profound influence on nutritional quality and the content of bioactive compounds in berries (Olsson et al., 2004; Anttonen and Karjalainen, 2005). Besides genotype variation, fruit maturation, preharvest conditions (such as environmental conditions, cultural practice techniques) and postharvest handling (such as storage conditions, controlled atmospheres, heat treatment, irradiation treatment, ozone, and treatment with natural compounds) could all affect antioxidant profiles and their activities. This chapter discusses the relationship among antioxidants, antioxidant enzymes, and oxygen radical scavenging activities in berry fruits.

2 Correlation Related to Species and Genotype Variation

It is well known that levels of phenolics and antioxidant capacity of berry fruits vary greatly among cultivars. There are wide differences in their components and their activities within and across genera of berry fruits. Genotype and species of berry fruits have a profound influence on the content of bioactive compounds. Different berry crops contain different major phenolic compounds and anthocyanins. For example, chlorogenic acid is a major contributor to antioxidant activity in blueberries (Wang et al., 2008a). Peonidin 3-galactoside serves as a main constituent in cranberry extract and comprises 20.8% of the total oxygen radical absorbance capacity (ORAC) value. Cyanidin 3-galactoside is the most dominant anthocyanin in lingonberries. Caffeic acid and its derivative are the two major phenolic acids in chokeberries and both have high antioxidant activities with 20.6 and 17.6%, respectively (Zheng and Wang, 2003). Black raspberries and blackberries are high in cyanidin glycosides, which are strong antioxidants (Macheix et al., 1990), while strawberries, rich in pelargonidin 3-glucoside (Gil et al., 1997) and ascorbic acid, are relatively weak antioxidants (Wang et al., 1997). The majority of glutathione in the cell is maintained in the reduced state (GSH). GSH in blackberries ranged from 63.9 to 78.7 nmol/g fresh weight. The oxidized state of glutathione (GSSG) was found to be present in low quantities with a concentration below 17.0 nmol/g fresh weight. A high GSH/GSSG ratio is necessary for several physiological functions. These functions include activation and inactivation of redox-dependent enzyme systems (Ziegler, 1985). In blackberry fruit, high ORAC values were correlated to high GSH content ($r = 0.90$) and high GSH/GSSH ratio ($r = 0.83$) (Jiao and Wang, 2000).

Anthocyanins and phenolics are secondary plant metabolites. They protect the plant against damaging photodynamic reactions by quenching the excited state of active oxygen species. A linear correlation exists between total phenolic content and ORAC activity for fruits of blackberry, raspberry, and strawberry (Wang and Lin, 2000). Zheng and Wang (2003) reported that the correlation coefficient for ORAC vs. anthocyanins was 0.951 and ORAC vs. total phenolics was 0.998 for various berry crops. Prior et al. (1998) also showed that the correlation coefficient of ORAC and total phenolic content was higher than that of ORAC and anthocyanin in fruit of *Vaccinium* species. These results suggest that the antioxidant activity of fruit is mainly derived from the contribution of phenolics.

Tulipani et al. (2008) found that a significant correlation was found between trolox equivalent antioxidant capacity (TEAC) and phenolic content in strawberries ($r = 0.95$). Moyer et al. (2002) found that the correlation coefficients of total anthocyanins, total phenolics, and ORAC or ferric reducing antioxidant power (FRAP) vary among different genotypes of *Vaccinium, Rubus* and *Ribes*. In blueberries, Connor et al. (2002a, b) showed that total phenolics correlated better with antioxidant activity ($r = 0.82$) compared to total anthocyanins ($r = 0.73$).

In raspberries, the antioxidant capacity also appears to be directly related to the total phenolic content (Wang and Lin, 2000; Anttonen and Karjalainen, 2005). Tosun et al. (2009) found that antioxidant activities analyzed by the β-carotene bleaching assay or FRAP values were highly correlated with phenol content in red raspberries ($R^2 = 0.96$ for β-carotene and $R^2 = 0.83$ for FRAP). The antioxidant capacity of black raspberries was correlated with cyanidin 3-rutinoside ($r = 0.63$) and cyanidin 3-xylosylrutinoside ($r = 0.76$) (Tulio et al., 2008). Anttonen and Karjalainen (2005) also found a very high correlation coefficient (0.98) between the content of total phenolics and ellagic acid in red raspberries and suggested that breeders could use the total phenolic content as a reliable parameter for selecting genotypes for increasing the antioxidant capacity of the fruit.

Pantelidis et al. (2007) showed that in raspberries, blackberries, red currants, and gooseberries, the FRAP values were highly correlated with phenolic content ($r = 0.95$), whereas a less linear correlation between total antioxidant capacity and anthocyanin content was recorded ($r = 0.64$). Similar results have been reported by other researchers (Wang and Lin, 2000) who found a linear correlation between total antioxidant capacity and phenolic content both in blackberries ($r = 0.96$) and raspberries ($r = 0.91$). In addition, Deighton et al. (2000) reported that there were linear relationships between FRAP and total phenolic acids ($r = 0.97$), whereas anthocyanin content had a minor influence on antioxidant capacity ($r = 0.59$) and ascorbic acid contributed only minimally to the antioxidant potential of *Rubus* juices. Kalt et al. (1999) reported that antioxidant capacity in small fruits was strongly correlated with the total phenol and anthocyanin content, but ascorbic acid only made a small contribution.

Wang and Fordham (2007) and Wang et al. (2007b) showed that different genotypes of autumn olive (*Elaeagnus umbellata*) had a high content of carotenoids and high scavenging radical activities and there was a good correlation between antioxidant activities and anti-cancer activity (antiproliferation and inducing apoptosis of human cancer cells). Hukkanen et al. (2006) showed sweet rowanberries were among the berries with the highest antioxidant activity. Cultivar Rubinovaja had the highest antioxidant activity in FRAP and 2, 2-Di (4-tert-octylphenyl) -1-picrylhydrazyl (DPPH) assays. Again, the correlation coefficient was higher for total phenolics vs. antioxidant capacity compared to total anthocyanins *vs.* antioxidant capacity.

Wild berries have significantly higher antioxidant activities and phenolic content than domestic berries (Halvorsen et al., 2002; Scalzo et al., 2005; Wang and Lewers, 2007; Cheel et al., 2007). Scalzo et al. (2005) found that *F. vesca* fruits were 2.5 times more active in antioxidant activity than cultivated strawberries in the TEAC assay. A similar finding was reported by Halvorsen et al. (2002) on FRAP assay. Wang and Lewers (2007) found that at the species level, *F. virginiana* fruit had significantly higher antioxidant capacity, total phenolics, and total anthocyanins than *F. chiloensis* and *F. x ananassa* fruit. Individual wild progenitor accessions that were higher in antioxidant capacity, total anthocyanins, and total phenolics than the top-ranking *F. x ananassa* accession tested were all *F. virginianna* accessions. *F. x ananassa* had higher ratios of pelargonidin 3-glucoside (PG) to cyanidin 3-glucoside (CG) compared to *F. chiloensis* and *F. virginiana*. ORAC correlated highly with total anthocyanins ($R^2 = 0.87$) and total phenolics ($R^2 = 0.99$). Wang and Lin (2000) also reported significant correlations between antioxidant capacity and both total phenolics and anthocyanins; however, there was little correlation between antioxidant activity and the levels of individual flavonoids. Therefore, the individual concentration of CG, PG or the ratios of PG to CG or any individual phytochemical may not be a sole index to reflect antioxidant activity (Wang and Lewers, 2007). The total antioxidant activity should be measured in order to select the optimum genotypes for breeding.

Antioxidant enzymes have the capacity to lower the free radical burden and neutralize excess free radicals created by stress conditions. In blackberries, there were close correlations between ORAC values and the activities of superoxide dismutase (SOD) ($r = 0.90$), glutathione peroxidase (GSH-POD) ($r = 0.86$), ascorbate peroxidase (AsA-POD) ($r = 0.90$), ascorbate (AsA) content ($r = 0.84$), ratio of AsA to dehydroascorbate (DHAsA) ($r = 0.97$) and glutathione reductase (GR) ($r = 0.86$) (Jiao and Wang, 2000). AsA-POD activity was also positively correlated with ascorbic acid content with $r = 0.83$. Similarly, in autumn olive, Wang and Fordham (2007) found that antioxidant activity was correlated with antioxidant enzymes and non-enzyme components, such as AsA and GSH.

Different cultivars of deerberry (*Vaccinium stamineum* L.) fruit exhibited varying degrees of antioxidant content, radical scavenging capacity, and antioxidant enzyme activity as well as non-enzyme components, AsA, and GSH. Antioxidant content was highly correlated with antioxidant enzyme activities of SOD, GSH-POD, AsA-POD, MDAR, DHAR, and GR (Wang and Ballington, 2007). Genotypes with high antioxidant activities had high AsA and GSH content (Wang and Ballington, 2007). Fruit extracts of deerberry also inhibited proliferation of human leukemia HL-60 cancer cells and human lung epithelial cancer A549 cells and induced apoptosis of HL-60 cells (Wang et al., 2007c). There was a positive correlation between inhibition of A549 lung epithelial cancer cell proliferation and antioxidant components in strawberries (Wang et al., 2007e) such as AsA-POD ($R^2 = 0.95$) and GR ($R^2 = 0.90$). Among individual genotypes, there was also a high positive correlation between inhibition of A549 cancer cell proliferation and antioxidant enzymes, non-enzyme components and antioxidant activities against free radicals ($ROO^{\bullet}$, $O_2^{\bullet-}$, $^{\bullet}OH$, and $^1O_2$). The antioxidant enzyme defense system consists of hundreds of different substances and mechanisms in which antioxidant enzymes could facilitate the prevention of cellular and tissue damage. Different species and genotypes have varying degrees of antioxidant enzyme activities and scavenging capacities on various active oxygen species. Therefore, correlation between antioxidant enzymes *vs.* radical scavenging activities varies with different genotypes.

3 Correlation Related to Specific Tissues

Several investigations have reported significant differences in phenolic content and antioxidant activity among different parts of berry fruits (Maas et al., 1991; Wang et al., 1995; Williner et al., 2003; Aaby et al., 2005; Cheel et al., 2007). Therefore, correlations among phenolics, antioxidant activities, and scavenging capacities vary with different tissues. In cranberries, outer pericarp tissue contained a higher concentration of ellagic acid compared to pulp and seeds (Wang et al., 1995). In blackberries, differences in ellagic acid were also observed between pulp and seeds. Strawberry achenes, on average, contributed to 50% of total phenolics, 43% of total flavonoids, and 37% of total anthocyanin content of the whole fruit. These results show that the achenes should be taken into account as important phenolic contributors for strawberries (Cheel et al., 2007). According to Aaby et al. (2005), phenolic content as well as antioxidant activity in strawberries were higher in achenes than in thalamus. The achenes contributed about 14% of the antioxidant activity in strawberries in spite of comprising only 1% fresh weight of the total fruit, and the main contribution was from ellagic acid and its derivatives. Maas et al. (1991) showed the highest level of total ellagic acid was found in strawberry achenes, rather than the thalamus. Williner et al. (2003) similarly reported that the total ellagic acid content in strawberry thalamus with achenes was about six-fold higher than that of thalamus without achenes. Meanwhile, resveratrol was also found to be higher in achenes than in thalamus (Wang et al., 2007d). Cheel et al. (2007) found that in both the achenes and thalamus of strawberries, total phenolic content, and total flavonoid content were correlated to DPPH activity.

4 Correlation Affected by Maturation

There is evidence that flavonoid biosynthesis is tightly associated with the developmental stage of fruits. In all berry fruits, anthocyanin content increases as the berries mature. For example, in cranberries, increases in levels of flavonols and anthocyanins during fruit ripening were observed (Vvedensksya and Vorsa, 2004). In blackberries and strawberries, total phenolic content significantly decreased as the fruit matured from the green to ripe stages (Wang and Lin, 2000). Interestingly, in raspberries, total phenolic content decreased from the green to pink stages followed by a significant increase from the pink stage to the ripe stages.

Maas et al. (1991) found that in strawberries, the content of ellagic acid was higher in the thalamus of green fruit than red fruit in 90% of 36 clones. Williner et al. (2003) also found that there were significant differences in ellagic acid content among ripening stages. The ellagic acid content in unripe fruit was higher (1.42 mg g^{-1} dry weight) than that in mid-ripe fruit (0.72 mg g^{-1} dry weight) and full-ripe fruit (0.37 mg g^{-1} dry weight). However, advancing maturation increased reservatrol content in strawberries (Wang et al., 2007d).

Antioxidant capacity varies considerably with different levels of maturity. In blueberries, increased maturity at harvest increased ORAC and anthocyanins (Prior et al., 1998; Kalt et al., 2003). Castrejón et al. (2008) studied the antioxidant capacity of blueberry fruits at five stages of maturation and ripening and found that antioxidant activity was strongly related to the total phenolic content in all stages. Antioxidant activity was higher at early maturation and during initial pigmentation than at full ripeness. This may be attributed to the higher concentrations of hydroxycinnamic acids and flavonols before ripening, whereas lower antioxidant activity of horticulturally mature berries may suggest that anthocyanins have less antioxidant potential than other phenolic compounds such as flavonols (Castrejón et al., 2008). Anthocyanins of all varieties of blueberry increased during successive harvest stages. Meanwhile, flavonols and hydroxycinnamic acids decreased from the unripe green to ripe blue stage of berry ripening. Blueberry antioxidant activity, as well as total phenolic content tended to decrease during ripening (Castrejón et al., 2008). Kahkonen et al. (2001) and Kalt et al. (2003) also showed that the ORAC values were higher in less ripened fruit compared to fully ripened fruit.

Lingonberries have a high content of antioxidants, and significant differences were found in antioxidant activity, total anthocyanin, and total phenolic contents among different maturities of lingonberry. Lingonberry fruit harvested during their green stage consistently yielded the highest ORAC values, DPPH radical scavenging activity, and total phenolic contents, followed by the pink stage fruit, and finally, the red fruit. This may be due to abundant procyanidin contents in the green fruit. There was a positive correlation between total phenolic contents and free radical scavenging activity in lingonberries (Wang et al., 2005). The ORAC value correlated with the total phenolic content at green, pink, and ripe stages with $R^2 = 0.90$, 0.85, and 0.90, respectively. Similar to blackberries and raspberries, there appeared to be an increasing correlation between the ORAC value and anthocyanin content as lingonberry fruit matured from the pink stage to the ripe stage. The DPPH radical scavenging activity was also correlated to the ORAC value with R^2 equal to 0.80. This indicates that the antioxidant capacity of lingonberries could be measured by either the ORAC or the DPPH radical scavenging assay.

Wang et al. (2009b) found that anthocyanin content steadily increased with fruit maturity in red raspberries, but the total phenolic content showed a decrease from green stage to ripe stage. Fruit harvested at their greener stages (5 and 20%) consistently yielded higher antioxidant activities and total phenolics than those harvested during the 50–80% mature stages. Fruit harvested at the pink stage (50% maturity) had the lowest ORAC and DPPH values. Following the pink stage, many phytonutrients are synthesized in parallel with the overall development and maturation of the fruit. The fully mature red raspberries (100% maturity) had stronger antioxidant activities compared to 50% mature fruit but still lower than the greener stages fruit (5 and 20%) as shown by higher ORAC and DPPH values and total anthocyanin content (Wang et al., 2009b). These findings were in agreement with findings from Rommel and Wrolstad (1993) who found that in red raspberries, the concentrations of ellagic acid and its derivatives decreased with increasing ripeness in the cultivar.

In blackberries, the total anthocyanin content increased considerably during ripening, while total phenolic content and antioxidant properties did not show such pronounced changes (Siriwoharn et al., 2004). Wang and Jiao (2001) studied the change of oxygen scavenging enzyme systems in four stages of maturities (green, pink, ripe, and over-ripe) of four blackberry cultivars and found that maturation and ripening of blackberry (*Rubus* sp.) fruit was accompanied by decreased activities of oxygen-scavenging enzymes (SOD, G-POD, catalase) and enzymes in the ascorbate-glutathione cycle [(AsA-POD), monodehydroascorbate reductase (MDAsAR), dehydroascorbate reductase (DAsAR) and GR]. Non-enzyme components in the ascorbate-glutathione cycle such as AsA, DHAsA, GSH, and GSSG and the ratios of AsA/DHAsA, GSH/GSSG also decreased.

5 Correlation Affected by Preharvest Conditions

5.1 Environmental Conditions

Environmental factors play an important role in determining the phenolic composition and content in berry fruits. Growing temperatures, light intensity, and illumination can all affect phytochemical and antioxidant capacity in berry fruits. In strawberries, increased light intensity resulted in higher ascorbic acid content (Kader, 1998) High temperature growing conditions resulted in strawberries with significantly higher content of resveratrol, flavonoids, and antioxidant capacities compared to strawberries grown under low temperature conditions. Fruit grown in cool day and night temperatures generally had the lowest antioxidant capacity (Wang and Zheng, 2001; Wang et al., 2007d). One explanation for this difference could be related to different flavonoid concentrations (Wang and Zheng, 2001).

Connor et al. (2002b) examined correlations among fruit antioxidant activity, total phenolic, and total anthocyanin content among a set of 16 highbush and interspecific hybrid blueberry cultivars grown in three different geographic locations (Minnesota [MN], Michigan [MI], and Oregon [OR]) for over 2 years. Correlation of antioxidant activity with total phenolic content was high in MN and MI ($r =$ 0.88 and 0.89, respectively), and moderate in OR ($r = 0.75$). Antioxidant activity correlated to a lesser degree with anthocyanins compared to total phenolics at all three locations. Similarly, Häkkinen and Törrönen (2000) found that when strawberry and blueberry cultivars were grown in different parts of Poland and Finland, their phenolic concentrations and antioxidant activities were different. Howard et al. (2003) evaluated total phenolics, total anthocyanins, total hydroxycinnamic acids, total flavonols, and ORAC in blueberry fruits in five commercial cultivars and 13 breeding selections grown at the same locations over two growing seasons and found that environmental growing conditions impacted levels of phenolics and ORAC in blueberries. Seasonal variation also affected the correlations among antioxidant activities and various phenolics. This study demonstrated that there is significant genotype–environment interactions for antioxidants in berry fruits and that evaluation of fruit over several years and locations appears necessary. Therefore, berry genotypes should be screened over multiple seasons in order to identify antioxidant capacity, anthocyanin- and phenolic-rich germplasm for breeding.

5.2 Cultural Practices

Cultural practices such as ground cover, organic or conventional cultivations, use of compost as a soil supplement, enriching the atmosphere with carbon dioxide, or applying naturally occurring compounds can all affect phytochemical and antioxidant capacity in berry fruits. Strawberries from a hill plasticulture (HC) production system were found to have higher flavonoid content and antioxidant capacities compared with fruit from plants grown in a matted row (MR) system (Wang et al., 2002).

In general, phenolic acid and flavonol content, as well as cyanidin-and pelargonidin-based anthocyanins and total flavonoids are greatest in the HC system. Fruits from plants grown in the MR system generally have the lowest content of phenolic acids, flavonols, and anthocyanins, but fruit grown under HC conditions have the highest ORAC values (Wang et al., 2002). Additionally, compost applied to the soil enhanced oxygen absorbance capacity for $ROO^{\bullet}$, $O_2^{\bullet-}$, H_2O_2, $^{\bullet}OH$, and $^1O_2$ radicals in strawberries (Wang and Lin, 2003). Compost and fertilizer significantly enhanced flavonoid content in strawberry fruit. The total flavonoid content positively correlated with antioxidant activities against $ROO^{\bullet}$, $O_2^{\bullet-}$, H_2O_2, $^{\bullet}OH$, and $^1O_2$ radicals with $r = 0.90$–0.98 (Wang and Lin, 2003).

Wang and Millner (2009) found that strawberries grown in a compost socks system had significantly higher ORAC, flavonoids, and anthocyanins than fruit produced in black plastic mulch or matted row systems. The correlation coefficients (R^2) for ORAC vs. total anthocyanins and total phenolics were high. The correlation coefficients were also high for the level of individual antioxidant components vs. antioxidant activity ranging from 0.90 to 0.99 (Wang and Millner, 2009).

Asami et al. (2003) showed that higher levels of total phenolics were consistently found in organically and sustainably grown cultivations of marionberry and strawberry as compared to those produced by conventional agricultural practices. In blueberries, Wang et al. (2008a) also showed that ORAC, total anthocyanins, and total phenolic content were higher in fruit from organic culture than from conventional culture. Organic culture also produced fruit with high chlorogenic acid and flavonoid content.

Plants grown in low-organic-matter and low-cation-exchange-capacity sandy soil amended with calcium, magnesium, and nitrogen produced more ascorbic acid in their fruit than plants without supplemental fertilizer (Penalosa et al., 1994). Carbon dioxide concentrations in the atmosphere also have an effect on antioxidant capacity. Higher CO_2 concentrations in the field resulted in an increase of anthocyanins, phenolics, and antioxidants in strawberry fruit. Strawberries grown in CO_2-enriched conditions had higher scavenging capacity for reactive oxygen than fruit grown under normal environments without CO_2 enrichment (Wang et al., 2003).

Pre-harvest spray of naturally occurring methyl jasmonate (MJ) significantly enhanced anthocyanin, total phenolic, flavonoid content, and antioxidant capacity in raspberries (Wang and Zheng, 2005). In blackberries, MJ treatment also significantly enhanced the anti-cancer activity (apoptosis and anti-proliferation of cancer cell lines) associated with antioxidant capacity (Wang et al., 2007a).

6 Correlation Affected by Postharvest Handling

6.1 Storage Conditions

Postharvest handling can affect antioxidant capacity and phytonutrient levels in fruits depending upon the type of fruit, temperature, and storage environment.

Increases in phenolic content during storage have been reported. Kalt et al. (1999) reported that storage of fresh small fruits (strawberries, raspberries, and highbush and lowbush blueberries) at temperatures higher than 0°C increased antioxidant capacity, anthocyanins, and total phenolic content. Anthocyanin content was strongly correlated with the total phenolic content of the fruit ($R^2 = 0.91$). Phenolics and anthocyanins were both strongly correlated to antioxidant capacity. Kalt et al. (2003) also found during ripening and storage of three highbush blueberry cultivars that ORAC was positively correlated with total phenolic content ($R^2 = 0.78$). Connor et al. (2002a) reported that antioxidant activity, total phenolic, and anthocyanin content in blueberry were strongly correlated with each other ($r = 0.87$–0.99) and their increases during cold storage were variety-dependent.

Cranberries stored at temperatures greater than 0°C had increased antioxidant capacity, anthocyanins, and total phenolic content (Wang and Stretch, 2001). Among a variety of cultivars at different storage temperatures (0–20°C), high correlation coefficients were seen between ORAC and anthocyanin content (0.88–0.93) and ORAC and total phenolic contents (0.90–0.95), indicating that the changes of ORAC in response to various temperatures were significantly correlated to the changes of total anthocyanin and phenolic contents in cranberries.

Ayala-Zavala et al. (2004) also found that storage temperatures significantly affected the ORAC of strawberry fruit. Strawberries Chandler stored at 5 or 10°C had higher antioxidant capacity, total phenolics, and anthocyanins than those stored at 0°C. Cordenunsi et al. (2005) found that as storage temperatures increased, ORAC values and anthocyanin accumulation in strawberries also increased, while flavonols (quercetin and kaempferol derivatives), ellagic acid, and total phenolic contents were not affected by storage temperatures. There was a significant increase in the ratio between pelargonidin and cyanidin for strawberries during storage, showing a preferential synthesis of pelargonidin over cyanidin (Cordenunsi et al., 2005).

6.2 Controlled Atmospheres

The controlled atmosphere (CA) storage technique is considered a supplement to refrigeration. The potential benefits of controlled atmospheres are retardation of senescence, suppression of physiological changes and microbial growth, maintenance of quality and extension of storage life of fresh produce. The magnitude of potential benefit of using controlled atmosphere is dependent upon commodity, variety, physiological age, atmosphere composition, and temperature and duration of storage.

Carbon dioxide-enriched atmospheres (10–20%) are especially effective in retarding decay and softening of strawberries (Gil et al., 1997). However, exposure to high concentrations of CO_2 could adversely affect the color change in strawberry fruit. High CO_2 caused a reduction in red color intensity and a decrease in anthocyanin content of strawberry fruit. As CO_2 levels increased, the concentration of pelargonidin glycosides in the internal tissue decreased (Gil et al., 1997). Agar et al.

(1997) found a decrease in vitamin C content in strawberries and red raspberries associated with 10–30% CO_2 storage. This suggests that high CO_2 concentrations may have a stimulating effect on the oxidation of ascorbic acid and/or an inhibition of mono- or dehydroascorbic acid reduction to ascorbic acid. Gunes et al. (2002) reported that total antioxidant activity increased by about 45% when cranberries were stored in air; however, this increase was not seen when the fruits were stored in 30% CO_2 plus 21% O_2. This may be because CA storage conditions prevent the release of bound phenolics and flavonoids from the cell matrix of cranberry fruits, resulting in lower antioxidant activities. Holcroft and Kader (1999) reported that the concentrations of ellagic acid, catechin, quercetin and kaempferol derivatives in strawberries increased during air storage but remained constant during high CO_2 storage. Remberg et al. (2003) evaluated the total antioxidant capacity of five cultivars of blueberries after 1 month of controlled atmosphere (10% O_2 + 10% CO_2) and found that the total antioxidant capacity in treated samples decreased considerably more than those stored in air at 1°C. Shin et al. (2008) showed that the increases in total and reduced ascorbic acid concentrations in cultivar Northeaster and Earliglow strawberries during air storage were prevented by 20% CO_2 storage at 3°C for 20 days. Anthocyanins and flavonoids, and total antioxidant activity of both cultivars were higher in air-stored fruit than in CO_2-stored fruit. It appears that high CO_2 storage generally decreases total phenolics, total anthocyanins and ORAC values and extent of the effect depended upon the commodity, CO_2 concentration, storage time and temperature.

Elevated O_2 atmospheres have been shown to delay microbial growth (Zeng et al., 2003, 2006; Ayala-Zavala et al., 2007). Zheng et al. (2003) studied the effects of superatmospheric O_2 treatments (40, 60, 80, or 100% O_2 at 5°C) on "Duke" highbush blueberries and showed that antioxidant levels were markedly increased by 60–100% O_2 treatments as compared with 40% O_2 treatment or air control during 35 days of storage. Elevated O_2 between 60 and 100% also promoted increases in total phenolics and total anthocyanins, especially malvidin-based anthocyanins as well as the individual phenolic compounds (Zheng et al., 2003). High O_2 ($\geq$40% at 5°C) storage of strawberries showed higher antioxidant capacity, total phenolics, less decay and longer shelf life (Zheng et al., 2006; Ayala-Zavala et al., 2007). In comparison with fruits stored in air, strawberries held in 80% O_2 + 20% CO_2 had higher levels of total anthocyanins during the first 4 days of storage at 8°C but significantly lower levels at the end of 9-day storage (Pérez and Sanz, 2001). Thus, correlations among antioxidants and various other phytochemicals are affected by controlled atmospheres since the levels of these phytochemicals change with increases or decreases of O_2 and/or CO_2 concentrations in the storage atmospheres.

6.3 Heat Treatment

Heat treatment has been demonstrated to effectively retard senescence and degradative processes to maintain quality of fresh fruits, control diseases and insect infestation, and suppress pathogens. Civello et al. (1997) found that heat treatments

(1–5 h at temperatures ranging from 39 to 50°C) can delay ripening and postharvest decay of strawberry fruit. However, heat treatments reduced anthocyanin accumulation and phenylalanine ammonia-lyase (PAL) activity compared to controls. Moreover, anthocyanin content of cultivar Selva strawberries treated at 48°C was significantly lower than that of fruit treated at 42°C. On the other hand, Yoshikawa et al. (1992) treated cultivar Chandler strawberries in 43% humidified air at 46°C for 80 min and found severe damage in the fruits. These contradictory results could be due to cultivar-dependent responses of strawberries to heat treatments. Reduction of anthocyanin and other bioactive compounds by heat treatment could alter the relationships of these compounds and affect their correlations.

6.4 Illumination

Light is one of the most important environmental factors influencing anthocyanin biosynthesis in plants. Red pigmentation of cranberries and red raspberries can be improved after harvest using artificial illumination (Zhou and Singh, 2004; Wang et al., 2009b). In submerged, harvested cranberries, red light and far-red light increased the total anthocyanin level by 41.5 and 34.7%, respectively. The level of each individual anthocyanin increased differently under different light exposures such as natural light, red light, and far-red light (Zhou and Singh, 2004).

Wang et al. (2009b) found high light intensity (photosynthetically active radiation [PAR] level of 56 ± 0.5 μmol m^{-2} $s^{-1)}$ enhanced red color development, especially for immature red raspberry fruit (5 and 20%). This indicates that red raspberries harvested before full maturity could synthesize pigment during storage under favorable conditions. Kalt et al. (1993) observed that light increased the surface color rating of white Blomidon strawberries; however, the harvested white and pink stages of highbush blueberries never attained a pigment level as high as that of the 100% blue or ripe fruit at harvest. Red raspberries harvested at different developmental stages continued their red color development during storage, even in darkness. For immature berries (5 and 20% maturities), fruit exposed to higher light intensities had higher flavonoids than those exposed to lower light intensities during storage (Wang et al., 2009b). The synthesis of both anthocyanins and other flavonoids may have contributed to the increase in antioxidant activity in red raspberries after storage. A positive relationship existed between antioxidant activities and anthocyanin content in raspberries, strawberries, and blueberries under various light conditions. These results indicate that anthocyanin biosynthesis and their composition may be manipulated by different light exposure to obtain antioxidant-richer berries.

UV irradiation as a postharvest treatment has been shown to induce and activate decay-resistance mechanisms, delay fruit softening, and extend storage life of fruits and vegetables. UV treatment reduced fruit softening and enhanced anthocyanin levels in strawberries (Baka et al., 1999). UV-C (9.2 kJ m^{-2}) and heat treatments (45°C) retained boysenberry fruit quality and antioxidant activity better compared to controls (Vicente et al., 2004). Erkan et al. (2008) found that UV-C at doses of 2.15 and

4.30 kJ m^{-2} promoted antioxidant capacity and enzyme activities and significantly reduced the severity of decay in strawberries after storage at 10°C for 15 days compared to controls. UV-C also increased content of anthocyanins and total phenolics, and enhanced the activities of antioxidant enzymes including GSH-POD, GR, SOD, AsA-POD, G-POD, MDAR, and DHAR. Non-enzyme components such as GSH and GSSG and ratio of GSH to GSSG also were increased by UV-C exposure. Wang et al. (2009a) found higher flavonoid content and antioxidant capacity in blueberries treated with 2.15 or 4.30 or 6.45 kJ m^{-2} compared with control fruit. The increases of total phenols and anthocyanins in blueberries by UV-C illumination appeared to be dose-dependent at lower doses (0.43∼2.15 kJ m^{-2}); however, higher doses (4.30∼6.45 kJ m^{-2}) tended to suppress these increases. This phenomenon has also been reported in strawberries where high doses of UV-C exposure caused too much stress and possibly resulted in injury (Baka et al., 1999). These results indicate that appropriate UV irradiation of berry fruits can be beneficial in terms of increasing the levels of antioxidant activity and potentially health-promoting nutraceutical compounds.

6.5 Ozone

Ozone (O_3) is an unstable compound which produces hydroxyl radicals and other free radical species. Ozone has been used in different applications in the food industry as a disinfectant or sanitizer. Barth et al. (1995) and Pérez et al. (1999) reported that blackberries and strawberries stored in an atmosphere containing ozone (0.3–0.35 L/L) resulted in a sharp decrease in ascorbic and anthocyanin levels. Anthocyanins or ascorbic acid might be oxidized by direct interaction with ozone, which may degrade the aromatic rings of anthocyanin. Ozone also results in the formation of other high-reactive species, such as $^{\bullet}OH$, $O_2^{\bullet -}$, and $\bullet O_3$ which facilitates degradation (Xue et al., 2008). Thus, the correlation between anthocyanins or ascorbic acid and other antioxidants could be affected because of this oxidation and degradation by ozone treatment. The effects of ozonation on the nutritional properties of berry fruits should be considered prior to its adoption as a postharvest technique.

6.6 Treatment with Naturally Occurring Compounds

Fungal decay is one of the major causes of rapid and extensive postharvest deterioration of fresh fruits and vegetables. The most effective prevention of fungal decay is the application of fungicidal substances. However, there have been increasing concerns regarding the use of synthetic fungicides in agricultural products and about their presence in the environment due to health risks. Therefore, the use of natural compounds with antimicrobial properties would be preferable. Natural antimicrobial compounds such as methyl jasmonate (MJ), essential oils, and other natural volatile compounds have been investigated as alternative methods to reduce postharvest deterioration and to prolong storage life of fresh fruits and vegetables. Some of these natural compounds have been found to affect the levels of antioxidants and antioxidant enzyme activities and to alter their correlations with radical scavenging capacities.

6.6.1 Methyl Jasmonate

Methyl jasmonate (MJ), a naturally occurring compound, has been found to maintain high levels of total anthocyanins and total phenolic content and increased antioxidant activities from tests including ORAC, $O_2^{\bullet-}$, H_2O_2, $^{\bullet}OH$, $^1O_2$, DPPH$^{\bullet}$ and ABTS$^+$ in cranberries, strawberries, raspberries, blueberries and blackberries (Changjirakul et al., 2006, 2007). Ayala-Zavala et al. (2005) found that cultivar Allstar strawberry fruit treated with MJ, in conjunction with ethanol, showed higher antioxidant capacity, total phenolics, and anthocyanins than those treated with ethanol alone or controls (non-treated) during the postharvest period. In raspberries, treatment with MJ enhanced the activity of several antioxidant enzymes, including SOD, G-POD, AsA-POD, GSH-POD, GR, MDAR, and DHAR. Moreover, raspberries treated with MJ showed the highest amount of AsA, DHAsA, GSH, and GSSG compared to controls and other treatments. These results indicate that MJ may increase the resistance of tissues to decay by enhancing their antioxidant system and their free radical scavenging capability.

6.6.2 Essential Oils and Other Natural Volatile Compounds

Essential oils or natural volatile compounds are aromatic oily extracts obtained from plant materials such as buds, flowers, seeds, leaves, barks, roots, fruits, and other parts of the plants. These compounds include thymol, menthol, eugenol, carvacrol, anethole, cinnamaldehyde, cinnamic acid, perillaldehyde, linalool, and *p*-cymene. Essential oils have been demonstrated to be effective in inhibiting microbial growth and reducing fruit decay. Strawberries treated with thymol, menthol, or eugenol and blueberries treated with carvacrol, anethole, and perillaldehyde enhanced total phenolics, total anthocyanins, and flavonoid content and free radical scavenging capacity (Wang et al., 2007f; Wang et al., 2007e; Wang et al., 2008b). Electron spin resonance showed that higher radical scavenging capacities were found against DPPH$^{\bullet}$ and $^{\bullet}OH$ in berries treated with thymol, eugenol, or menthol, compared to those in control groups (Wang et al., 2007f).

Chanjirakul et al. (2006, 2007) also found that the treatment with essential oil of *Melaleuca alternifoli* (tea tree oil or TTO) or ethanol (EtOH) enhanced free radical scavenging capacities and activity of antioxidant enzymes, including SOD, G-POD, AsA-POD, GSH-POD, GR, MDAR, DHAR and ascorbic acid and glutathione in strawberries, blackberries and raspberries. These results indicate that TTO and EtOH may increase the resistance of tissue decay by enhancing their antioxidant system and their free radical scavenging capability. Thus, these natural products have the potential to enhance flavonoid contents, change their correlations to radical scavenging activities, increase the resistance of tissues against oxidative damage, and preserve the quality and safety of berry fruits.

Allyl isothiocyanate (AITC) is a natural compound which is present in all plants belonging to the *Cruciferae* family and is generally considered safe for human consumption and believed to be conducive to health (Kermanshai et al., 2001; Shin et al., 2004). AITC has been shown to have various biological effects including anti-bacterial, anti-fungal, anti-nematode and anti-insect activities (Kermanshai et al., 2001; Shin et al., 2004). Chanjirakul et al. (2006, 2007) and Wang et al. (2010) have also shown that AITC reduced decay of strawberries, blackberries, and raspberries. However, the mechanism of AITC in reducing microbial growth is different from that of MJ and other essential oils. AITC treated fruits did not increase the amounts of phenolic compounds, anthocyanins, flavonoids, antioxidant enzyme activities or the capacity to scavenge free reactive oxygen species (ROS) in fruit tissue. The reduction of decay in fruit tissue by AITC may be due to its pro-oxidant action by paradoxically generating and accumulating additional amounts of ROS to inhibit the growth and proliferation of microbial cells (Wang et al., 2010). This treatment may be a potential substitute for commercial fungicides to control pathological rot on berry fruits.

7 Conclusion

Berry fruits are one of the most important sources of bioactive compounds with high antioxidant activity. Several genetic and environmental factors affect the production and accumulation of bioactive compounds in berry fruits. The correlations of antioxidants and antioxidant enzyme activities to radical scavenging activities in berry fruits are also affected by maturity, type of tissues, cultural practices and postharvest handling techniques. The content of phenolics and anthocyanins in fruits reported in the literature normally refers to extractable compounds analyzed in aqueous-organic extracts as presented in this chapter. However, significant amounts of bioactive compounds that are usually not considered in nutritional studies remain in the residue. Adding these aqueous-organic, non-extractable but bioavailable phenolic compounds to the equation would certainly change the correlations of antioxidants to radical scavenging activities. Further research in this aspect is warranted.

References

Aaby K, Skrede G, Wrolstad RE (2005) Phenolic composition and antioxidant activities in flesh and achenes of strawberries (*F. x ananassa*). J Agric Food Chem 53:4032–4040

Agar IT, Streif J, Bangerth F (1997) Effect of high CO_2 and controlled atmosphere on the ascorbic and dehydroascorbic acid content of some berry fruits. Postharvest Biol Technol 11:47–55

Ames BM, Shigena MK, Hagen TM (1993) Oxidants, antioxidants and the degenerative diseases of aging. Proc Natl Acad Sci USA 90:7915–7922

Anttonen MJ, Karjalainen RO (2005) Environmental and genetic variation of phenolic compounds in red raspberry. J Food Compost Anal 18:759–769

Asami DK, Hong Y, Barrett DM et al (2003) Comparison of the total phenolic and ascorbic acid content of freeze-dried and air-dried marionberry, strawberry, and corn grown using conventional, organic, and sustainable agricultural practices. J Agric Food Chem 51:1237–1341

Ayala-Zavala JF, Wang SY, Wang CY, Gonzalez-Aguilar G (2004) Effect of storage temperatures on antioxidant capacity and aroma compounds in strawberry fruit. Food Sci Technol 37: 687–695

Ayala-Zavala JF, Wang SY, Wang CY, Gonzalez-Aguilar G (2005) Methyl jasmonate in conjunction with ethanol treatment increases antioxidant capacity, aroma compounds and postharvest life of strawberry fruit. Eur Food Res Technol 221:731–738

Ayala-Zavala JF, Wang SY, Wang CY, Gonzalez-Aguilar G (2007) Response of strawberry fruit to high oxygen treatment. Food Technol Biotechnol 45:166–173

Baka M, Mercier J, Corcuff R et al (1999) Photochemical treatment to improve storability of fresh strawberries. J Food Sci 64:1068–1072

Barth MM, Zhou C, Mercier J et al (1995) Ozone storage effects on anthocyanin content and fungal growth in blackberries. J Food Sci 60:1286–1288

Castrejón ADR, Eichholz I, Rohn S et al (2008) Phenolic profile and antioxidant activity of highbush. Food Chem 109:564–572

Chanjirakul K, Wang SY, Wang CY et al (2006) Effect of natural volatile compounds on antioxidant capacity and antioxidant enzymes in raspberries. Postharvest Biol Technol 40:106–115

Chanjirakul K, Wang SY, Wang CY et al (2007) Natural volatile treatments increase free radical scavenging capacity of strawberries and blackberries. J Sci Food Agric 87:1463–1472

Cheel J, Theoduloz C, Rodríguez JA et al (2007) Free radical scavenging activity and phenolic content in achenes and thalamus from *Fragaria chiloensis* ssp. Chiloensis, *F. Vesca* and *F. x ananassa* cv. Chandler. Food Chem 102:36–44

Civello PM, Martinez GA, Chaves AR et al (1997) Heat treatments delay ripening and postharvest decay of strawberry fruit. J Agric Food Chem 45:4589–4594

Connor AM, Luby JJ, Hancock JF et al (2002a) Changes in fruit antioxidant activity among blueberry cultivars during cold-temperature storage. J Agric Food Chem 50:893–898

Connor AM, Luby JJ, Tong CBS et al (2002b) Genotypic and environmental variation in antioxidant activity, total phenolic content, and anthocyanin content among blueberry cultivars. J Am Soc Hortic Sci 127:89–97

Cordenunsi BR, Genovese MI, Nascimento JR et al (2005) Effects of temperature on the chemical composition and antioxidant activity of three strawberry cultivars. Food Chem 91:113–121

Deighton N, Brennan R, Finn C et al (2000) Antioxidant properties of domesticated and wild Rubus species. J Sci Food Agric 80:1307–1313

Erkan M, Wang SY, Wang CY (2008) Effect of UV treatment on antioxidant capacity, antioxidant enzyme activity and decay in strawberry fruit. Postharvest Biol Technol 48:163–171

Gil MI, Holcroft DM, Kader AA (1997) Changes in strawberry anthocyanins and other polyphenols in response to carbon dioxide treatments. J Agric Food Chem 45:1662–1667

Gunes G, Liu RH, Watkins CB (2002) Controlled-atmosphere effects on postharvest quality and antioxidant activity of cranberry fruits. J Agric Food Chem 50:5932–5938

Häkkinen S, Törrönen AR (2000) Content of flavonols and selected phenolic acids in strawberries and Vaccinium species: influence of cultivar, cultivation site and technique. Food Res Int 33:517–524

Halvorsen BL, Holte K, Myhrstad MCW et al (2002) Systematic screening of total antioxidants in dietary plants. J Nutr 132:461–471

Heinonen IM, Meyer AS, Frankel EN (1998) Antioxidant activity of berry phenolics on human low-density lipoprotein and liposome oxidation. J Agric Food Chem 46:4107–4112

Holcroft DM, Kader AA (1999) Carbon dioxide-induced changes in color and anthocyanin synthesis of stored strawberry fruit. HortScience 34:1244–1248

Howard L, Clark J, Brownmiller C (2003) Antioxidant capacity and phenolic content in blueberries as affected by genotype and growing season. J Sci Food Agric 83:1238–1248

Hukkanen AT, Pölönen SS, Kärenlampi SO et al (2006) Antioxidant capacity and phenolic content of sweet rowanberries. J Agric Food Chem 54:112–119

Jiao HJ, Wang SY (2000) Correlation of antioxidant capacities to oxygen radical scavenging enzyme activities in blackberry. J Agri Food Chem 48:5672–5676

Kader AA (1998) Influence of preharvest and postharvest environment on nutritional composition of fruits and vegetables. In: Quebedeaux B, Bliss FA (eds) Horticulture and human health: contributions of fruits and vegetables. Prentice Hall, Englewood Cliffs, NJ

Kahkonen MP, Hopia AI, Heinonen M (2001) Berry phenolics and their antioxidant activity. J Agric Food Chem 49:4076–4082

Kalt W, Forney CF, Martin A et al (1999) Antioxidant capacity, vitamin C, phenolics, and anthocyanins after fresh storage of small fruits. J Agric Food Chem 47:4638–4644

Kalt W, Lawand C, Ryan DAJ et al (2003) Oxygen radical absorbing capacity, anthocyanin and phenolic content of highbush blueberries (*Vaccinium corymbosum* L.) during ripening and storage. J Am Soc Hortic Sci 128:917–923

Kalt W, Prange RK, Lidster PD (1993) Postharvest color development of strawberries: influence of maturity, temperature and light. Can J Plant Sci 73:541–548

Kermanshai R, McCarry BE, Rosenfeld J et al (2001) Benzyl isothiocyanate is the chief or sole anthelmintic in papaya seed extracts. Phytochemistry 57:427–435

Lila MA, Raskin I (2005) Health-related interactions of phytochemicals. J Food Sci 70:R20–R27

Maas JL, Wang SY, Galletta GJ (1991) Evaluation of strawberry cultivars for ellagic acid content. HortScience 26:66–68

Macheix JJ, Fleuriet A, Billot J (1990) Fruit phenolics. CRC Press, Boca Raton, FL

Moyer RA, Hummer KE, Finn CE et al (2002) Anthocyanins, phenolics, and antioxidant capacity in diverse small fruits: *Vaccinium*, *Rubus*, and *Ribes*. J Agric Food Chem 50:519–525

Olsson ME, Ekvall J, Gustavsson K et al (2004) Antioxidants, low molecular weight carbohydrates, and total antioxidant capacity in strawberry (*Fragaria x ananassa*): effects of cultivar, ripening, and storage. J Agric Food Chem 52:2490–2498

Pantelidis GE, Vasilakakis M, Manganaris GA et al (2007) Antioxidant capacity, phenol, anthocyanin and ascorbic acid contents in raspberries, blackberries, red currants, gooseberries and cornelian cherries. Food Chem 102:777–783

Penalosa JM, Cadahia C, Sarro MJ et al (1994) Improvement of strawberry nutrition in sandy soil by addition of manure, calcium and magnesium. J Plant Nutr 17:147–153

Pérez AG, Sanz C (2001) Effect of high-oxygen and high-carbon-dioxide atmospheres on strawberry flavor and other quality traits. J Agric Food Chem 49:2370–2375

Pérez AG, Sanz C, Ríos JJ et al (1999) Effects of ozone treatment on postharvest strawberry quality. J Agric Food Chem 47:1652–1656

Prior RL, Cao G, Martin A et al (1998) Antioxidant capacity as influenced by total phenolic and anthocyanin content, maturity and variety of *Vaccinium* species. J Agric Food Chem 46:2686–2693

Remberg SF, Haffnier K, Blomhoff R (2003) Total antioxidant capacity and other quality criteria in blueberries cvs Bluecrop, Hardyblue, Patriot, Putte and Aron after storage in cold store and controlled atmosphere. Acta Hortic 600:595–598

Rommel A, Wrolstad R (1993) Ellagic acid content of red raspberry juice as influenced by cultivar, processing, and environmental factors. J Agric Food Chem 41:1951–1960

Scalzo J, Politi A, Pellegrini N (2005) Plant genotype affects total antioxidant capacity and phenolic contents in fruit. Nutrition 21:207–213

Shin IS, Masuda H, Naohide K (2004) Bactericidal activity of wasabi (*Wasabia japonica*) against *Helicobacter pylori*. Int J Food Microbiol 94:255–261

Shin Y, Ryu JA, Liu RH et al (2008) Fruit quality, antioxidant contents and activity, and antiproliferative activity of strawberry fruit stored in elevated CO_2 atmospheres. J Food Sci 72:S339–S344

Siriwoharn T, Wrolstad RE, Finn CE et al (2004) Influence of cultivar, maturity, and sampling on blackberry (*Rubus* L. Hybrids) anthocyanins, polyphenolics, and antioxidant properties. J Agric Food Chem 52:8021–8030

Tosun M, Ercisli S, Karlidag H et al (2009) Characterization of red raspberry (*Rubus idaeus* L.) genotypes for their physicochemical properties. J Food Sci 74:C575–C579

Tulio AZ Jr, Reese RN, Faith J et al (2008) Cyanidin 3-rutinoside and cyanidin 3-xylosylrutinoside as primary phenolic antioxidants in black raspberry. J Agric Food Chem 56:1880–1888
Tulipani S, Mezzetti B, Capocasa F et al (2008) Antioxidants, phenolic compounds, and nutritional quality of different strawberry genotypes. J Agric Food Chem 56:696–704
Velioglu YS, Mazza G, Gao L (1998) Antioxidant activity and total phenolics in selected fruits, vegetables, and grain products. J Agric Food Chem 46:4113–4117
Vicente AR, Repice B, Martinez GA et al (2004) Maintenance of fresh boysenberry fruit quality with UV-C light and heat treatments combined with low storage temperature. J Hortic Sci Biotechnol 79:246–251
Vvedensksya IO, Vorsa N (2004) Flavonoid composition over fruit development and maturation in American cranberry, *Vaccinium macrocarpon* Ait. Plant Sci 167:1043–1054
Wang SY, Ballington JR (2007) Free radical scavenging capacity and antioxidant enzyme activity in deerberry (*Vaccinium stamineum* L.). LWT Food Sci Technol 40:1352–1361
Wang SY, Bowman L, Ding M (2007a) Methyl jasmonate enhances antioxidant activity and flavonoid content in blackberries (*Rubus* spp.) and promotes antiproliferation of human cancer cells. Food Chem 107:1261–1269
Wang SY, Bowman L, Ding M (2007b) Variations in free radical scavenging capacity and antiproliferative activity among different genotypes of autumn olive (*Elaeagnus umbellate* thunb). Planta Med 73:468–477
Wang SY, Bunce JA, Maas JL (2003) Elevated carbon dioxide increases contents of antioxidant compounds in field-grown strawberries. J Agric Food Chem 51:4315–4350
Wang H, Cao G, Prior RL (1997) Oxygen radical absorbing capacity of anthocyanins. J Agric Food Chem 45:304–309
Wang SY, Chen CT, Sciarappa W et al (2008a) Fruit quality, antioxidant capacity, and flavonoid content of organically and conventionally grown blueberries. J Agric Food Chem 56: 5788–5794
Wang SY, Chen CT, Wang CY et al (2007d) Resveratrol content in strawberry fruit is affected by preharvest conditions. J Agric Food Chem 55:8269–8274
Wang CY, Chen CT, Wang SY (2009a) Changes of flavonoid content and antioxidant capacity in blueberries after illumination with UV-C. Food Chem 117:426–431
Wang SY, Chen CT, Wang CY (2009b) The influence of light and maturity on fruit quality and flavonoid content of red raspberries. Food Chem 112:676–684
Wang SY, Chen CT, Yin JJ (2010) Effect of allyl isothiocyanate on antioxidants and fruit decay of blueberries. Food Chem 120:199–204
Wang SY, Feng R, Bowman L et al (2005) Antioxidant activity in lingonberries (*Vaccinium vitis-idaea* L) and its inhibitory effect on activator protein 1, nuclear factor-κB, and MAPK-activated protein kinases activation. J Agric Food Chem 53:3156–3166
Wang SY, Feng R, Bowman L et al (2007c) Antioxidant activity of *Vaccinium Stamineum* L. exhibits anticancer capability in human lung and leukemia cells. Planta Medica 73:451–460
Wang SY, Fordham IM (2007) Differences in chemical composition and antioxidant capacity among different genotypes of autumn olive (*Elaeagnus umbellate* Thunb). Food Technol Biotechnol 45:402–409
Wang SY, Jiao HJ (2000) Scavenging capacity of berry crops on superoxide radicals, hydrogen peroxide, hydroxyl radicals, and singlet oxygen. J Agric Food Chem 48:5677–5684
Wang SY, Jiao HJ (2001) Changes in oxygen-scavenging systems and membrane lipid peroxidation during maturation and ripening in blackberry. J Agric Food Chem 49:1612–1619
Wang SY, Lewers KS (2007) Antioxidant capacity and flavonoid content in wild strawberries. J Am Soc Hortic Sci 132:647–658
Wang SY, Lewers KS, Bowman L et al (2007e) Antioxidant activities and inhibition of cancer cell proliferation in wild strawberries. J Am Soc Hortic Sci 132:629–637
Wang SY, Lin HS (2000) Antioxidant activity in fruit and leaves of blackberry, raspberry, and strawberry varies with cultivar and developmental stage. J Agric Food Chem 48: 140–146

Wang SY, Lin HS (2003) Compost as a soil supplement increases the level of antioxidant compounds and oxygen radical absorbance capacity in strawberries. J Agric Food Chem 51:6844–6850
Wang SY, Maas JL, Payne JA et al (1995) Ellagic acid content in small fruits, mayhaws, and other plants. J Small Fruit Vitic 2:39–49
Wang SY, Millner P (2009) Effect of different cultural systems on antioxidant capacity, phenolic content, and fruit quality of strawberries (*Fragaria x aranassa* Duch.). J Agric Food Chem 57:9651–9657
Wang SY, Stretch AW (2001) Antioxidant capacity in cranberry is influenced by cultivar and storage temperature. J Agric Food Chem 49:969–974
Wang CY, Wang SY, Chen CT (2008b) Increasing antioxidant activity and reducing decay of blueberries by essential oil. J Agric Food Chem 56:3587–3592
Wang CY, Wang SY, Yin JJ et al (2007f) Enhancing antioxidant, antiproliferation, and free radical scavenging activities in strawberries with essential oils. J Agric Food Chem 55:6527–6532
Wang SY, Zheng W (2001) Effect of plant temperature on antioxidant capacity in strawberry. J Agric Food Chem 49:4977–4982
Wang SY, Zheng W (2005) Preharvest application of methyl jasmonates increases fruit quality and antioxidant capacity in raspberries. Int J Food Sci Technol 40:187–195
Wang SY, Zheng W, Galletta G (2002) Cultural system affects fruit quality and antioxidant capacity in strawberries. J Agric Food Chem 50:6534–6542
Williner MR, Pirovani ME, Güemes DR (2003) Ellagic acid content in strawberries of different cultivars and ripening stages. J Sci Food Agric 83:842–845
Xue J, Chen L, Wang H (2008) Degradation mechanism of alizarin red in hybrid gas–liquid phase dielectric barrier discharge plasmas: experimental and theoretical examination. Chem Eng J 138:120–127
Yoshikawa FT, Gordon MF, Mayer G (1992) Moist heat treatment of strawberries are studied. Calif Agric 46:26
Zheng W, Wang SY (2003) Oxygen radical absorbing capacity of flavonoids and phenolic acids in blueberries, cranberries, chokeberries and lingonberries. J Agric Food Chem 51:502–509
Zheng Y, Wang CY, Wang SY et al (2003) Effect of high oxygen atmospheres on blueberry phenolics, anthocyanins and antioxidant capacity. J Agric Food Chem 51:7162–7169
Zheng Y, Wang CY, Wang SY et al (2006) Changes in strawberry phenolics, anthocyanins, and antioxidant capacity in response to high oxygen treatments. Food Sci Technol 40:49–57
Zhou Y, Singh BR (2004) Effect of light on anthocyanin levels in submerged, harvested cranberry fruit. J Biomed Biotechnol 5:259–263
Ziegler DM (1985) Role of reversible oxidation-reduction of enzyme thiols-disulfides in metabolic regulation. Annu Rev Biochem 54:305–329

Part III
Chemopreventive Effects of Berries and Berry Components in Animal Model Systems

Chapter 5
Berries in the Prevention of Esophageal Adenocarcinoma

Laura A. Kresty, Amy Exum, and Bree Zeyzus-Johns

Abstract Worldwide esophageal cancer is the eighth most commonly diagnosed cancer, with squamous cell carcinoma and adenocarcinoma representing the two major histological types. In the United States, rates of esophageal adenocarcinoma (EAC) have increased over 500% in the last 30 years resulting in EAC being identified as the fastest increasing of all cancer types. Esophageal adenocarcinoma represents the major type of esophageal cancer in the western world today, while rates of squamous cell carcinoma, which is tightly linked to tobacco use, have been steadily declining. The precise reasons for the rapid increase in EAC and the only known precursor lesion, Barrett's esophagus (BE), are still being unraveled. Persistent, symptomatic, reflux of gastric and duodenal contents, known as gastroesophageal disease (GERD), have long been known to correlate with the development of Barrett's esophagus and EAC. Other risk factors for EAC include obesity, animal-based diets, tobacco use, and excess alcohol intake. Conversely, plant-based diets have generally been associated with a reduction of risk for EAC, thereby supporting evaluations of fruits, vegetables, or plant constituents as potential inhibitors of EAC or BE. Esophageal cancer mortality statistics nearly parallel the incidence statistics reflecting the insidious nature of this disease, one in which the 5-year survival rates consistently remain under 20%. Clearly, new treatment and preventive strategies are needed to combat the increase of this deadly malignancy. This chapter will cover the epidemiology of BE and EAC, berries as potential inhibitors of EAC or BE, and specific issues posing challenges to chemoprevention against EAC.

Keywords Berry · Black raspberry · Cranberry · Esophageal adenocarcinoma · Barrett's esophagus · Esophageal cancer · Chemoprevention · Food-based cancer prevention · Biomarker · Preclinical models

---

L.A. Kresty (✉)
Department of Epidemiology and Public Health, Miller School of Medicine,
University of Miami Sylvester Cancer Center, Miami, FL 33136, USA
e-mail: lkresty@med.miami.edu

G.D. Stoner, N.P. Seeram (eds.), *Berries and Cancer Prevention*,
DOI 10.1007/978-1-4419-7554-6_5, © Springer Science+Business Media, LLC 2011

1 Esophageal Adenocarcinoma and Related Precursor Lesions

1.1 Epidemiology of Barrett's Esophagus and Esophageal Adenocarcinoma

Worldwide esophageal cancer is the eighth most commonly diagnosed cancer (Lambert and Hainaut, 2007) with squamous cell carcinoma and adenocarcinoma representing the two major histological types. Esophageal adenocarcinoma represents the major type of esophageal cancer in the western world today, while rates of squamous cell carcinoma, which is tightly linked to tobacco use, have been steadily declining in all race and gender groups in recent decades (Holmes and Vaughan, 2007). In the United States, rates of esophageal adenocarcinoma (EAC) have increased over 500% in the last 30 years resulting in EAC being identified as the fastest increasing of all cancer types particularly in White males (Devesa et al., 1998; Poh and Welch, 2005; Brown et al., 2008; Corley et al., 2009). The precise reasons for the rapid increase in EAC and the only known precursor lesion, Barrett's esophagus (BE), are still being unraveled. Barrett's esophagus is defined as a premalignant condition in which the normal stratified squamous epithelium lining the esophagus is replaced by columnar lined epithelium with goblet cells (Spechler et al., 2010) and this lesion imparts increased risk for EAC development. Persistent, symptomatic reflux of gastric and duodenal contents, known as gastroesophageal disease (GERD), have long been known to correlate with the development of Barrett's esophagus and EAC (Friedenberg et al., 2008; Hampel et al., 2005; El-Serag, 2008). The presence of GERD or BE results in a 30–40 fold increased risk for EAC, which is very similar to the increased risk for lung cancer associated with smoking. Heartburn is the primary symptom of GERD and is estimated to impact approximately 60 million Americans (Locke et al., 1997). This represents a large population at increased risk for the development of Barrett's esophagus and EAC, thereby illustrating the potential global health significance of this growing problem. Also alarming is the fact that rates of esophageal adenocarcinoma have been rising throughout Western Europe and Australia, as well (Botterweck et al., 2000; Stavrou et al., 2009). Esophageal cancer is the fourth leading cause of cancer-related mortality in UK males and the sixth leading cause of cancer-related deaths in UK females (CancerResearchUK.org, 2009). In the United States, 16,640 new incident cases of esophageal cancer are estimated to occur in 2010 alongside 14,500 deaths which represent the 7th leading cause of cancer-related deaths among US males (ACS Cancer Facts and Figures, 2010). Esophageal cancer mortality statistics nearly parallel the incidence statistics reflecting the insidious nature of this disease, one in which the 5-year survival rates consistently remain under 20% (ACS Cancer facts and Figures, 2010). Clearly, new treatment and preventive strategies are needed to combat the increase of this deadly malignancy.

1.1.1 Obesity as a Risk Factor

In addition to GERD, other factors leading to increased risk for EAC include obesity, tobacco use, poor diet, and to a lesser extent, alcohol intake. Elevated BMI or obesity has recently emerged as a strong, consistent, and dose-dependent risk factor for EAC. Obesity is reported to impart a 2 to 2.5-fold increased risk for EAC and a 1.5 to 2-fold increased risk for GERD (El-Serag, 2008). Furthermore, epidemiological evidence indicates that obesity is a factor in over 50% of the EAC cases in the US and 40% of the cases in the UK (Fair and Montgomery, 2009; Ryan et al., 2008; Merry et al., 2007). Postulated reasons for the linkage between obesity and EAC include: obesity induced changes in gastroesophageal physiology, including reduced lower esophageal sphincter (LES) pressure; the presence of hiatal hernia; increased gastric pressure among the obese, in turn increasing GERD (Friendenberg et al., 2008; Pandolfino et al., 2008); and finally, that obesity may alter circulating levels of pro-proliferative or pro-inflammatory molecules supporting carcinogenesis (Ryan et al., 2008; Moayyedi, 2008). However, the fact that obesity has been associated with EAC independently of reflux suggests a more complex relationship than simply increased intra-abdominal pressure (Chow et al., 1998; Lagergren et al., 1999). Further mechanistic research is needed to improve understanding of this complex relationship.

1.1.2 Tobacco and Alcohol as EAC Risk Factors

Tobacco and alcohol are well established risk factors for esophageal SCC, increasing risk by 3 to 8 and 3 to 5-fold, respectively (Holmes and Vaughan, 2007; Doll et al., 1994; McLaughlin et al., 1995; Ishikawa et al., 2006; Freedman et al., 2007). In contrast, alcohol consumption appears to be a weak risk factor for EAC with some studies reporting no positive correlation (Holmes and Vaughan, 2007). Recent reports also indicate that total alcohol is not a strong risk for BE and that an inverse association may exist for BE among wine drinkers (Kubo et al., 2009). Smoking increases EAC risk the range of 1.5 to 4-fold. Interestingly, although the magnitude of risk associated with AEC and tobacco use is lower compared to SCC, the duration of risk reportedly remains elevated for 30 years after tobacco cessation (Gammon et al., 1997), thus providing a logical window for chemopreventive interventions.

1.1.3 Dietary Factors and Supplementation Relative to EAC Risk

A number of case control, cohort, and intervention studies have examined the role of dietary factors, dietary patterns and supplement intake related to esophageal cancer risk. In summary, diets rich in fruits and vegetables have consistently been associated with reduced risk, whereas those of animal origin characterized by high meat intake and saturated fat consumption generally increase risk (World Cancer Research Fund/American Institute for Cancer Research, 2007) In addition, recent research by Corley et al. (2009) investigated a number of dietary factors in BE patients including the "Western" dietary pattern (high in fast food and meat) compared to the "health conscious" (high in fruit, vegetables, and non-fried fish). Their findings reported that a health conscious dietary pattern was inversely associated with BE and that a diet of fast food and meat may adversely impact BE (Kubo et al., 2008b). Another study of BE patients utilizing a case-control study design reported that dietary antioxidants, fruits, and vegetables were inversely associated with BE

(Kubo and Corley 2007); however, the group found no modification of risk for BE with supplement intake (Kubo et al., 2008a). In contrast, a prospective study conducted by the Seattle Barrett's Esophagus Program revealed that BE patients who took one or more multivitamins per day had a significantly decreased risk of EAC and tetrapoidy compared to patients not taking vitamins (Dong et al., 2008). The authors reported current NSAID use, high consumption of fruits and vegetables, and low fat intake to be associated with lower incidence of EAC and fewer alterations in ploidy, a marker of neoplastic progression. Intake of supplemental vitamin C, E, β-carotene and selenium were associated with reduced risk for EAC and ploidy. The different results of these studies may be attributed to a number of factors. The case control study by Kubo et al. (2008b) focused on BE risk, whereas the prospective study evaluated risk of progression to EAC suggesting that the protective impact of supplemental vitamins may be specific to a later phase of neoplastic progression or that the differences are due to other factors. Divergent study methods or true differences in the population cohorts themselves may have resulted in the reported outcomes. An earlier chemopreventive intervention focused on patients at increased risk for esophageal SCC found that the long-term response to supplementation may be age dependent as well. The intervention trial was conducted in an area of high esophageal cancer rates in an undernourished population in China reported that the long-term impact of vitamin and mineral supplementation depended on the age of the population. Those 55 years of age and younger benefited, while those over 55 years of age actually experienced increased risk for esophageal SCC (Qiao et al., 2009). The baseline nutritional status of the population, as well as risk behaviors and age of the population, may be important considerations for conducting interventions aimed at decreasing esophageal cancer risk. Another recent study evaluated diet, multivitamin use, and gene promoter methylation among smokers reported that multivitamin intake, consumption of green, leafy vegetables and folate significantly protected against altered methylation of cancer-related genes (Stidley et al., 2010). A significant amount of work remains with regard to our knowledge of how, when, and where to intervene in specific high risk patients cohorts for improved patient outcomes, namely cancer prevention. Still, the body of research continues to support an inverse association between BE, EAC and high levels of fruit and vegetable consumption which in turn has led to a number of preclinical evaluations as well as early phase clinical trials evaluating food-based chemopreventives, including berries.

1.1.4 Additional Risk Factors for EAC

Esophageal cancer rates generally increase with age, peaking between 75 and 79 years of age (El-Serag et al., 2002; van Blankenstein et al., 2005) and more slowly thereafter. El-Serag et al. (2002) also noticed an increase in EAC among both younger and older patients. Other non-modifiable risk factors for EAC development include race and gender. Men are diagnosed with EAC 6–8 times more frequently than women and whites 3–4 times more than blacks (Crew and Neugut, 2004; Lagergren, 2005; Pera et al., 2005; Corley et al., 2009) for reasons that are not completely understood. A study conducted by Corley et al. (2009) in a large, ethnically diverse population of patients with Barrett's esophagus supports that the demographic patterns seen in patients with EAC closely reflect the patterns of patients diagnosed with BE leading the authors to conclude that EAC risk is largely driven by BE distribution versus differential rates of neoplastic progression among different demographic groups.

1.1.5 Summary of Molecular Alterations

Figure 5.1 is an attempt to summarize some of the many molecular alterations which are documented to occur as the normal squamous esophageal epithelium changes to metaplastic BE, dysplasia, and progresses to EAC in about 10% of BE patients. The specific molecular alterations have been comprehensively reviewed by others (Reid et al., 2010; Hormi-Carver and Souza, 2009; Prasad et al., 2010; Barbera and Fitzgerald, 2009). In brief, reflux of acid and bile into the lower esophagus leads to inflammation, the generation of reactive oxygen and nitrogen species which in turn damages lipids, proteins, and DNA supporting molecular and concomitant histopathologic changes as the esophageal epithelium attempts to adapt. Molecular changes that occur early in the process which are linked to EAC progression include changes in ploidy and alterations of the tumor suppressor genes p53 and p16 (Reid et al., 2010). Esophageal cells become increasingly resistant to apoptosis with repeated or chronic exposure to injurious refluxant via inappropriate activation of the MAP kinase, NF-κB and cytokine signaling pathways (Jaiswal et al., 2006;

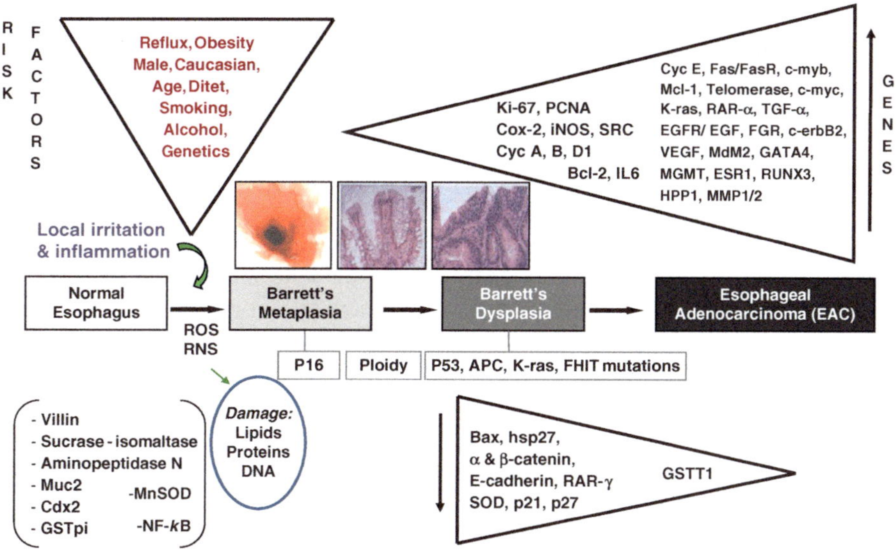

Fig. 5.1 Development of EAC, risk factors, molecular alterations and histologic progression

Hormi-Carver et al., 2009; Souza et al., 2009; Duggan et al., 2010). Thus, evaluations of chemopreventive agents such as berries which counteract reflux-induced alterations in key cancer signaling pathways may prove especially promising.

2 Methodological Challenges

2.1 Preclinical Assessments Utilizing Animal Models and In Vitro Systems

Preclinical models with human relevancy are valuable for evaluating chemopreventive and therapeutic efficacy, unraveling agent specific mechanisms of cancer inhibition and improving our understanding of complex gene environment interactions in the context of cancer development. Similar to other cancers of epithelial origin, the latency period for esophageal adenocarcinoma development is long supporting the need for validated preclinical models to rapidly access new preventive agents, treatment regimens, risk factors, as well as the biological trajectory of cancer development and the molecular mechanisms involved. Rat surgical models represent the most frequently utilized models for research on esophageal adenocarcinoma, Barrett's esophagus, and esophagitis. Multiple rat models exist (Li and Martin, 2007; Lu and Wang, 2008; Attwood et al., 2008) which involve the application of various surgical techniques to induce reflux of stomach acid and/or bile, known risk factors for esophageal premalignancy and esophageal adenocarcinoma. Commonly utilized models include: the esophagogastroduodenal anastamosis (EGDA) model (Chen et al., 1999; Su et al., 2004; Chen et al., 2008; Hao et al., 2009b; Szentpáli et al., 2010), the esophagogastrojejunostomy (EGJ) model (Lu et al., 2009), the esophagoduodenal anastomosis (ED or EDA) model (Goldstein et al., 1997; Li and Martin, 2007; Aiyer et al., 2009), the esophagojejunostomy (EJ) model (Buttar et al., 2002; Cheng et al., 2005) and variations of the mentioned surgical models with total gastrectomy (Miyashita et al., 2008). The EGDA and EGJ models are among the most promising for assessments of dietary factors or for dietary delivery of chemopreventive agents due to the fact that relatively normal stomach function is maintained resulting in the maintenance of normal nutritional status. Many of the other models report significantly decreased weight gain (Aiyer et al., 2009) or where total gastrectomy has been performed alterations in normal digestive processes. The EGDA and EGJ differ by the type and location of the anastomosis as illustrated in Fig. 5.2; however, both preserve stomach function, maintain the normal anatomic location of the esophagus, and result in reflux of gastric acid and bile into the distal esophagus leading to esophageal premalignancy and esophageal adenocarcinoma.

Additional model development is ongoing, utilizing both surgical and genetically altered mouse models; however, success has been limited to date. Hao et al. (2009a) performed EGDA and EGDA with gastrectomy surgery on wild-type, *p53A135V* transgenic, and *INK4a/Arf+/-* mice of the A/J strain and reported that

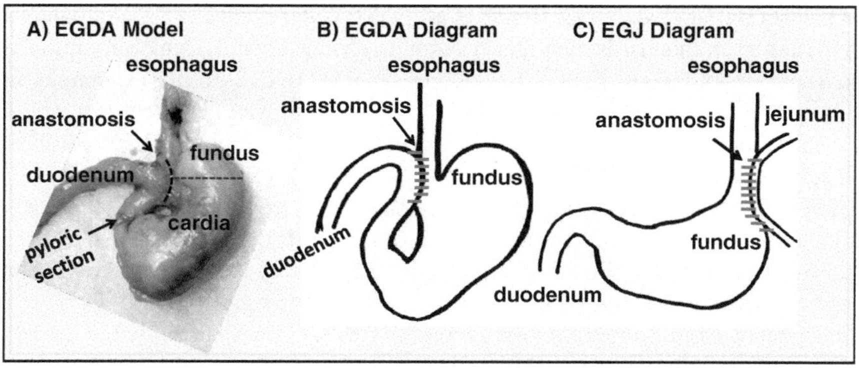

Fig. 5.2 Rat anastomosis models for studies of esophageal adenocarcinoma. **A**) Esophageal-gastroduodenal-anastomosis (EGDA) model 6 weeks following the surgical anastomosis between the gastroesophageal junction and the duodenum on the antimesenteric border with mucosa to mucosa opposition. **B**) A diagram illustrating the EGDA model for comparison to the **C**) EGJ model in which the anastomosis occurs between the jejunum and the gastroesophageal junction

esophageal adenocarcinoma was not induced after 80 weeks of follow-up; however, squamous cell lesions were induced. Earlier attempts to induce EAC in p53 knockout mice via EJ and total gastrectomy resulted in poor survival, thus limiting the utility of the model (Fein et al., 1999). In contrast, Raggi et al. (2010) recently reported that performing EJ on BALB-C mice induced intestinal metaplasia in 60% 4 months post-surgery and adenocarcinoma in 55% 5 months post-surgery. This data is promising, but the relevancy of this particular model in terms of histopathologic and molecular changes needs to be investigated. Also, the authors reported higher surgical-related mortality compared to that in most of the rat models, which is not surprising given the inherent surgical challenges with working at a smaller scale.

Rat models have proven extremely useful for screening chemopreventive agents and improving our understanding of genetic changes associated with the metaplasia-dysplasia-adenocarcinoma sequence despite the fact that rodent models differ from humans in terms of their natural propensity to develop Barrett's esophagus and EAC and given evident differences between these model systems and humans in terms of anatomy and physiology. Moreover, the rat surgical models induce histopathologic changes similar to those reported in humans and a number of shared molecular alterations have been identified. Similar to the human scenario, rodent surgical models have shown progressive histopathologic changes with concomitant gene expression alterations (Su et al., 2004; Bonde et al., 2007; Cheng et al., 2005; Hao et al., 2006). Disruptions in cell cycle regulatory pathways, stimulation of markers of inflammation, oxidative and nitrosative stress, altered expression of transcription factors, changes in markers of differentiation, and decreased DNA repair capacity have been reported in rat reflux models, mimicking the human situation (Cheng et al., 2005; Hao et al., 2006; Chen et al., 2008; Bonde et al., 2007; Hao et al., 2009a; Souza et al., 2009). Molecular alterations reported in rodent reflux models with perhaps the greatest human relevancy include p53, cyclin D1, Cox-2, PGE2, IGF, Cdx2, Sox2 and Gata4 (Buttar et al., 2002; Bonde et al., 2007; Chen et al., 2008; Szentpáli et al., 2010); however, this list is continually evolving. Work toward developing improved transgenic or knockout models for studies of EAC and Barrett's esophagus will likely continue and further move the field foward; however, currently available rat surgical models offer imperfect, albeit extremely useful, models for research in a holistic system.

Cell based in vitro model systems represent another tool for initial hypotheses testing and rapid screening of new agents. However, cell lines derived from Barrett's precursor lesions or esophageal adenocarinoma are sorely lacking. Moreover, many of the esophageal cell lines (SEG-1, BIC-1, SK-GT-5) heavily relied upon by the esophageal research community for the past two decades have recently been verified to be contaminated (Boonstra et al., 2010) which calls into question the relevance of results from hundreds of studies and raises concerns regarding research based on results obtained from the misidentified cell lines. Ongoing research in our laboratory assessing berry extracts' inhibitory potential have pointed to differential inhibitory effects based on the target organ from which the cells originated as well as the specific cell line in terms of modulating global gene expression patterns and pathway specific markers, thus placing additional emphasis on the importance of conducting research in authentic cell lines. We have previously published that a cranberry proanthocyanidin rich extract (PAC) inhibits cancer cell proliferation, including acid-induced proliferative events in SEG-1 and BIC-1 cells thought at the time to be EAC cells; however, it has since been determined that these lines are actually lung and colon cancer cells, respectively. Studies with berry extracts are currently ongoing in authenticated esophageal adenocarcinoma cell lines. As illustrated in Fig. 5.3, black raspberry extracts (BRB 80:20 and BRB-ETOH) and proanthocyanidin rich cranberry extract (PAC) significantly inhibit OE19 EAC cellular viability in a dose dependent manner with maximum inhibition at 72 h post-treatment. Specifics regarding extract isolation and characterization have previously been reported (Howell, 2007; Kresty et al., 2008; Wang et al., 2009; Stoner, 2009). Higher concentrations of BRB extracts had to be utilized to inhibit OE19 cellular viability compared to PAC. In addition, a single treatment with BRB 80:20 imparted greater inhibition compared to daily or multiple doses, suggesting that active metabolites of the parent extract are likely inhibitory. In contrast, BRB-ETOH was significantly more inhibitory when administered daily compared to a single administration; yet, 200 μg/mL was equally inhibitory as 400 μg/mL. OE19 cell viability was inhibited to a greater extent by the cranberry extract compared to the two black raspberry extracts tested. The PAC inhibited OE19 cell viability at a lower concentration (50 and 100 μg/mL compared to 200 and 400 μg/mL). Our earlier work showed cell cycle arrest at the G1 checkpoint and cells reducing the percentage of cells in S-phase; however, recent evaluations of PAC in authenticated esophageal adenocarcinoma cell lines has actually resulted in cells stacking up at the G2/M checkpoint and potent effects on cell death via apoptosis and at higher concentrations of PAC or upon daily treatment rapid necrosis is evident. Lower [50 μg/mL] concentration of PAC induced morphological changes consistent with apoptosis induction, whereas the higher concentration in a single exposure

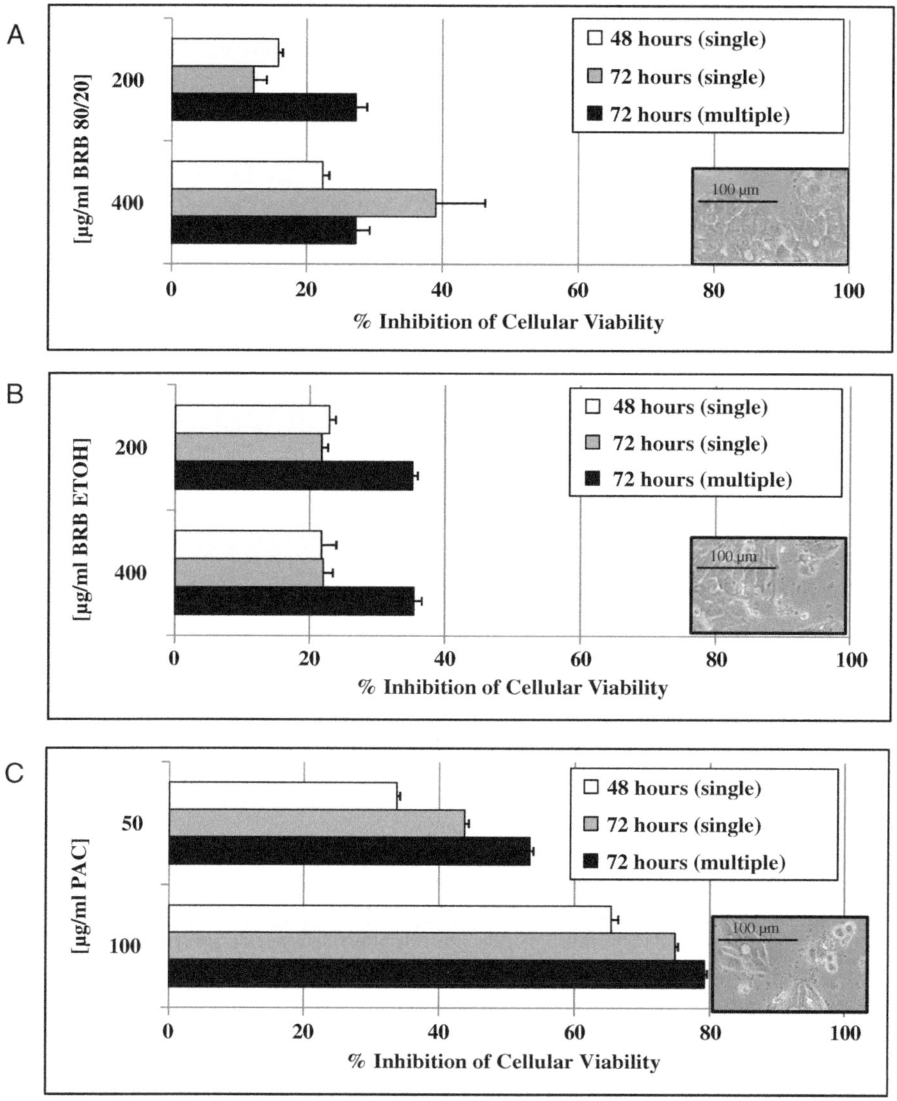

Fig. 5.3 Berries inhibit viability of OE19 EAC cells

or daily exposure appears to cause cytoplasmic swelling consistent with necrosis induction. Ultimately, multiple berry types may possess cancer inhibitory potential but the mechanisms of inhibition are likely to vary, as does the composition of the berries. Thus, evaluation of a mixture of well characterized berries eliciting inhibition through different mechanisms may prove most efficacious.

Boonstra et al. (2010) verified that 10 of 14 esophageal adenocarcinoma cell lines evaluated were authentic based on genotyping results comparing the original archival tissues to the cell lines established. However, few of the cell lines are commercially available, further limiting widespread use of authentic esophageal adenocarcinoma cell lines for research purposes. To our knowledge, only the OE33 and OE19 esophageal carcinoma cell lines (Rocket et al., 1997) are currently commercially available for purchase via the European Collection of Cell Cultures (ECACC, 2010). In contrast to esophageal adenocarcinoma cell lines, six esophageal cell lines of squamous origin are available through ECACC. Het-1A, an SV40 immortalized normal human esophageal cell line, remains the only human cell line of esophageal origin available through the American Type Culture Collection (ATCC, 2010). According to Dr. Peter Rabinovitch, a number of esophageal premalignant cell lines have been submitted to ATCC and may be available in the near future. Ultimately, the report findings illustrate the importance of validating the authenticity of all cell lines and the need for improved access to authentic esophageal cell lines of adenocarcinoma and Barrett's origin prior to embarking on research.

Other methodological issues unique to esophageal research include surveillance challenges associated with esophageal tissue heterogeneity. The esophagus is basically a dynamic tube and the lesions formed are frequently not circumferential, making for a challenging biopsy situation that is time consuming, labor intensive, and error prone with rather poor sensitivity and specificity (Egger et al., 2003). Thus, research incorporating immunohistochemical markers must carefully address this by evaluating biomarker variation thoroughly to ensure valid results.

3 Berries as Chemopreventive Agents Targeting BE or EAC

As previously summarized there is good evidence to suggest that plant-based diets lower esophageal cancer risk; however, evidence for specific foods, fruits, or vegetables is more difficult to ascertain. Diets and even specific fruits and vegetables are really complex mixtures whose constituents vary based upon a plethora of factors including growing conditions (soil, water, and specific variety), time of harvest, storage, processing and preparation. In addition, we are limited by the capacity of our evaluation tools. Numerous food frequency questionnaires have been created and validated to differing extents for evaluation of diet as it relates to cancer risk; however, limitations persist particularly for assessing multidimensional exposures in free living populations. However, development of new tools to address previously unmeasured intakes may provide additional insight with regard to specific foods or categories of foods with cancer inhibitory properties. For example, recent reports have linked proanthocyanidins or anthocyanidins to risk reduction for colon, stomach, and esophageal cancers (Rossi et al., 2010a, b; Bobe et al., 2009). The three referenced studies utilized a proanthocyanidins (PAC) database developed by the US Department of Agriculture in 2004 which quantifies PACs in multiple foods.

This type of tool enables new dietary comparisons to be explored in a more specific way and may better inform our understanding of the relative cancer inhibitory contribution that specific categories of foods impart. The data base does not, however, attempt to separately quantify PACs based on their chemical linkage type, but only according to their oligomeric fraction. Linkage type has proven very important for urinary tract health effects. Howell (2007) have shown that it is specifically the A-type linkages of cranberries that inhibit adhesion of p-fimbriated uropathogenic *Escherichia coli* to uroepithelial cells inhibiting infection. Other types of PACs with mainly B-type linkages such as those found in apple juice were not significantly inhibitory. The importance of the linkage type is not currently known in terms of cancer prevention, but important to consider if incorporating the survey tool cited.

The berry type most extensively studied for cancer inhibitory effects in the esophagus is the black raspberry, comprehensively reviewed recently by Dr. Gary Stoner (2009). In brief, black raspberries and black raspberry extracts have shown inhibitory effects in multiple preclinical models of epithelial cancers, including esophageal SCC. Mechanisms of inhibition include reduced cell proliferation, induction of apoptosis, alteration of inflammatory markers, and effects on angiogenesis (Kresty et al., 2006). In addition, a recent publication by Stoner et al. (2010) reported that various berry types including black and red raspberries, strawberries, blueberries, noni, acai, and wolfberry all significantly inhibited carcinogen induced squamous cell cancer in the rat F344 model and select serum cytokines were altered. It is promising that all the berries investigated significantly inhibited NMBA-induced esophageal SCC given the differences among the berries in terms of composition of bioactive constituents pointing potentially to the involvement of multiple mechanisms.

In contrast to esophageal SCC, very limited research utilizing berries or berry-derived extracts has been completed in validated preclinical models for esophageal adenocarcinoma. Based on positive preclinical data, we conducted a pilot study administering black raspberries (BRB) to patients with Barrett's esophagus and found that daily consumption of BRB significantly reduced urinary excretion of markers linked to oxidative damage, urinary 8-iso prostaglandin $F_{2\alpha}$, and 8-hydroxy-2-deoxyguanosine. In addition, about one-third of the patients responded with increased levels of the important detoxification enzyme glutathione *S*-transferase pi, at the tissue level following the 6 month BRB intervention (unpublished results). Additional studies are warranted with regard to characterizing the various berries, expanding mechanistic studies, and evaluating combinations of berries for improved efficacy in high risk cohorts, such as those with Barrett's esophagus or esophageal dysplasia.

References

Aiyer HS, Li Y, Martin RC (2009) Diet Composition Affects Surgery-Associated Weight Loss in Rats with a Compromised Alimentary Tract. [Epub ahead of print]
American Cancer Society (2010) Cancer Facts & Figures. Atlanta: American Cancer Society; 2010
American Type Culture Collection (2010) http://www.atcc.org/. Accessed 23 Apr 2010

Attwood SE, Harrison L-E, Preston SL et al (2008) Esophageal adenocarcinoma in "mice and men" back to basics! Am J Gastroenterol 103:2367–2372

Barbera M, Fitzgerald RC (2009) Cellular mechanisms of Barrett's esophagus development. Surg Oncol Clin N Am 18(3):393–410

Bobe G, Peterson JJ, Gridley G, et al (2009) Flavonoid consumption and esophageal cancer among black and white men in the United States. Int J Cance 125(5):1147–1154

Bonde P, Gao D, Chen L, et al (2007) Duodenal reflux leads to down regulation of DNA mismatch repair pathway in an animal model of esophageal cancer. Ann Thorac Surg 83(2):433–440

Boonstra JJ, Marion Rv, Beer DG et al (2010) Verification and unmasking of widely used human esophageal adenocarcinoma cell lines. J Natl Cancer Inst 102:271–274

Botterweck AA, Schouten LI, Volovics A et al (2000) Trends in incidence of adenocarcinoma of the oesophagus and gastric cardia in ten European countries. Int J Epidemiol 29:645–654

Brown LM, Devesa SS, Chow WH (2008) Incidence of adenocarcinoma of the esophagus among white Americans by sex, stage, and age. J Natl Cancer Inst 100:1184–1187

Buttar NS, Wang KK, Leontovich O et al (2002) Chemoprevention of esophageal adenocarcinoma by COX-2 inhibitors in an animal model of Barrett's esophagus. Gastroenterology 122(4):1101–1112

Cancer in the UK Summary (2009) http://info.cancerresearchuk.org/cancerstats/. Accessed 23 Apr 2010

Chen X, Qin R, Liu B et al (2008) Multilayered epithelium in a rat model and human Barrett's esophagus: similar expression patterns of transcription factors and differentiation markers. BMC Gastroenterol 8:1–9

Chen X, Yang G, Ding WY et al (1999) An esophagogastroduodenal anastomosis model for esophageal adenocarcinoma in rats and enhancement by iron overload. Carcinogenesis 20:1801–1808

Cheng P, Gong J, Wang T et al (2005) Gene expression in rats with Barrett's esophagus and esophageal adenocarcinoma induced by gastroduodenoesophageal reflux. World J Gastroenterol 11:5117–5122

Chow WH, Blot WJ, Vaughan TL, Risch HA, Gammon MD et al (1998) Body mass index and risk of adenocarcinomas of the esophagus and gastric cardia. J Natl Cancer Inst 90:150–155

Corley DA, Kubo A, Levin TR et al (2009) Race, ethnicity, sex and temporal differences in Barrett's oesophagus diagnosis: a large community-based study, 1994-2006. Gut 58:182–188

Crew KD, Neugut AI (2004) Epidemiology of upper gastrointestinal malignancies. Semin Oncol 31:450–464

Devesa SS, Blot WJ, Fraumeni JF (1998) Changing patterns in the incidence of esophageal and gastric carcinoma in the United States. Cancer 83:2049–2053

Doll R, Peto R, Wheatley K et al (1994) Mortality in relation to smoking: 40 years observations on male British doctors. BMJ 309:901–911

Dong LM, Kristal AR, Peters U et al (2008) Dietary supplement use and risk of neoplastic progression in esophageal adenocarcinoma. Nutr Cancer 60:39–48

Duggan SP, Behan FM, Kirca M, Smith S, Reynolds JV, Long A, Kelleher D (2010) An integrative genomic approach in oesophageal cells identifies TRB3 as a bile acid responsive gene, downregulated in Barrett's oesophagus, which regulates NF-kappaB activation and cytokine levels. Carcinogenesis 31:936–945

Egger K, Meining A, Ott R et al (2003) Biopsy surveillance is still necessary in patients with Barrett's oesophagus despite new endoscopic imaging techniques. Gut 52:18–23

El-Serag H (2008) The association between obesity and GERD: a review of the epidemiological evidence. Dig Dis Sci 53:2307–2312

El-Serag HB, Mason AC, Peterson N et al (2002) Epidemiological differences between adenocarcinoma of the esophagus and adenocarcinoma of the gastric cardia in the USA. Gut 50:368–372

European Collection of Cell Cultures (2010) http://www.hpacultures.org.uk/collections/ecacc.jsp. Accessed 23 Apr 2010

Fair AM, Montgomery K (2009) Energy balance, physical activity, and cancer risk. Methods Mol Biol 472:57–88

Fein M, Peters JH, Baril N et al (1999) Loss of function of Trp53, but not Apc, leads to the development of esophageal adenocarcinoma in mice with jejunoesophageal reflux. J Surg Res 83:48–55

Freedman ND, Abnet CC, Leitzmann MF et al (2007) A prospective study of tobacco, alcohol, and the risk of esophageal and gastric cancer subtypes. Am J Epidemiol 165:1424–1433

Friedenberg FK, Xanthopoulos M, Foster GD, Richter JE (2008) The association between gastroesophageal reflux disease and obesity. Am J Gastroenterol 103:2111–2122

Gammon MD, Schoenberg JB, Ahsan H et al (1997) Tobacco, alcohol, and soceconomic status and adenocarcinoma of the esophagus and gastric cardia. J Natl Cancer Inst 89:1277–1284

Goldstein SR, Yang G-y, Curtis SK et al (1997) Development of esophageal metaplasia and adenocarcinoma in a rat surgical model without the use of a carcinogen. Carcinogenesis 18:2265–2270

Hampel H, Abraham NS, El-Serag HB (2005) Meta-analysis: obesity and the risk for gastroesophageal reflux disease and its complications. Ann Intern Med 2:199–211

Hao J, Liu B, Yang CS et al (2009a) Gastroesophageal reflux leads to esophageal cancer in a surgical model with mice. BMC Gastroenterol 9:59

Hao Y, Triadafilopoulos G, Sahbaie P et al (2006) Gene expression profiling reveals stromal genes expressed in common between Barrett's esophagus and adenocarcinoma. Gastroenterol 131:925–933

Hao J, Zhang B, Liu B et al (2009b) Effect of α-tocopherol, *N*-acetylcysteine and omeprazole on esophageal adenocarcinoma formation in a rat surgical model. Int J Cancer 124:1270–1275

Holmes RS, Vaughan TL (2007) Epidemiology and pathogenesis of esophageal cancer. Semin Radiat Oncol 17:2–9

Hormi-Carver K, Souza RF (2009) Molecular markers and genetics in cancer development. Surg Oncol Clin N Am 18(3):453–467

Hormi-Carver K, Zhang X, Zhang HY et al (2009) Unlike esophageal squamous cells, Barrett's epithelial cells resist apoptosis by activating the nuclear factor-kappaB pathway. Cancer Res 69(2):672–677

Howell AB (2007) Bioactive compounds in cranberries and their role in prevention of urinary tract infections. Mol Nutr Food Res. 51:732–737

Ishikawa A, Kuriyama S, Tsubono Y et al (2006) Smoking, alcohol drinking, green tea consumption and the risk of esophageal cancer in Japanese men. J Epidemiol 16:185–192

Jaiswal K, Lopez-Guzman C, Souza RF et al (2006) Bile salt exposure increases proliferation through p38 and ERK MAPK pathways in a non-neoplastic Barrett's cell line. Am J Physiol Gastrointest Liver Physiol 290:335–342

Kresty LA, Frankel WL, Hammond CD et al (2006) Transitioning from preclinical to clinical chemopreventive assessments of lyophilized black raspberries: interim results show berries modulate markers of oxidative stress in Barrett's esophagus patients. Nutr Cancer. 54:148–156

Kresty LA, Howell AB, Baird M (2008) Cranberry proanthocyanidins induce apoptosis and inhibit acid-induced proliferation of human esophageal adenocarcinoma cells. J Agric Food Chem 56:676–680

Kubo A, Corley DA (2007) Meta-analysis of antioxidant intake and the risk of esophageal and gastric cardia adenocarcinoma. Am Gastroenterol 102:2323–2330

Kubo A, Levin TR, Block G et al (2008a) Dietary antioxidants, fruits, and vegetables and the risk of Barrett's esophagus. Am Gastroenterol 103:1614–1623

Kubo A, Levin TR, Block G et al (2008b) Dietary patterns and the risk of barrett's esophagus. Am J Epidemiol 167:839–846

Kubo A, Levin TR, Block G et al (2009) Alcohol types and sociodemographic characteristics as risk factors for Barrett's esophagus. Gastroenterology 136(3):806–815

Lagergren J (2005) Adenocarcinoma of oesophagus: what exactly is the size of the problem and who is at risk? Gut 54(Suppl 1):1–5

Lagergren J, Bergstrom R, Nyren O (1999) Association between body mass and adenocarcinoma of the esophagus and gastric cardia. Ann Intern Med 130:883–890
Lambert R, Hainaut P (2007) The multidisciplinary management of gastrointestinal cancer. Epidemiology of oesophagogastric cancer. Best Pract Res Clin Gastroenterol. 21:921–945
Li Y, Martin RCG (2007) Reflux injury of esophageal mucosa: experimental studies in animal models of esophagitis, Barrett's esophagus and esophageal adenocarcinoma. Dis Esophagus 20:372–378
Locke GR 3rd, Talley NJ, Fett SL et al (1997) Prevalence and clinical spectrum of gastroesophageal reflux: a population-based study in Olmsted County
Lu S, Lowe AW, Triadafilopoulos G et al (2009) Endoscopic evaluation of esophago-gastro-jejunostomy in rat model of Barrett's esophagus. Dis Esophagus 22:323–330
Lu S, Wang TD (2008) In vivo cancer biomarkers of esophageal neoplasia. Cancer Biomark 4: 341–350
McLaughlin JK, Hrubec Z, Blot WJ et al (1995) Smoking and cancer mortality among US veterans: a 26-year follow-up. Int J Cancer 60(2):190–193
Merry AH, Schouten LJ, Goldbohm RA, van den Brandt PA (2007) Body mass index, height and risk of adenocarcinoma of the oesophagus and gastric cardia: a prospective cohort study. Gut 56:1503–1511
Miyashita T, Shah FA, Marti G et al (2008) Vaccine impedes the development of reflux-induced esophageal cancer in a surgical rat model: efficacy of the vaccine in a Pre-Barrett's esophagus setting. J Gastrointest Surg 12(1):2–7
Moayyedi P (2008) Barrett's esophagus and obesity, the missing part of the puzzle. Am J Gastroenterol 103:301–303
Pandolfino JE, Kwiatek MA, Kahrilas PJ (2008) The pathophysiologic basis for epidemiologic trends in gastroesophageal reflux disease. Gastroenterol Clin North Am 37(4):827–843
Pera M, Manterola C, Vidal O et al (2005) Epidemiology of esophageal adenocarcinoma. J Surg Oncol 92:151–159
Poh H, Welch HG (2005) The role of overdiagnosis and reclassification in the marked increase of esophageal adenocarcinoma incidence. J Natl Cancer Inst 97:142–146
Prasad GA, Bansal A, Sharma P, Wang KK. (2010) Predictors of Progression in Barrett's Esophagus: Current Knowledge and Future Directions. Am J Gastroenterol 105(7):1490–1502
Qiao YL, Dawsey SM, Kamangar F et al (2009) Total and cancer mortality after supplementation with vitamins and minerals: follow-up of the Linxian general population nutrition intervention trial. J Natl Cancer Inst 101:507–518
Raggi M, Langer R, Feith M et al (2010) Successful evaluation of a new animal model using mice for esophageal adenocarcinoma. Langenbecks Arch Surg 395:347–350
Reid BJ, Li X, Galipeau PC, Vaughan TL (2010) Barrett's oesophagus and oesophageal adenocarcinoma: time for a new synthesis. Nat Rev Cancer 10(2):87–101
Rocket JC, Larkin K, Darton SJ et al (1997) Five newly established oesophageal carcinoma cell lines: phenotypic and immunological characterization. Br J Cancer 75:258–263
Rossi M, Negri E, Parpinel M et al (2010a) Proanthocyanidins and the risk of colorectal cancer in Italy. Cancer Causes Control 2:243–250
Rossi M, Negri E, Parpinel M et al (3 June 2010b) Flavonoids, proanthocyanidins, and the risk of stomach cancer. Cancer Causes Control 21(10):1597–1604
Ryan AM, Healy LA, Power DG et al (2008) Barrett's esophagus: prevalence of central adiposity, metabolic syndrome, and a proinflammatory state. Ann Surg 247:909–915
Souza RF, Huo X, Schuler CM et al (2009) Gastroesophageal reflux might cause esophagitis through a cytokine-mediated mechanism rather than caustic acid injury. Gastroenterology 137:1776–1784
Spechler SJ, Fitzgerald RC, Prasad GA et al (2010) History, molecular mechanisms, and endoscopic treatment of Barrett's esophagus. Gastroenterology 138:854–869
Stavrou EP, McElroy HJ, Baker DF, Smith G, Bishop JF (2009) Adenocarcinoma of the oesophagus: incidence and survival rates in New South Wales, 1972–2005. Med J Aust 191(6):310–314

Stidley CA, Picchi MA, Leng S et al (2010) Multivitamins, folate, and green vegetables protect against gene promoter methylation in the aerodigestive tract of smokers. Cancer Res 70: 568–574

Stoner GD (2009) Foodstuffs for preventing cancer: the preclinical and clinical development of berries. Cancer Prev Res 2(3):187–194

Stoner GD, Wang L-S, Seguin C et al (2010) Multiple berry types prevent N-nitrosomethylbenzylamine-induced esophageal cancer in rats. Pharm Res 27(6):1138–1145

Su y, Chen X, Klein M et al (2004) Phenotype of columnar-lined esophagus in rats with esophagogastroduodenal anastomosis:similarity to human Barrett's esophagus. Lab Invest 84:753–765

Szentpáli K, Széll M, Paszt A et al (2010) Simultaneous adeno- and squamous cell carcinoma with different phenotypic profiles in a rat model of chronic gastroesophageal reflux. Dis Esophagus 20:305–310

U.S. Department of Agriculture (2004) USDA database for the proanthocyanidin content of selected foods. USDA, Beltsville, MD

van Blankenstein M, Looman CW, Hop WC (2005) The incidence of adenocarcinoma and squamous cell carcinoma of the esophagus. Barrett's esophagus makes a difference. Am J Gastroenterol 100:766–774

Wang L-S, Hecht SS, Carmella SG et al (2009) Anthocyanins in black raspberries prevent esophageal tumors in rats. Cancer Prev Res 2:84–93

World Cancer Research Fund/American Institute for Cancer Research (2007) Food, nutrition, physical activity, and prevention of cancer: a global perspective. Washington DC: AICR

Chapter 6
Endothelial Cell Tumor Prevention with Berry Extracts: Clinical Problems, Molecular Mechanisms and Therapeutic Opportunities

Gayle M. Gordillo and Chandan K. Sen

Abstract Endothelial cell tumors are the most common soft tissue tumors in infants. The majority of these tumors occur in the head and neck region, so even a small tumor causes an obvious physical deformity. Approximately 10% of these lesions can threaten normal development or even the life of the affected child when they are located near vital structures such as the eyes, neck, or mouth. The most effective treatment options are high dose steroids, interferon-α, and propanolol. All of them are used over the course of several months, all have potentially life-threatening side effects, and none have defined mechanisms of action in endothelial cell tumors. This chapter will review mechanistic studies that show how the production of reactive oxygen species by the nox-4 subunit of NADPH oxidase stimulates expression of monocyte chemoattractant protein-1 to drive endothelial cell tumor formation. It will also discuss how blueberry extract can inhibit tumorigenic responses of EOMA cells in vitro and inhibit endothelial cell tumor formation in vivo.

Keywords Hemangioma · Hemangioendothelioma · Endothelial cell tumor · Monocyte chemoattractant protein -1 · Nox-4 · Blueberry extract · Activator protein-1 · Nuclear factor-kappaB · Hydrogen peroxide

1 Endothelial Cell Tumors: The Clinical Problem

1.1 Incidence

Endothelial cell (EC) tumors are the most common soft tissue tumors in children. They occur in 1–2% of all children and up to 10% of Caucasian children (Mulliken et al., 2004). The spectrum of malignant behavior in endothelial cell

G.M. Gordillo (✉)
Division of Plastic Surgery, Davis Heart Lung Research Institute, The Ohio State University, Columbus, OH 43212, USA
e-mail: gayle.gordillo@osumc.edu

G.D. Stoner, N.P. Seeram (eds.), *Berries and Cancer Prevention*,
DOI 10.1007/978-1-4419-7554-6_6,

tumors includes infantile hemangiomas, which make up the vast majority of EC tumors and are classified as benign. However, in 10% of children with hemangiomas, the location (i.e., near the eye) can threaten normal development and in 1% of affected children it can affect their life, as with airway or liver involvement (see Fig. 6.1). Kaposiform Hemangioendotheliomas (KHE) are considered an intermediate grade malignancy primarily due to the potential to develop Kassabach-Merritt phenomenon in which the tumor sequesters blood and platelets resulting in anemia, heart failure, and excessive bleeding. The mortality rate of KHE can be as high as 30% when the Kassabach-Merritt phenomenon occurs (Fernandez et al., 2009). Hemangioendotheliomas can be difficult to distinguish from hemangiomas (Cohen, 2002; Hand and Frieden, 2002). Although there are some differences between KHE and hemangiomas, they share one overriding and very important similarity. When pharmacologic interventions are used, both types of EC tumors are treated with the same medications (Mulliken et al., 2004; Gruman et al., 2005). Because the pharmacologic approach to both forms of EC tumors is the same, new treatment strategies devised for one form of these EC tumors will be applied to the other.

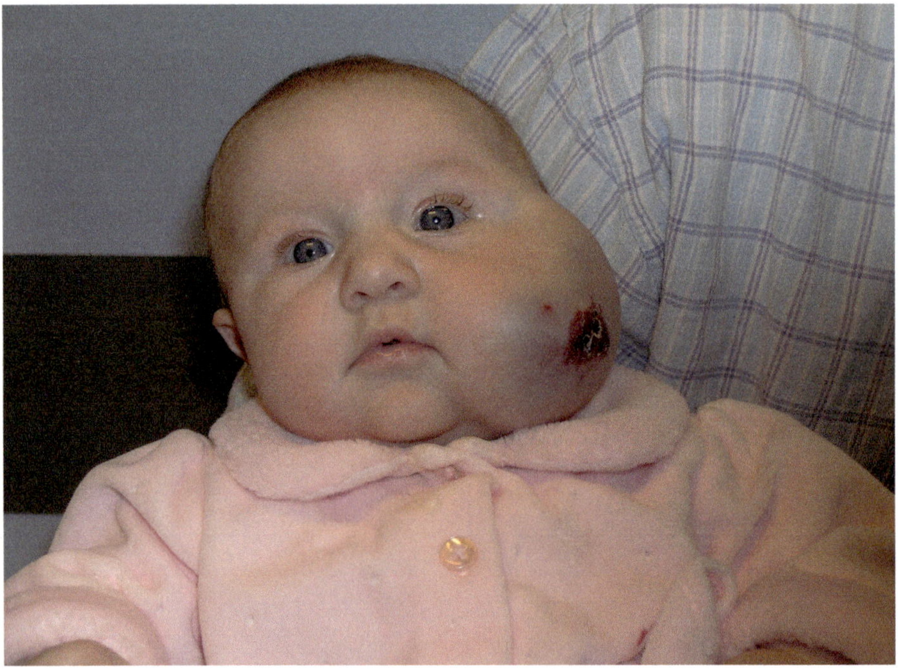

Fig. 6.1 Four month old child with a parotid hemangioma treated with high dose steroid therapy. This lesion threatened to occlude the child's airway and required aggressive treatment

1.2 Indications for Treatment

The most common form of treatment for EC tumors is "benign neglect" because most are hemangiomas that will resolve spontaneously over the course of 5–9 years.

Since the majority of these EC tumors occur in the head and neck area, even a small tumor causes an obvious deformity. Furthermore, once the tumors regress, 50% of children are left with residual deformity (Mulliken, 1997). Patients with threatening lesions have tumors that interfere with the function of vital structures and require treatment with pharmacologic agents to avoid permanent disability or loss of life (Fig. 6.1). Surgery is generally not an option for threatening lesions due to the potential for life-threatening hemorrhage, the risk of injury to vital structures such as the facial nerve, and in many instances excision would result in an unacceptable residual deformity. The families of those patients who do not have threatening lesions must either choose less effective treatments, such as lasers or intralesional steroids, opt for surgery with the inherent scarring as a result of tumor excision, or accept a long period of deformity as these lesions frequently take 5–9 years to resolve.

1.3 Current Treatment Options

Currently, the most effective treatment options are high dose steroids, interferon-α, and propanolol. All of these treatments are used over the course of several months, all have potentially life-threatening side effects, and none have defined mechanisms of action in endothelial cell tumors. Complications associated with the use of these drugs include: femur fractures, gastric ulcers, life-threatening infections, hypotension, hypoglycemia, respiratory distress, and spastic diplegia, a generalized neurologic insult with symptoms similar to cerebral palsy. Because of the high risks associated with using these drugs, their use is limited to those patients with threatening tumors. The goal in developing new treatment options is to provide a safe, non-invasive treatment alternative that is available to all children with EC tumors, not just those with threatening lesions. Treating these lesions at a very early stage before there is extensive growth could limit the potential for residual deformity.

1.4 Experimental Models of Endothelial Cell Tumors

EOMA cells are endothelial cells arising from a spontaneously arising KHE in the 129 P/3 mouse (Hoak et al., 1971; Warner et al., 1971). The power of this model for EC tumors is that manipulations can be done to EOMA cells in vitro and the effects observed in vivo. When injected subcutaneously into 129 P/3 mice, they form KHE with 100% efficiency (Gordillo et al., 2004, 2002). Mice with KHE develop Kassabach-Merritt phenomenon, which is also observed in humans with KHE (Warner et al., 1971). EOMA cells injected into mice establish a connection with the host vasculature to create blood-filled, perfused tumors through the process of angiogenesis. The expression of endothelial cell markers and proteins to confirm the endothelial cell phenotype of EOMA cells is well documented (Felbor et al., 2000; O'Reilly et al., 1997; Obeso et al., 1990; Sage and Bornstein, 1982; Wei et al., 1999). This validated mouse model of EC tumor growth and angiogenesis has also been used by many other investigators to test the effectiveness of anti-angiogenic compounds (Albini et al., 2001; Lannutti et al., 1997; O'Reilly et al., 1995; Taraboletti et al., 1995; Wang et al., 1999).

There is another EC tumor model that entails the use of brain endothelial (b.END3) cells transformed using the oncogenic papovavirus polyoma middle T antigen (Bautch et al., 1987; Montesano et al., 1990; Taraboletti et al., 1995; Bhandarkar et al., 2009). The bEND 3 cells are on a mixed MHC background ($H\text{-}2^d$ / $H\text{-}2^b$) making them suitable for use only in SCID mice (Bhandarkar et al., 2009; Bautch et al., 1987). The EOMA model is preferred because it can be used in syngeneic 129 P/3 mice with complete immunocompetence. Since EOMA cells are on an MHC $H\text{-}2^b$ background, they can be used in other mice such as C57Bl/6 with only minor histocompatibility mismatch and can readily be used with commercially available knockout mice on the C57Bl/6 background.

2 Molecular Mechanisms – Oxidant Production Promotes Endothelial Cell Tumor Growth

There is increasing evidence that the function of metabolic enzymes contribute to the pathogenesis of cancer (DeBerardinis et al., 2008; Thompson, 2009; Yan et al., 2009). NADPH oxidase is an enzyme originally identified in phagocytic cells with cytosolic subunits consisting of p47 phox, p67 phox, p40 phox, rac-1 or rac-2, and a membrane bound catalytic core consisting of p22phox and gp91. The function of NADPH oxidase is to perform a 1 electron reduction to convert molecular oxygen to superoxide (O_2^-) and the gp91 subunit is the catalytic component that mediates the electron transfer. NADPH oxidase is the major source of reactive oxygen species (ROS) in ECs, and NADPH oxidase activity is recognized as regulating cell signaling for angiogenesis and inflammation resulting in atherosclerosis (Cave, 2009; Diebold et al., 2009; Muller and Morawietz, 2009; Roy et al., 2008; Violi et al., 2009; Xia et al., 2007). Since the neoplastic process for solid tumors frequently co-opts the signaling pathways for inflammation and angiogenesis, this makes NADPH oxidase a logical target for mediating HE formation.

2.1 Contribution of Nox-4 Derived Oxidants

There are 7 homologs for gp91 in humans depending on the cell type (nox1-5 and duox 1&2) and 6 homologs in mice, which do not have nox 5 (Lambeth et al., 2007). The nox-2 and nox-4 homologs are found in endothelial cells. When EOMA cells were screened by real-time PCR for all 6 murine homologs of gp91, only nox-4 was present and it was present in levels 69-fold greater than detected in a non-tumor forming transformed murine aortic endothelial (MAE) cell line (Gordillo et al., 2010). Detection of nox-4 by immunohistochemistry on human hemangioma, kaposiform hemangioendothelioma, arteriovenous malformation, and normal blood vessel showed significantly elevated levels of nox-4 tumor forming ECs versus non-tumor forming ECs (GG unpublished data). These results validate two important concepts: the mouse model accurately represents the human condition; and high levels of nox-4 expression occur in both hemangiomas and kaposiform hemangioendotheliomas. These 2 EC tumors share pathologic mechanisms. For the sake of clarity, these two forms of EC tumors will collectively be referred to as HE throughout the rest of the chapter.

Experiments were performed to determine the significance of nox-4 activity on HE formation by using post-transcriptional gene silencing techniques targeting nox-4 in EOMA cells. Specifically, knockdown of nox-4 resulted in decreased cell proliferation, decreased angiogenic responses of EOMA cells grown on Matrigel, and decreased tumor size in vivo. We also demonstrated that the biologically active form of ROS produced by nox-4 was hydrogen peroxide (H_2O_2), which is produced through dismutation of superoxide (Gordillo et al., 2010). This finding is consistent with previously published results regarding the bioactive product of nox-4 activity (Dikalov et al., 2008). Live cell imaging was used to show that the H_2O_2 production was occurring in the nucleus, indicating that the nox-4 was located in a peri-nuclear membrane, which is also consistent with other published results (Gordillo et al., 2010; Hilenski et al., 2004; Pendyala et al., 2009).

There is no catalase in the nucleus, therefore elevated H_2O_2 production from increased levels of nox-4 expression would significantly alter redox homeostasis, especially since nox-4 is constitutively expressed (Bedard and Krause, 2007; Martyn et al., 2006). Excess H_2O_2 production in the nucleus would make DNA and cell cycling proteins targets for oxidative modifications. Injection of EOMA cells into mice resulted in a significant increase in the amount of oxidized DNA excreted in the urine (Gordillo et al., 2010). Nox-4 inhibition in melanoma cells resulted in cell cycle arrest with accumulation at the G2-M checkpoint. These results were attributed to nox-4 mediated effects on the phosphorylation status of cdc25 and cyclin dependent kinase 1, which regulate the G2-M transition in the cell cycle (Yamaura et al., 2009). Knockdown of nox-4 activity in EOMA cells also results in cell cycle inhibition at the G2-M transition (Gordillo et al., 2010). Nox-4 activity has also been shown to promote solid tumor growth in other models. Nox-4 activity in pancreatic cancer cells has been shown to inhibit protein tyrosine phosphatases resulting in sustained activation of kinases that inhibit apoptosis and promote cell survival and mitogenic signaling (Lee et al., 2007; Mochizuki et al., 2006). Thus, nox-4 activity may play a role in tumor promotion and initiation and it may serve as the source of "oxidative stress" that is inherent in the neoplastic transformation process.

2.2 The Role of AP-1 and NF-kB

NF-kB is constitutively expressed in many solid tumors and cancers of hematologic origin (Baud and Karin, 2009; Shen and Tergaonkar, 2009). AP-1 stimulates cell proliferation, is constitutively expressed in many cancers, and is required for tumor promotion (Arrigo, 1999; Bernstein and Colburn, 1989; Domann et al., 1994; Droge, 2006; Karin and Gallagher, 2005, 2009; Piechaczyk and Farras, 2008; Sen and Packer, 1996; Vesely et al., 2009; Young et al., 1999). Both of these transcription factors are also known to be redox sensitive and H_2O_2 inducible (Sen and Packer, 1996; Surh et al., 2005). There is evidence to support the concept that nox-4 derived H_2O_2 may serve as a stimulus for aberrant NF-kB and AP-1 activation in HE. We have found that H_2O_2 production is increased in transformed tumor forming endothelial (EOMA) cells compared to transformed non-tumor forming endothelial (MAE) cells (Gordillo et al., 2010). We have also shown that treatment of EOMA cells with blueberry extract (BBE), which has potent antioxidant properties, can decrease NF-kB transcriptional activation and nuclear DNA binding, as well as AP-1 transcriptional activation and c-Jun nuclear DNA binding (Atalay et al., 2003; Gordillo et al., 2009). Thus, nox-4 may be an upstream regulator of AP-1 and NF-kB activities that represent the nexus of inflammatory, angiogenic, and tumorigenic pathways that has been observed in many cancers.

2.3 MCP-1 Is Required for Endothelial Cell Tumor Formation

In endothelial cell tumors, one of the downstream targets of NF-kB and AP-1 transcription factors is MCP-1. Both of these transcription factors have been shown to bind to the MCP-1 promoter in endothelial cells (Martin et al., 1997; Sica et al., 1990). MCP-1 recruitment of macrophages is thought to facilitate angiogenesis required for tumor growth. We have shown that MCP-1 expression in EOMA cells is oxidant inducible, stimulated by nox-4, and inhibited by treatment with BBE (Gordillo et al., 2002, 2010, 2009). When EOMA cells were injected into MCP-1 knockout mice, half the mice developed tumors, the result of which was attributed to the expression of MCP-1 by EOMA cells that exceeded a critical threshold level sufficient to stimulate tumor formation. However, when neutralizing antibody to MCP-1 was co-injected with EOMA cells into 129 P/3 mice or MCP-1 knockout mice, it completely inhibited tumor formation in all mice. When EOMA cells, neutralizing antibody to MCP-1 and macrophages were co-injected, the tumor formation response was completely restored (Gordillo et al., 2004).

The requirement for MCP-1 and macrophage recruitment to promote EC tumor growth is consistent with the increasing recognition of the role that MCP-1 plays in mediating the growth of many cancers including breast (Leek et al., 1996; Saji et al., 2001; Ueno et al., 2000), thyroid (Tanaka et al., 2009), ovarian (Hefler et al., 1999), malignant melanoma (Torisu et al., 2000) and prostate cancers. The extent of macrophage infiltration correlates directly with tumor progression as macrophages are obligate partners in making angiogenesis, malignant cell migration, invasion, and metastases happen (Condeelis and Pollard, 2006; Pollard, 2004). These conclusions are not just based on correlations observed in clinical studies, but also on experimental evidence that shows that ablation of macrophage function or infiltration into experimental tumors inhibits growth and metastases (Gordillo et al., 2004; Lin et al., 2001; Lu et al., 2009).

3 Therapeutic Opportunities Using Blueberry Extract

Establishing the central role of the nox-4/MCP-1 axis in the growth of endothelial cell tumors provides a clear rationale for using antioxidant approaches as a potential therapeutic intervention. Nutritional interventions are particularly appealing for this problem given the young age of the affected population and the inherent safety with this approach. Blueberry extract was selected as a possible therapeutic intervention because it has high oxygen radical absorbance capacity and is rich in anthocyanins, which are antiangiogenic and can inhibit AP-1 stimulated neoplastic transformation (Bagchi et al., 2004; Chow et al., 2003; Ding et al., 2004; Hou et al., 2004; Roy et al., 2002). Thus, BBE appears to have properties that address significant promoters of EC tumor growth. Specifically, nox-4 derived oxidant production and AP-1 activity that can induce MCP-1 expression. Efforts have been made to identify biomarkers that measure the effects of BBE on these two stimuli for EC tumor growth.

3.1 Oxidant Derived Biomarkers to Monitor Response to Treatment

Urinary 8-Hydroxy-2′-deoxyguanosine (8-OHdG) is gaining increasing recognition as a marker for oxidative stress and as an indicator for cancer risk as the formation of 8-OHdG is known to be pro-mutagenic (Cheng et al., 1992; Collins et al., 2003; Fraga et al., 1990; Kasai, 1997, 2002; Marnett, 2000; Zhou et al., 2005). Urinary 8-OHdG levels have been found to be elevated in patients with lung and breast cancers (Kuo et al., 2007; Yano et al., 2009). An ELISA assay that detects 8-OHdG was used to show EC tumor formation following EOMA cell injection in mice, resulting in increased excretion of oxidatively modified DNA in the urine (Gordillo et al., 2010). These results may be due to the expression of nox-4 derived oxidants directly in the nucleus of EOMA cells. The Fenton reaction would convert H_2O_2 expressed in the nucleus to a hydroxyl radical capable of oxidatively modifying DNA (Bergeron et al., 2010; Cadet et al., 2003). The Fenton reaction is catalyzed by iron, and iron chelators have been shown to modulate production of DNA strand breaks and 8-OHdG (Toyokuni and Sagripanti, 1999). When mice injected with EOMA cells were treated with the iron chelator deferoxamine, they developed significantly smaller EC tumors (Gordillo et al., 2010). Collectively, this data suggests that oxidative modification of DNA may be clinically significant and merits consideration as a possible biomarker.

Elevated MCP-1 protein levels have been observed for many other tumors including breast (Leek et al., 1996; Saji et al., 2001; Ueno et al., 2000), thyroid (Tanaka et al., 2009), ovarian (Hefler et al., 1999), and malignant melanoma (Torisu et al., 2000). MCP-1 expression levels have also been shown to correlate with mortality in breast cancer (Leek et al., 1996; Bingle et al., 2002). In the EOMA model, MCP-1 expression in the tumor peaks at 7 days after EOMA cell injection, which corresponds with peak tumor growth. By 14 days, MCP-1 levels are lower than at 7 days, but growth of tumor parenchyma subsides and changes in tumor size are due to sequestration of blood within the tumor (Gordillo et al., 2004). Data from human hemangioma specimens has also shown that MCP-1 expression is seen only during tumor proliferation. MCP-1 is not detectable in the urine of mice with EC tumor, but it is detectable in the serum. Measurement of serum MCP-1 levels represents another possible biomarker approach for EC tumors.

3.2 Effects of BBE on Pro-tumorigenic Responses In Vitro

We have shown that BBE effectively targets MCP-1 expression by EOMA cells. BBE treatment inhibited both MCP-1 protein expression and transcriptional activation of the MCP-1 promoter in EOMA cells (Atalay et al., 2003). Transwell assay was used to show that BBE treatment of EOMA cells placed in the lower chambers inhibited macrophage migration from the upper chamber, confirming the functional effects of MCP-1 inhibition (Gordillo et al., 2009). The decreased transcriptional activation of the MCP-1 promoter may be due to decreased NF-kB and AP-1 DNA binding as described in Section 2.2. AP-1 activation in EOMA cells occurs through the c-Jun N-terminal kinase (JNK) pathway and its ability to phosphorylate c-Jun. Both of these reactions are oxidant inducible (Lo et al., 1996; Park et al., 2000). JNK activation, c-Jun phosphorylation and nuclear DNA binding were all inhibited by BBE treatment of EOMA cells. BBE treatment also inhibited EOMA cell proliferation and angiogenic responsiveness in a Matrigel assay, both of which are key indicators for tumorigenic capacity in vivo (Gordillo et al., 2009).

3.3 Effects of BBE Treatment on Endothelial Cell Tumor Growth In Vivo

An extensive series of experiments has been performed to demonstrate that BBE treatment of EOMA cells can effectively inhibit HE growth in vivo. When EOMA cells were treated with BBE prior to injection into mice, the incidence of HE formation was decreased by 50% and the tumors that did form were significantly smaller. Immunohistochemistry was used to document decreased macrophage recruitment to HE treated with BBE compared to cells treated with vehicle control (Atalay et al., 2003).

Additional experiments were performed to evaluate the effectiveness of BBE treatment in a more clinical context. Mice injected with EOMA cells were given BBE administered by oral gavage feedings starting on the day of injection. Toxicity studies were performed in conjunction with a veterinary pathologist to determine the effects of oral BBE given to mice at a 1,000 mg/kg dose. Serum levels of liver transaminases were not elevated nor were serum creatinine levels indicating normal liver and renal function. Histologic evaluation of heart, lung, brain, adrenal glands, and skin also failed to reveal any abnormalities. A BBE dose response study was performed and all doses resulted in a significant decrease in HE size, but there was no significant difference in HE size between mice receiving 20 mg/kg of BBE and those receiving a higher dose. To determine whether oral administration of BBE had any systemic antioxidant effects, serum levels of lipid peroxidation were assessed using a thiobarbituric acid reactive substances assay to measure malondialdehyde (MDA) and high pressure liquid chromatography (HPLC) was used to measure the ratios of reduced glutathione (GSH) to oxidized glutathione (GSSG) as an indicator of oxidative stress. There was a dose dependent decrease in MDA with BBE dosing and a dose dependent increase in the GSH/GSSG up to the 20 mg/kg dose, but above that there was a decrease in GSH/GSSG. Finally, Kaplan-Meier analysis demonstrated that mice given BBE at 20 mg/kg had a significantly increased length of survival compared to mice given vehicle control (water) (Gordillo et al., 2009).

4 Summary

Collectively, the findings presented herein provide clear evidence to establish the importance of the nox-4/MCP-1 axis in promoting the development of HE through

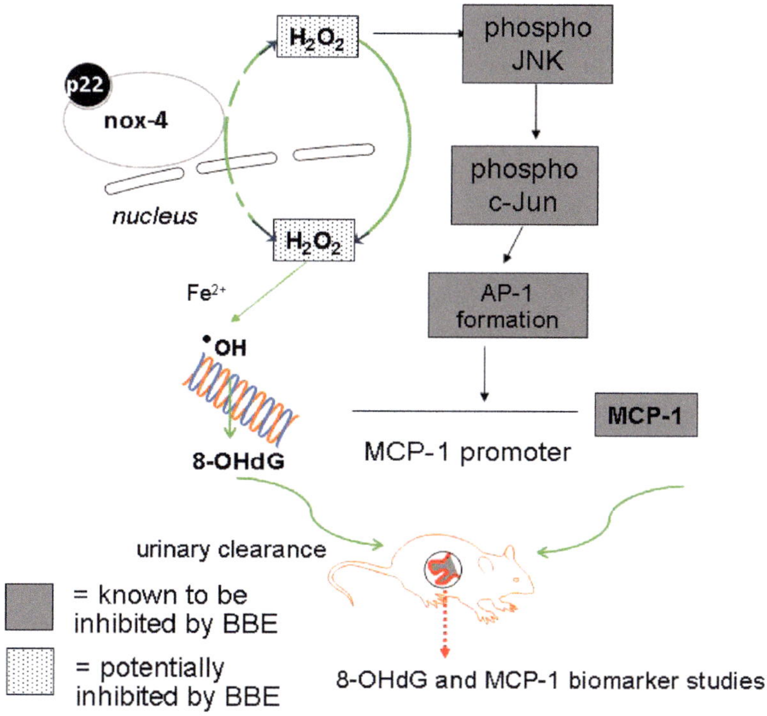

Fig. 6.2 Schematic showing mechanisms that promote HE growth and the proposed mechanisms of BBE treatment. The *grey boxes* show signaling mechanisms that are known to be inhibited by BBE and the *dotted boxes* show potential areas of BBE inhibition

the production of reactive oxygen species as shown in Fig. 6.2. Blueberry extract has very high oxygen radical absorbance capacity and is rich in anthocyanins and both of these properties can potentially inhibit the stimuli for endothelial cell tumor formation. The effects of BBE extract on HE growth have been published using a validated mouse model of HE. BBE treatment can inhibit HE growth in vivo with the most dramatic results noted after direct application of BBE to EOMA cells. Thus, a nutritional intervention using BBE represents a viable therapeutic approach that could be available to all children with endothelial cell tumors.

Acknowledgments Supported by R01GM095657 to GMG and RO1 HL073087, GM 077185, and GM 069589 to CKS.

References

Albini A, Morini M, D'Agostini F, Ferrari N, Campelli F et al (2001) Inhibition of angiogenesis-driven Kaposi's sarcoma tumor growth in nude mice by oral N-acetylcysteine. Cancer Res 61:8171–8178

Arrigo AP (1999) Gene expression and the thiol redox state. Free Radic Biol Med 27:936–944

Atalay M, Gordillo G, Roy S, Rovin B, Bagchi D et al (2003) Anti-angiogenic property of edible berry in a model of hemangioma. Febs Lett 544:252–257

Bagchi D, Sen C, Bagchi M, Atalay M (2004) Anti-angiogenic, antioxidant, and anti-carcinogenic properties of a novel anthocyanin-rich berry extract formula. Biochemistry 69:75–80

Baud V, Karin M (2009) Is NF-kappab a good target for cancer therapy? Hopes and pitfalls. Nat Rev Drug Discov 8:33–40

Bautch VL, Toda S, Hassell JA, Hanahan D (1987) Endothelial cell tumors develop in transgenic mice carrying polyoma virus middle t oncogene. Cell 51:529–537

Bedard K, Krause KH (2007) The NOX family of ROS-generating NADPH oxidases: physiology and pathophysiology. Physiol Rev 87:245–313

Bergeron F, Auvre F, Radicella JP, Ravanat JL (2010) HO$*$ radicals induce an unexpected high proportion of tandem base lesions refractory to repair by DNA glycosylases. Proc Natl Acad Sci USA 107:5528–5533

Bernstein LR, Colburn NH (1989) AP1/Jun function is differentially induced in promotion-sensitive and resistant JB6 cells. Science 244:566–569

Bhandarkar SS, Jaconi M, Fried LE, Bonner MY, Lefkove B et al (2009) Fulvene-5 potently inhibits NADPH oxidase 4 and blocks the growth of endothelial cell tumors in mice. J Clin Invest 119:6

Bingle L, Brown NJ, Lewis CE (2002) The role of tumour-associated macrophages in tumour progression: implications for new anticancer therapies. J Pathol 196:254–265

Cadet J, Douki T, Gasparutto D, Ravanat JL (2003) Oxidative damage to DNA: formation, measurement and biochemical features. Mutat Res 531:5–23

Cave A (2009) Selective targeting of NADPH oxidase for cardiovascular protection. Curr Opin Pharmacol 9:208–213

Cheng KC, Cahill DS, Kasai H, Nishimura S, Loeb LA (1992) 8-Hydroxyguanine, an abundant form of oxidative DNA damage, causes G—t and A—c substitutions. J Biol Chem 267:166–172

Chow LM, Chui CH, Tang JC, Lau FY, Yau MY et al (2003) Anti-angiogenic potential of Gleditsia sinensis fruit extract. Int J Mol Med 12:269–273

Cohen MM Jr (2002) Vasculogenesis, angiogenesis, hemangiomas, and vascular malformations. Am J Med Genet 108:265–274

Collins C, Awada MM, Zhou X, Dedon PC (2003) Analysis of 3′-phosphoglycolaldehyde residues in oxidized DNA by gas chromatography/negative chemical ionization/mass spectrometry. Chem Res Toxicol 16:1560–1566

Condeelis J, Pollard JW (2006) Macrophages: obligate partners for tumor cell migration, invasion, and metastasis. Cell 124:263–266
DeBerardinis RJ, Lum JJ, Hatzivassiliou G, Thompson CB (2008) The biology of cancer: metabolic reprogramming fuels cell growth and proliferation. Cell Metab 7:11–20
Diebold I, Djordjevic T, Petry A, Hatzelmann A, Tenor H et al (2009) Phosphodiesterase 2 mediates redox-sensitive endothelial cell proliferation and angiogenesis by thrombin via Rac1 and NADPH oxidase 2. Circ Res 104:1169–1177
Dikalov SI, Dikalova AE, Bikineyeva AT, Schmidt HH, Harrison DG et al (2008) Distinct roles of Nox1 and Nox4 in basal and angiotensin II-stimulated superoxide and hydrogen peroxide production. Free Radic Biol Med 45:1340–1351
Ding M, Lu Y, Bowman L, Huang C, Leonard S et al (2004) Inhibition of AP-1 and neoplastic transformation by fresh apple peel extract. J Biol Chem 279:10670–10676
Domann FE Jr, Levy JP, Finch JS, Bowden GT (1994) Constitutive AP-1 DNA binding and transactivating ability of malignant but not benign mouse epidermal cells. Mol Carcinog 9:61–66
Droge W (2006) Redox regulation in anabolic and catabolic processes. Curr Opin Clin Nutr Metab Care 9:190–195
Felbor U, Dreier L, Bryant R, Ploegh H, Olsen B et al (2000) Secreted cathepsin l generates endostatin from collagen XVIII. The EMBO J 19:1187–1194
Fernandez Y, Bernabeu-Wittel M, Garcia-Morillo JS (2009) Kaposiform hemangioendothelioma. Eur J Intern Med 20:106–113
Fraga CG, Shigenaga MK, Park JW, Degan P, Ames BN (1990) Oxidative damage to DNA during aging: 8-hydroxy-2′-deoxyguanosine in rat organ DNA and urine. Proc Natl Acad Sci USA 87:4533–4537
Gordillo GM, Atalay M, Roy S, Sen CK (2002) Hemangioma model for in vivo angiogenesis: inducible oxidative stress and MCP-1 expression in EOMA cells. Meth Enzymol 352:422–432
Gordillo G, Fang H, Khanna S, Harper J, Phillips G et al (2009) Oral administration of blueberry inhibits angiogenic tumor growth and enhances survival of mice with endothelial cell neoplasm. Antioxid Redox Signal 11:47–58
Gordillo G, Fang H, Park HA, Roy S (2010) Nox-4 dependent nuclear H2O2 drives DNA oxidation resulting in 8-ohdg as urinary biomarker and hemangioendothelioma formation. Antioxid Redox Signal 12:10
Gordillo G, Onat D, Stockinger M, Roy S, Atalay M et al (2004) A key angiogenic role of monocyte chemoattractant protein-1 in hemangioendothelioma proliferation. Am J Physiol (Cell) 287:C866–C873
Gruman A, Liang MG, Mulliken JB, Fishman SJ, Burrows PE et al (2005) Kaposiform hemangioendothelioma without Kasabach-Merritt phenomenon. J Am Acad Dermatol 52:616–622
Hand JL, Frieden IJ (2002) Vascular birthmarks of infancy: resolving nosologic confusion. Am J Med Genet 108:257–264
Hefler L, Tempfer C, Heinze G, Mayerhofer K, Breitenecker G et al (1999) Monocyte chemoattractant protein-1 serum levels in ovarian cancer patients. Br J Cancer 81:855–859
Hilenski LL, Clempus RE, Quinn MT, Lambeth JD, Griendling KK (2004) Distinct subcellular localizations of Nox1 and Nox4 in vascular smooth muscle cells. Arterioscler Thromb Vasc Biol 24:677–683
Hoak JC, Warner ED, Cheng HF, Fry GL, Hankenson RR (1971) Hemangioma with thrombocytopenia and microangiopathic anemia (Kasabach-Merritt syndrome): an animal model. J Lab Clin Med 77:941–950
Hou DX, Kai K, Li JJ, Lin S, Terahara N et al (2004) Anthocyanidins inhibit activator protein 1 activity and cell transformation: structure-activity relationship and molecular mechanisms. Carcinogenesis 25:29–36
Karin M, Gallagher E (2005) From JNK to pay dirt: jun kinases, their biochemistry, physiology and clinical importance. Iubmb Life 57:283–295

Karin M, Gallagher E (2009) TNFR signaling: ubiquitin-conjugated traffic signals control stop-and-go for MAPK signaling complexes. Immunol Rev 228:225–240

Kasai H (1997) Analysis of a form of oxidative DNA damage, 8-hydroxy-2′-deoxyguanosine, as a marker of cellular oxidative stress during carcinogenesis. Mutat Res 387:147–163

Kasai H (2002) Chemistry-based studies on oxidative DNA damage: formation, repair, and mutagenesis. Free Radic Biol Med 33:450–456

Kuo HW, Chou SY, Hu TW, Wu FY, Chen DJ (2007) Urinary 8-hydroxy-2′-deoxyguanosine (8-OHdG) and genetic polymorphisms in breast cancer patients. Mutat Res 631:62–68

Lambeth JD, Kawahara T, Diebold B (2007) Regulation of Nox and Duox enzymatic activity and expression. Free Radic Biol Med 43:319–331

Lannutti B, Gately S, Quevedo M, Soff G, Paller A (1997) Human angiostatin inhibits murine hemangioendothelioma tumor growth in vivo. Cancer Res 57:5277–5280

Lee JK, Edderkaoui M, Truong P, Ohno I, Jang KT et al (2007) NADPH oxidase promotes pancreatic cancer cell survival via inhibiting JAK2 dephosphorylation by tyrosine phosphatases. Gastroenterology 133:1637–1648

Leek RD, Lewis CE, Whitehouse R, Greenall M, Clarke J et al (1996) Association of macrophage infiltration with angiogenesis and prognosis in invasive breast carcinoma. Cancer Res 56: 4625–4629

Lin EY, Nguyen AV, Russell RG, Pollard JW (2001) Colony-stimulating factor 1 promotes progression of mammary tumors to malignancy. J Exp Med 193:727–740

Lo YY, Wong JM, Cruz TF (1996) Reactive oxygen species mediate cytokine activation of c-Jun NH2-terminal kinases. J Biol Chem 271:15703–15707

Lu Y, Chen Q, Corey E, Xie W, Fan J et al (2009) Activation of MCP-1/CCR2 axis promotes prostate cancer growth in bone. Clin Exp Metastasis 26:161–169

Marnett LJ (2000) Oxyradicals and DNA damage. Carcinogenesis 21:361–370

Martin T, Cardarelli PM, Parry GC, Felts KA, Cobb RR (1997) Cytokine induction of monocyte chemoattractant protein-1 gene expression in human endothelial cells depends on the cooperative action of NF-kappa B and AP-1. Eur J Immunol 27:1091–1097

Martyn KD, Frederick LM, von Loehneysen K, Dinauer MC, Knaus UG (2006) Functional analysis of nox4 reveals unique characteristics compared to other NADPH oxidases. Cell Signal 18: 69–82

Mochizuki T, Furuta S, Mitsushita J, Shang WH, Ito M et al (2006) Inhibition of NADPH oxidase 4 activates apoptosis via the AKT/apoptosis signal-regulating kinase 1 pathway in pancreatic cancer PANC-1 cells. Oncogene 25:3699–3707

Montesano R, Pepper M, Mohle-Steinlein U, Risau W, Wagner E et al (1990) Increased proteolytic activity is responsible for the aberrant morphogenetic behavior of endothelial cells expressing middle T oncogene. Cell 62:435–445

Muller G, Morawietz H (2009) NAD(P)h oxidase and endothelial dysfunction. Horm Metab Res 41:152–158

Mulliken JB (1997) In: Aston S, Beasley R, Thorne C (eds) Grabb and Smith's plastic surgery, 5th edn. Lippincott-Raven, Philadelphia, PA, pp 191–203

Mulliken JB, Anupindi S, Ezekowitz RA, Mihm MC Jr (2004) Case records of the Massachusetts General Hospital. Weekly clinicopathological exercises. Case 13-2004. A newborn girl with a large cutaneous lesion, thrombocytopenia, and anemia. N Engl J Med 350:1764–1775

Obeso J, Weber J, Auerbach R (1990) A hemangioendothelioma-derived cell line: its use as a model for the study of endothelial cell biology. Lab Invest 63:259–269

O'Reilly M, Boehm T, Shing Y, Fukai N, Vasios G et al (1997) Endostatin: an endogenous inhibitor of angiogenesis and tumor growth. Cell 88:277–285

O'Reilly M, Brem H, Folkman J (1995) Treatment of murine hemangioendotheliomas with the angiogenesis inhibitor AGM-1470. J Pediatr Surg 30:325–330

Park HS, Park E, Kim MS, Ahn K, Kim IY et al (2000) Selenite inhibits the c-Jun N-terminal kinase/stress-activated protein kinase (JNK/SAPK) through a thiol redox mechanism. J Biol Chem 275:2527–2531

Pendyala S, Gorshkova IA, Usatyuk PV, He D, Pennathur A et al (2009) Role of Nox4 and Nox2 in hyperoxia-induced reactive oxygen species generation and migration of human lung endothelial cells. Antioxid Redox Signal 11:747–764
Piechaczyk M, Farras R (2008) Regulation and function of JunB in cell proliferation. Biochem Soc Trans 36:864–867
Pollard JW (2004) Tumour-educated macrophages promote tumour progression and metastasis. Nat Rev Cancer 4:71–78
Roy S, Khanna S, Alessio HM, Vider J, Bagchi D et al (2002) Anti-angiogenic property of edible berries. Free Radic Res 36:1023–1031
Roy S, Khanna S, Sen CK (2008) Redox regulation of the VEGF signaling path and tissue vascularization: hydrogen peroxide, the common link between physical exercise and cutaneous wound healing. Free Radic Biol Med 44:180–192
Sage H, Bornstein P (1982) Endothelial cells from umbilical vein and hemangioendothelioma secrete basement membrane largely to the exclusion of interstitial procollagens. Arteriosclerosis 2:27–36
Saji H, Koike M, Yamori T, Saji S, Seiki M et al (2001) Significant correlation of monocyte chemoattractant protein-1 expression with neovascularization and progression of breast carcinoma. Cancer 92:1085–1091
Sen CK, Packer L (1996) Antioxidant and redox regulation of gene transcription. FASEB J 10:709–720
Shen HM, Tergaonkar V (2009) NfkappaB signaling in carcinogenesis and as a potential molecular target for cancer therapy. Apoptosis 14:348–363
Sica A, Wang JM, Colotta F, Dejana E, Mantovani A et al (1990) Monocyte chemotactic and activating factor gene expression induced in endothelial cells by IL-1 and tumor necrosis factor. J Immunol 144:3034–3038
Surh YJ, Kundu JK, Na HK, Lee JS (2005) Redox-sensitive transcription factors as prime targets for chemoprevention with anti-inflammatory and antioxidative phytochemicals. J Nutr 135:2993S–3001S
Tanaka K, Kurebayashi J, Sohda M, Nomura T, Prabhakar U et al (2009) The expression of monocyte chemotactic protein-1 in papillary thyroid carcinoma is correlated with lymph node metastasis and tumor recurrence. Thyroid 19:21–25
Taraboletti G, Garofalo A, Belotti D, Drudis T, Borsotti P et al (1995) Inhibition of angiogenesis and murine hemangioma growth by batimastat, a synthetic inhibitor of matrix metalloproteinases. J Natl Cancer Inst 87:293–298
Thompson CB (2009) Metabolic enzymes as oncogenes or tumor suppressors. N Engl J Med 360:813–815
Torisu H, Ono M, Kiryu H, Furue M, Ohmoto Y et al (2000) Macrophage infiltration correlates with tumor stage and angiogenesis in human malignant melanoma: possible involvement of TNFalpha and IL-1alpha. Int J Cancer 85:182–188
Toyokuni S, Sagripanti JL (1999) Iron chelators modulate the production of DNA strand breaks and 8-hydroxy-2′-deoxyguanosine. Free Radic Res 31:123–128
Ueno T, Toi M, Saji H, Muta M, Bando H et al (2000) Significance of macrophage chemoattractant protein-1 in macrophage recruitment, angiogenesis, and survival in human breast cancer. Clin Cancer Res 6:3282–3289
Vesely PW, Staber PB, Hoefler G, Kenner L (2009) Translational regulation mechanisms of AP-1 proteins. Mutat Res 682:7–12
Violi F, Basili S, Nigro C, Pignatelli P (2009) Role of NADPH oxidase in atherosclerosis. Future Cardiol 5:83–92
Wang C, Quevedo ME, Lannutti BJ, Gordon KB, Guo D et al (1999) In vivo gene therapy with interleukin-12 inhibits primary vascular tumor growth and induces apoptosis in a mouse model. J Invest Dermatol 112:775–781
Warner ED, Hoak JC, Fry GL (1971) Hemangioma, thrombocytopenia, and anemia. The Kasabach-Merritt syndrome in an animal model. Arch Pathol Lab Med 91:523–528

Wei W, Moses M, Wiederschain D, Arbiser J, Folkman J (1999) The generation of endostatin is mediated by elastase. Cancer Res 59:6052–6056

Xia C, Meng Q, Liu LZ, Rojanasakul Y, Wang XR et al (2007) Reactive oxygen species regulate angiogenesis and tumor growth through vascular endothelial growth factor. Cancer Res 67:10823–10830

Yamaura M, Mitsushita J, Furuta S, Kiniwa Y, Ashida A et al (2009) NADPH oxidase 4 contributes to transformation phenotype of melanoma cells by regulating G2-M cell cycle progression. Cancer Res 69:2647–2654

Yan H, Parsons DW, Jin G, McLendon R, Rasheed BA et al (2009) IDH1 and IDH2 mutations in gliomas. N Engl J Med 360:765–773

Yano T, Shoji F, Baba H, Koga T, Shiraishi T et al (2009) Significance of the urinary 8-OHdG level as an oxidative stress marker in lung cancer patients. Lung Cancer 63:111–114

Young MR, Li JJ, Rincon M, Flavell RA, Sathyanarayana BK et al (1999) Transgenic mice demonstrate AP-1 (activator protein-1) transactivation is required for tumor promotion. Proc Natl Acad Sci USA 96:9827–9832

Zhou X, Liberman RG, Skipper PL, Margolin Y, Tannenbaum SR et al (2005) Quantification of DNA strand breaks and abasic sites by oxime derivatization and accelerator mass spectrometry: application to gamma-radiation and peroxynitrite. Anal Biochem 343:84–92

Chapter 7
Effects of Black Raspberries on UV-Induced Cutaneous Inflammation and Tumor Development

Tatiana Oberyszyn

Abstract Sunlight is the most common carcinogen that we are exposed to on a daily basis. Unfortunately, the target of this complete carcinogen is our skin. In recent years, the frequency of skin cancer has increased due to both to a decrease in the ozone layer as well as changes in tanning practices, including increased tanning bed use. In fact these skin tumors are by far the most common form of cancer in humans, with over 1 million new cases identified in the United States each year. More Americans will be diagnosed with some form of skin cancer than all other cancers combined. Repeated severe sunburns or intense sun exposure in a short time period have been shown to be risk factors for development of both melanoma and nonmelanoma skin cancers (NMSC). Current treatment modalities for nonmelanoma skin cancers include surgical excision, cryotherapy, radiotherapy or topical treatment with chemotherapeutic drugs, immune response modifiers or anti-inflammatory agents. These treatments range in severity of side effects including (but not limited to); ulceration, scarring, long duration of inflammation and pain at site of application. In addition, long treatment periods reduce compliance, and often have limited clinical efficacy. Therefore, alternative preventive and treatment strategies are needed. Increasing evidence suggests that natural compounds derived from functional foods can be use as a safe alternative to prevent or treat diseases. This chapter discusses the efficacy of using black raspberry extracts as a potential chemopreventive/chemotherapeutic agent against NMSC.

Keywords Skin · Antioxidants · Natural compounds · Squamous cell carcinoma · Sunburn

---

T. Oberyszyn (✉)
Department of Pathology, The Ohio State University, Columbus, OH 43201, USA
e-mail: oberyszyn.1@osu.edu

G.D. Stoner, N.P. Seeram (eds.), *Berries and Cancer Prevention*,
DOI 10.1007/978-1-4419-7554-6_7,

1 The Skin

1.1 Structure/Function

The skin is the largest organ of our body. It is responsible for acting as both a barrier and a regulating influence between the outside world and the environment within our bodies. This organ plays a key role in protection against infection, prevention of excessive water loss or absorption, as well as temperature regulation. Our skin is made up of three distinct layers; the epidermis, dermis, and hypodermis. The outermost layer, the epidermis, is comprised primarily of keratinocytes, which proliferate in the basal layer and gradually migrate outwards towards the surface. As these cells migrate they gradually lose their internal organelles becoming essentially sacs of keratin. The structural component of the skin, the dermis, is made up of collagen and elastin fibers that provide the strength and elasticity that our skin needs to function. This layer also contains hair follicles, nerves, sweat glands as well as blood vessels that provide oxygen and nutrients to both the dermis and the epidermis. The lowest layer, the hypodermis, is a layer of fat and connective tissue that contains larger blood vessels and nerves. The size of this layer varies throughout the body and from person to person.

1.2 Malignancies

Exposure to sunlight has been linked with the development of basal cell carcinoma and squamous cell carcinoma, collectively known as non-melanoma skin cancers (NMSC). These skin tumors are by far the most common form of cancer in humans, with over 1 million new cases identified in the United States each year (Black et al., 1997; www.cancer.org). In fact, more Americans will be diagnosed with some form of skin cancer than all other cancers combined. NMSC occurs on sun-exposed sites and can be reduced by sun protection (English et al., 1997). Approximately 80% of skin cancers are basal cell carcinomas while 16% are the more dangerous type of NMSC, or squamous cell carcinoma of the skin. Although both cancers occur on sun-exposed sites, it is believed that cumulative lifetime sun exposure has a strong dose-response association with squamous-cell carcinoma, whereas for basal-cell carcinoma, intermittent sun exposure and exposure during childhood might be more important (Kricker et al., 1995; Rosso et al., 1996). While NMSC is mistakenly believed to be harmless, in reality even immunocompetent patients experience both morbidity and mortality from NMSC. A Danish case-control study found mortality rates of 0.12% for BCC and 4.3% for SCC (Osterlind et al., 1991). In the United States, The American Cancer Society estimated there would be about 2,940 deaths from NMSC in 2009 (www.cancer.org). Despite a relatively low mortality rate, the treatment of NMSC is the fifth most costly cancer in the Medicare population (Housman et al., 2003). The estimated cost in the United States in 2002 for the treatment and management of all NMSCs was 1.4 billion dollars, corresponding to

1.6 million office visits (Group, 2005). Although exposure to UV radiation can be minimized, it is unlikely that it will ever be completely eliminated. Clearly a better understanding of the development, growth, and treatment of this cancer is critical.

1.2.1 Susceptible Populations

Numerous studies have demonstrated an association of gender, age, race and immunosuppressive status with increased incidence of NMSC development. Epidemiological studies have reported the development of significantly more NMSC in men than in women, with the American Cancer Society reporting approximately twice the incidence in men compared to women (Armstrong and Kricker, 2001; Scrivener et al., 2002; www.cancer.org). Similarly murine studies have demonstrated that when exposed to equal amounts of sunlight, male mice develop tumors earlier, develop more tumors, and have a higher percentage of tumors of higher malignant grade (Thomas-Ahner et al., 2007). While UV radiation is known to be the major risk factor for the general population, the incidence and the mortality rate greatly increases in the immunosuppressed population such as transplant patients, HIV infected individuals, and patients suffering from chronic lymphocytic leukemia (CLL) (Bridges and Steinberg, 1986; Kaplan and Cook, 2005; Nguyen et al., 2002; Ramsay et al., 2002; Ulrich et al., 2008). In all of these patients, SCC is vastly over-represented compared with its frequency in non-immunosuppressed patients. The presence of signature p53 mutations in skin tumors arising in immunocompromised patients indicates that as seen in the general population, UV light is also an important etiologic factor for the development of these tumors (McGregor et al., 1997).

2 Ultraviolet Light

2.1 Wavelengths

Sunlight is composed of light with a range of wavelengths including those in the near ultraviolet range (320–400 nm) which have been designated as ultraviolet A light (UVA), and wavelengths of light that are within the 290–320 nm range termed ultraviolet B (UVB) light. Although less than 1–2% of the UV light from the sun is in the 290–320 nm spectral range (ultraviolet B, UVB), UVB radiation is responsible for the majority of cutaneous damage following both acute and long-term exposure (de Gruijl, 2000, 2002; Gerber et al., 2002). UVA rays constitute 90–95% of the ultraviolet light reaching the earth. They have a relatively long wavelength (320–400 nm) and penetrate the furthest into the skin. UVA tends to suppress the immune function and is implicated in premature aging of the skin (Council on Scientific Affairs, 1989; Fuller et al., 1992). While in the past UVA was considered less harmful, recent studies have found that it contributes to skin cancer development via the induction of reactive oxygen species within the skin, resulting in oxidative DNA damage (Agar et al., 2004; Marrot and Meunier, 2008).

2.2 Role in Cutaneous Inflammation and Carcinogenesis

Although UV radiation is known to be the major risk factor for both the general population as well as immunocompromised patients, significant information is lacking about the molecular mechanisms leading to skin cancer development. One immediate physiologic consequence of UVB exposure is the cutaneous acute inflammatory response, characterized by increased blood flow and vascular permeability which results in edema and erythema, the infiltration of neutrophils into the dermis, the induction of pro-inflammatory cytokines, and the production of reactive oxygen species (ROS) (Jung, 1991; Kripke, 1991; Rivas and Ullrich, 1994; Clydesdale et al., 2001; Scapini et al., 2000; Terui and Tagami, 2000). As part of the acute inflammatory response, prostaglandins are also increased (Black et al., 1978; Hruza and Pentland, 1993; Shreedhar et al., 1998). Epidemiological, as well as basic research studies, have demonstrated that the inflammatory response following both brief periods of high intensity sun exposure and chronic sun exposure plays a critical role in the formation of NMSC (Gallagher et al., 1995a, b; Marks et al., 1990; Strickland et al., 1989). This exposure induces functional changes in both resident skin cells as well as infiltrating cells of the immune system, which may ultimately contribute to the development of skin cancer (Elmets and Bergstresser, 1982; Kripke, 1984, 1991; Yamawaki et al., 1997). It is now clear that inflammatory cells have significant effects on tumor development. Early in the tumor development process, inflammatory cells such as neutrophils can be powerful tumor promoters. Neutrophils and other phagocytic cells induce DNA damage in proliferating cells through their generation of reactive oxygen and nitrogen species, which in normal circumstances are produced by these cells to fight infection (Maeda and Akaike, 1998). In addition, these cells mediate damage through the generation of arachidonic acid derivatives, including prostaglandins and leukotrienes, which are capable of producing an intense inflammatory response (Malech and Gallin, 1987). Exposure of epidermal cells to UVB light both in vivo and in vitro has been associated with increased release of arachidonic acid (AA) from membrane phospholipids (Cohen and DeLeo, 1993; Hruza and Pentland, 1993) as well as increased biosynthesis of prostaglandins from AA via the induction of the cyclooxygenase-2 (COX-2) enzyme (Gresham et al., 1996). These prostaglandins are now believed to contribute to the damage associated with the UVB induced inflammatory response in the skin. It is known that the production of prostaglandin E_2 (PGE_2) by the COX pathway contributes to ROS generation in two ways: first, oxygen radical generation during the catalytic conversion of prostaglandin G_2 to H_2 and second, prostaglandin-mediated oxidative alterations of the inflammatory process. As a byproduct of prostaglandin synthesis, reactive oxygen species that can induce the formation of oxidative DNA adducts such as 8-oxo-deoxyguanosine (8-oxo-dG) are formed (Eling and Curtis, 1992). A number of studies demonstrated that 8-oxo-dG is one of the major modified DNA base products after UVB irradiation and suggested that 8-oxo-dG may be associated with UVB-induced skin carcinogenesis (Beehler et al., 1992; Hattori et al., 1996; Wilgus et al., 2003a). Several studies suggest that reactive intermediates such as those produced following UVB exposure may also contribute to the mutation of genes such as p53, allowing for an increased rate of accumulation of genetic damage in the cell (Nakamura and Sakamoto, 2001; Yu et al., 2002). Therefore, an increase in PGE_2 production and function appears to be critical to the observed damaging effects of UVB light on the skin (Black et al., 1997; Fischer, 2002; Fischer et al., 2007; Seibert et al., 1994; Vane et al., 1994; Wilgus et al., 2000). Indeed, in mice, topical application of anti-inflammatory compounds after UVB exposure inhibit UVB-induced reactive oxygen species and prostaglandin synthesis (Nichols and Katiyar 2010; Wei et al., 2002), and COX-2 inhibitors inhibit formation of UVB-induced skin tumors when administered systemically (Fischer, 2002; Fischer et al., 1999) or topically (Wilgus et al., 2003a, b). Thus, early UVB-induced inflammation is a key step in skin cancer development, and blocking inflammation can be beneficial in the chemoprevention of skin tumors.

2.3 Murine Models of UV Induced Inflammation and Skin Cancer

Outbred SKH-1 hairless mice and inbred haired mice that are shaved prior to UVB exposure are used as murine models of UVB-induced skin cancer. Both hairless and haired mice can develop UV induced skin tumors (Daynes et al., 1986; Kripke, 1977; Morison et al., 1986). The main advantage of haired mouse models is that the mice are usually inbred, facilitating immunologic studies. However, haired mice have some distinct disadvantages in skin cancer research, including difficulty in measuring erythema and sunburn protection, the requirement for hair removal prior to UVB exposure, high UVB doses, a long period (>25 weeks) of chronic exposure and the development of fibrosacromas (Kim et al., 2003; Kripke, 1977; Martin et al., 2009; Ward et al., 1989). In contrast, SKH-1 mice are hairless and rapidly develop skin tumors in response to chronic, sub-erythemal UVB exposure developing SCC precursors and SCC similar to that observed in humans (de Gruijl and Forbes, 1995; Gallagher et al., 1984). In addition, SKH-1 mice, like humans, are outbred, making them very useful for chemoprevention and chemotherapy studies.

3 Black Raspberries

3.1 Background

Numerous studies suggest that consuming large amounts of fruits and vegetables can prevent the incidence of cancer in a number of organs (Potter, 2005). Berries contain a number of chemopreventive agents including vitamins A, C, E, ellagic acid and anthocyanins (Kresty et al., 2001). The anthocyanins, responsible for the color of fruit, have been shown to improve the overall antioxidant defense status of human plasma (Cao and Prior, 1999). Previous studies showed that a methanol fraction of black raspberries inhibited B(a)P induce transformation of Syrian hamster embryo cells in a dose-dependent manner (Xue et al., 2001). Furthermore, freeze dried black raspberries inhibited NMBA tumorigenesis in the rat esophagus and were shown to suppress the development of preneoplastic lesions into papillomas (Kresty et al., 2001). Pilot clinical trials in patients with Barrett's esophagus or oral dysplasia showed that topical black raspberry in a 10% bioadhesive gel was more effective against oral dysplasia than oral powder was against Barrett's esophagus, perhaps because the topical treatment allowed for the absorption of berry anthocyanins and other compounds into the oral lesions (Kresty et al., 2006; Mallery et al., 2008; Shumway et al., 2008).

3.2 Role as Chemopreventive/Chemotherapeutic Agents in Skin

Chemoprevention is defined as the administration of medicines, natural compounds, or other agents alone or in combination to prevent or delay the development of cancer (Dennis et al., 2009). A large body of evidence indicates that fruits and vegetables can protect against various types of cancers including skin cancer (Adhami et al., 2009; Gupta and Mukhtar, 2001; Katiyar, 2008; Siddiqui et al., 2009; Singh and Agarwal, 2005). While in vivo studies demonstrating the efficacy of black raspberries in the prevention and treatment of oral, colon, and esophageal cancer have been carried out (Casto et al., 2002; Harris et al., 2001; Kresty et al., 2001; Mallery et al., 2008; Stoner et al., 2006), the majority of studies examining the effects of black raspberries on skin cells following exposure to carcinogens have been carried out in vitro.

In vitro studies using JB6 murine epithelial cells have provided the majority of information about the effects of black raspberry methanol extracts on signaling in epidermal cells. Studies from Huang et al. (2002) have shown that specific methanol fractions of black raspberries differentially inhibited BaP diol-epoxide (BPDE) induced AP-1 and $NF_{k}B$ activity in these cells. This effect appeared to be mediated through the inhibition of MAPK activation and inhibitory subunit κB phosphorylation. These studies suggested that the ability of black raspberries to inhibit tumor development may be mediated by blocking signal transduction pathways that result in the activation of AP-1 and NFκB. Since previous studies showed that the phosphatidylinositol 3-kinase (PI-3 K)/Akt pathway is required for BPDE induced AP-1 activation (Li et al., 2004) and this pathway is involved in the induction of vascular endothelial growth factor (VEGF), further in vitro studies from the same group determined the effect of black raspberry extracts on VEGF and inducible nitric oxide synthase (iNOS) expression. They demonstrated that pretreatment of mouse epidermal cells with black raspberry extracts reduced the activation of AP-1 and the expression of VEGF, but did not affect iNOS levels, thus suggesting that a potential mechanism for chemopreventive capabilities of black raspberry extracts may occur via the inhibition of the PI-3 K/Akt/AP-1/VEGF pathway (Huang et al., 2006). Additional evidence for the protective effects of methanol extracts of black raspberries was recently demonstrated by the same group examining the efficacy of the extract to inhibit the induction of NFκB and AP-1 in mouse epidermal cells exposed to UVB. While the black raspberry methanol extract inhibited UVB induced activation of NFκB in a time and dose dependent manner, methanol extracts from other berries, specifically strawberries and blueberries were ineffective. Interestingly, none of the fractions from the three berries were able to inhibit UVB induction of AP-1 (Huang et al., 2007). These in vitro studies suggest that berries differ in their ability to affect UV induced signaling pathways in epidermal cells.

To date, few in vivo studies have been reported examining the efficacy of black raspberries on skin tumor development. Duncan et al., 2009 used the SKH-1 hairless mouse model to explore the efficacy of an ethanol/water (80:20) extract of black raspberries in modulating UV induced inflammation and skin carcinogenesis. They found that the topical application of 500 μg of the extract immediately following a single dose of UV exposure reduced hallmarks of an acute inflammatory response, notably edema, neutrophil infiltration, epidermal p53 levels, and oxidative DNA damage. To determine the potential efficacy of the extract on tumor development, animals were exposed to UV three times weekly on non-consecutive days and treated topically with the black raspberry extract or vehicle control immediately afterwards for 25 weeks. Topical treatment with the extract not only reduced the number of tumors but also resulted in the development of significantly smaller tumors over the course of 25 weeks. To determine if the application of the black raspberry extract to previously UV exposed skin could decrease tumor development, mice were exposed to only UV three times weekly for 10 weeks. UV exposure was continued for an additional 15 weeks with the addition of topical treatment with vehicle or black raspberry extract following each exposure. As seen previously, animals treated with the extract developed fewer tumors compared to vehicle controls; however, this treatment paradigm had no significant effect on tumor size (Duncan et al., unpublished data). Topical treatment of tumors that resulted from 14 weeks of only UV exposure was not effective in altering the growth of established tumors in this model (Duncan et al., unpublished data). These data suggest that black raspberry extract may be an effective chemopreventative but not chemotherapeutic option for skin cancer.

4 Conclusion

Until we can change our society's ideas about the dangers of sun exposure, we need to develop better chemopreventive and chemotherapeutic strategies aside from the use of sunscreen. In addition, alternative treatment modalities for populations, such as solid organ transplant recipients at the highest risk for developing multiple and aggressive NMSC, are needed. Numerous studies over the last several years have demonstrated that there is a role for natural compounds in the prevention and treatment of non-melanoma skin cancers. Singh and Agarwal (2002) have described the efficacy of silibinin, a non-toxic bioactive component of milk thistle, in preventing both UV and chemically induced skin cancers in murine models. Additionally, more

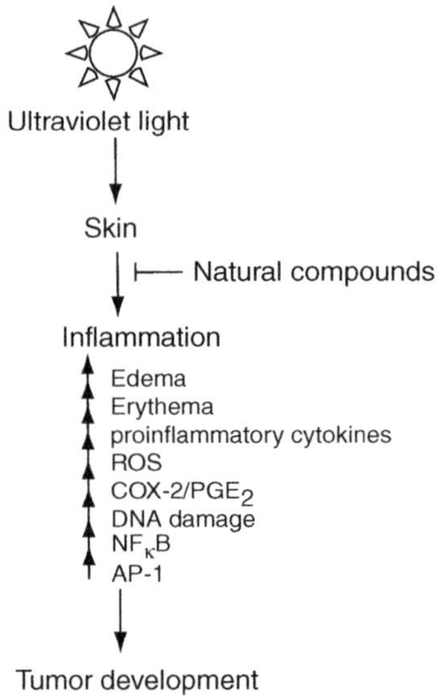

Fig. 7.1 Cutaneous consequences of ultraviolet light exposure

recent studies have described the preventative effects of broccoli sprout extracts, green tea polyphenols, goji berries, and topical isoflavanoids on UV on cutaneous damage and tumor formation (Bandara et al., 2010; Dinkova-Kostova et al., 2010; Katiyar et al., 2010; Reeve et al., 2010). As seen with black raspberry extract, these natural compounds decreased the UV-induced inflammatory response and levels of DNA damage. It is increasingly apparent that there is room for the use of natural compounds alongside, or instead of, traditional medicines. Based upon in vivo and in vitro studies carried out to date, further studies evaluating the efficiency of both topically applied or orally delivered black raspberries in modulating the deleterious effects of sunlight on the skin are warranted.

References

Adhami VM, Khan N, Mukhtar H (2009) Cancer chemoprevention by pomegranate: laboratory and clinical evidence. Nutr Cancer 61:811–815

Agar NS, Halliday GM, Barnetson RS, Ananthaswamy HN, Wheeler M, Jones AM (2004) The basal layer in human squamous tumors harbors more UVA than UVB fingerprint mutations: a role for UVA in human skin carcinogenesis. Proc Natl Acad Sci USA 101:4954–4959

Armstrong BK, Kricker A (2001) The epidemiology of UV induced skin cancer. J Photochem Photobiol B 63:8–18

Bandara M, Arun SJ, Allanson M, Widyarini S, Chai Z, Reeve VE (2010) Topical isoflavonoids reduce experimental cutaneous inflammation in mice. Immunol Cell Biol 88:727–733

Beehler BC, Przybyszewski J, Box HB, Kulesz-Martin MF (1992) Formation of 8-hydroxydeoxyguanosine within DNA of mouse keratinocytes exposed in culture to UVB and H2O2. Carcinogenesis 13:2003–2007

Black AK, Greaves MW, Hensby CN, Plummer NA (1978) Increased prostaglandins E2 and F2alpha in human skin at 6 and 24 h after ultraviolet B irradiation (290–320 nm). Br J Clin Pharmacol 5:431–436

Black HS, deGruijl FR, Forbes PD, Cleaver JE, Ananthaswamy HN, deFabo EC et al (1997) Photocarcinogenesis: an overview. J Photochem Photobiol B 40:29–47

Bridges N, Steinberg JJ (1986) Aggressive squamous cell carcinoma of the skin after chronic lymphocytic leukemia. J Surg Oncol 33:27–30

Cao G, Prior RL (1999) Anthocyanins are detected in human plasma after oral administration of an elderberry extract. Clin Chem 45:574–576

Casto BC, Kresty LA, Kraly CL, Pearl DK, Knobloch TJ, Schut HA et al (2002) Chemoprevention of oral cancer by black raspberries. Anticancer Res 22:4005–4015

Clydesdale GJ, Dandie GW, Muller HK (2001) Ultraviolet light induced injury: immunological and inflammatory effects. Immunol Cell Biol 79:547–568

Cohen D, DeLeo VA (1993) Ultraviolet radiation-induced phospholipase A2 activation occurs in mammalian cell membrane preparations. Photochem Photobiol 57:383–390

Council on Scientific Affairs (1989) Harmful effects of ultraviolet radiation. JAMA 262:380–384

Daynes RA, Samlowski WE, Burnham DK, Gahring LC, Roberts LK (1986) Immunobiological consequences of acute and chronic UV exposure. Curr Probl Dermatol 15:176–194

de Gruijl FR (2000) Photocarcinogenesis: UVA vs UVB. Methods Enzymol 319:359–366

de Gruijl FR (2002) Photocarcinogenesis: UVA vs. UVB radiation. Skin Pharmacol Appl Skin Physiol 15:316–320

de Gruijl FR, Forbes PD (1995) UV-induced skin cancer in a hairless mouse model. Bioessays 17:651–660

Dennis T, Fanous M, Mousa S (2009) Natural products for chemopreventive and adjunctive therapy in oncologic disease. Nutr Cancer 61:587–597

Dinkova-Kostova AT, Fahey JW, Benedict AL, Jenkins SN, Ye L, Wehage SL et al (2010) Dietary glucoraphanin-rich broccoli sprout extracts protect against UV radiation-induced skin carcinogenesis in SKH-1 hairless mice. Photochem Photobiol Sci 9:597–600

Duncan FJ, Martin JR, Wulff BC, Stoner GD, Tober KL, Oberyszyn TM et al (2009) Topical treatment with black raspberry extract reduces cutaneous UVB-induced carcinogenesis and inflammation. Cancer Prev Res 2:665–672

Eling TE, Curtis JF (1992) Xenobiotic metabolism by prostaglandin H synthase. Pharmacol Ther 53:261–273

Elmets CA, Bergstresser PR (1982) Ultraviolet radiation effects on immune processes. Photochem Photobiol 36:715–719

English DR, Armstrong BK, Kricker A, Fleming C (1997) Sunlight and cancer. Cancer Causes Control 8:271–283

Fischer SM (2002) Is cyclooxygenase-2 important in skin carcinogenesis? J Environ Pathol Toxicol Oncol 21:183–191

Fischer SM, Lo HH, Gordon GB, Seibert K, Kelloff G, Lubet RA et al (1999) Chemopreventive activity of celecoxib, a specific cyclooxygenase-2 inhibitor, and indomethacin against ultraviolet light-induced skin carcinogenesis. Mol Carcinog 25:231–240

Fischer SM, Pavone A, Mikulec C, Langenbach R, Rundhaug JE (2007) Cyclooxygenase-2 expression is critical for chronic UV-induced murine skin carcinogenesis. Mol Carcinog 46:363–371

Fuller CJ, Faulkner H, Bendich A, Parker RS, Roe DA (1992) Effect of beta-carotene supplementation on photosuppression of delayed-type hypersensitivity in normal young men. Am J Clin Nutr 56:684–690

Gallagher CH, Canfield PJ, Greenoak GE, Reeve VE (1984) Characterization and histogenesis of tumors in the hairless mouse produced by low-dosage incremental ultraviolet radiation. J Invest Dermatol 83:169–174

Gallagher RP, Hill GB, Bajdik CD, Coldman AJ, Fincham S, McLean DI et al (1995a) Sunlight exposure, pigmentation factors, and risk of nonmelanocytic skin cancer. II. Squamous cell carcinoma. Arch Dermatol 131:164–169

Gallagher RP, Hill GB, Bajdik CD, Fincham S, Coldman AJ, McLean DI et al (1995b) Sunlight exposure, pigmentary factors, and risk of nonmelanocytic skin cancer. I. Basal cell carcinoma. Arch Dermatol 131:157–163

Gerber B, Mathys P, Moser M, Bressoud D, Braun-Fahrlander C (2002) Ultraviolet emission spectra of sunbeds. Photochem Photobiol 76:664–668

Gresham A, Masferrer J, Chen X, Leal-Khouri S, Pentland AP (1996) Increased synthesis of high-molecular-weight cPLA2 mediates early UV-induced PGE2 in human skin. Am J Physiol 270:C1037–C1050

Group TL (2005) The burden of skin diseases. In: The society for investigative dermatology and the American academy of dermatology association. Cleveland, OH and Washington, DC, http://www.lewin.com/content/publications/april2005skindisease.pdf

Gupta S, Mukhtar H (2001) Chemoprevention of skin cancer through natural agents. Skin Pharmacol Appl Skin Physiol 14:373–385

Harris GK, Gupta A, Nines RG, Kresty LA, Habib SG, Frankel WL et al (2001) Effects of lyophilized black raspberries on azoxymethane-induced colon cancer and 8-hydroxy-2′-deoxyguanosine levels in the Fischer 344 rat. Nutr Cancer 40:125–133

Hattori Y, Nishigori C, Tanaka T, Uchida K, Nikaido O, Osawa T et al (1996) 8-hydroxy-2′-deoxyguanosine is increased in epidermal cells of hairless mice after chronic ultraviolet B exposure. J Invest Dermatol 107:733–737

Housman TS, Feldman SR, Williford PM, Fleischer AB Jr, Goldman ND, Acostamadiedo JM et al (2003) Skin cancer is among the most costly of all cancers to treat for the Medicare population. J Am Acad Dermatol 48:425–429

Hruza LL, Pentland AP (1993) Mechanisms of UV-induced inflammation. J Invest Dermatol 100:35S–41S

Huang C, Huang Y, Li J, Hu W, Aziz R, Tang MS et al (2002) Inhibition of benzo(a)pyrene diol-epoxide-induced transactivation of activated protein 1 and nuclear factor kappaB by black raspberry extracts. Cancer Res 62:6857–6863

Huang C, Li J, Song L, Zhang D, Tong Q, Ding M et al (2006) Black raspberry extracts inhibit benzo(a)pyrene diol-epoxide-induced activator protein 1 activation and VEGF transcription by targeting the phosphotidylinositol 3-kinase/Akt pathway. Cancer Res 66:581–587

Huang C, Zhang D, Li J, Tong Q, Stoner GD (2007) Differential inhibition of UV-induced activation of NF kappa B and AP-1 by extracts from black raspberries, strawberries, and blueberries. Nutr Cancer 58:205–212

Jung EG (1991) Photocarcinogenesis in the skin. J Dermatol 18:1–10

Kaplan AL, Cook JL (2005) Cutaneous squamous cell carcinoma in patients with chronic lymphocytic leukemia. Skinmed 4:300–304

Katiyar SK (2008) Grape seed proanthocyanidins and skin cancer prevention: inhibition of oxidative stress and protection of immune system. Mol Nutr Food Res 52(Suppl 1):S71–S76

Katiyar SK, Vaid M, van Steeg H, Meeran SM (2010) Green tea polyphenols prevent UV-induced immunosuppression by rapid repair of DNA damage and enhancement of nucleotide excision repair genes. Cancer Prev Res 3:179–189

Kim TH, Ananthaswamy HN, Kripke ML, Ullrich SE (2003) Advantages of using hairless mice versus haired mice to test sunscreen efficacy against photoimmune suppressions. Photochem Photobiol 78:37–42

Kresty LA, Frankel WL, Hammond CD, Baird ME, Mele JM, Stoner GD et al (2006) Transitioning from preclinical to clinical chemopreventive assessments of lyophilized black raspberries: interim results show berries modulate markers of oxidative stress in Barrett's esophagus patients. Nutr Cancer 54:148–156

Kresty LA, Morse MA, Morgan C, Carlton PS, Lu J, Gupta A et al (2001) Chemoprevention of esophageal tumorigenesis by dietary administration of lyophilized black raspberries. Cancer Res 61:6112–6119

Kricker A, Armstrong BK, English DR, Heenan PJ (1995) Does intermittent sun exposure cause basal cell carcinoma? A case-control study in Western Australia. Int J Cancer 60:489–494

Kripke ML (1977) Latency, histology, and antigenicity of tumors induced by ultraviolet light in three inbred mouse strains. Cancer Res 37:1395–1400

Kripke ML (1984) Immunological unresponsiveness induced by ultraviolet radiation. Immunol Rev 80:87–102
Kripke ML (1991) Immunological effects of ultraviolet radiation. J Dermatol 18:429–433
Li J, Tang MS, Liu B, Shi X, Huang C (2004) A critical role of PI-3 K/Akt/JNKs pathway in benzo[a]pyrene diol-epoxide (B[a]PDE)-induced AP-1 transactivation in mouse epidermal Cl41 cells. Oncogene 23:3932–3944
Maeda H, Akaike T (1998) Nitric oxide and oxygen radicals in infection, inflammation, and cancer. Biochemistry (Mosc) 63:854–865
Malech HL, Gallin JI (1987) Current concepts: immunology. Neutrophils in human diseases. N Engl J Med 317:687–694
Mallery SR, Zwick JC, Pei P, Tong M, Larsen PE, Shumway BS et al (2008) Topical application of a bioadhesive black raspberry gel modulates gene expression and reduces cyclooxygenase 2 protein in human premalignant oral lesions. Cancer Res 68:4945–4957
Marks R, Jolley D, Lectsas S, Foley P (1990) The role of childhood exposure to sunlight in the development of solar keratoses and non-melanocytic skin cancer. Med J Aust 152:62–66
Marrot L, Meunier JR (2008) Skin DNA photodamage and its biological consequences. J Am Acad Dermatol 58:S139–S148
Martin J, Duncan FJ, Keiser T, Shin S, Kusewitt DF, Oberyszyn T et al (2009) Macrophage Migration Inhibitory Factor (MIF) plays a critical role in pathogenesis of ultraviolet-B (UVB) -induced nonmelanoma skin cancer (NMSC). FASEB J 23:720–730
McGregor JM, Berkhout RJ, Rozycka M, ter Schegget J, Bouwes Bavinck JN, Brooks L et al (1997) p53 mutations implicate sunlight in post-transplant skin cancer irrespective of human papillomavirus status. Oncogene 15:1737–1740
Morison WL, Jerdan MS, Hoover TL, Farmer ER (1986) UV radiation-induced tumors in haired mice: identification as squamous cell carcinomas. J Natl Cancer Inst 77:1155–1162
Nakamura T, Sakamoto K (2001) Reactive oxygen species up-regulates cyclooxygenase-2, p53, and Bax mRNA expression in bovine luteal cells. Biochem Biophys Res Commun 284:203–210
Nichols JA, Katiyar SK (2010) Skin photoprotection by natural polyphenols: anti-inflammatory, antioxidant and DNA repair mechanisms. Arch Dermatol Res 302:71–83
Osterlind A, Hjalgrim H, Kulinsky B, Frentz G (1991) Skin cancer as a cause of death in Denmark. Br J Dermatol 125:580–582
Potter JD (2005) Vegetables, fruit, and cancer. Lancet 366:527–530
Ramsay HM, Fryer AA, Hawley CM, Smith AG, Harden PN (2002) Non-melanoma skin cancer risk in the Queensland renal transplant population. Br J Dermatol 147:950–956
Reeve VE, Allanson M, Arun SJ, Domanski D, Painter N (2010) Mice drinking goji berry juice (Lycium barbarum) are protected from UV radiation-induced skin damage via antioxidant pathways. Photochem Photobiol Sci 9:601–607
Rivas JM, Ullrich SE (1994) The role of IL-4, IL-10, and TNF-alpha in the immune suppression induced by ultraviolet radiation. J Leukoc Biol 56:769–775
Rosso S, Zanetti R, Martinez C, Tormo MJ, Schraub S, Sancho-Garnier H et al (1996) The multicentre south European study 'Helios'. II: Different sun exposure patterns in the aetiology of basal cell and squamous cell carcinomas of the skin. Br J Cancer 73:1447–1454
Scapini P, Lapinet-Vera JA, Gasperini S, Calzetti F, Bazzoni F, Cassatella MA (2000) The neutrophil as a cellular source of chemokines. Immunol Rev 177:195–203
Scrivener Y, Grosshans E, Cribier B (2002) Variations of basal cell carcinomas according to gender, age, location and histopathological subtype. Br J Dermatol 147:41–47
Seibert K, Zhang Y, Leahy K, Hauser S, Masferrer J, Perkins W et al (1994) Pharmacological and biochemical demonstration of the role of cyclooxygenase 2 in inflammation and pain. Proc Natl Acad Sci USA 91:12013–12017
Shreedhar V, Giese T, Sung VW, Ullrich SE (1998) A cytokine cascade including prostaglandin E2, IL-4, and IL-10 is responsible for UV-induced systemic immune suppression. J Immunol 160:3783–3789
Shumway BS, Kresty LA, Larsen PE, Zwick JC, Lu B, Fields HW et al (2008) Effects of a topically applied bioadhesive berry gel on loss of heterozygosity indices in premalignant oral lesions. Clin Cancer Res 14:2421–2430

Siddiqui IA, Tarapore RS, Mukhtar H (2009) Prevention of skin cancer by green tea: past, present and future. Cancer Biol Ther 8:1288–1291

Singh RP, Agarwal R (2002) Flavonoid antioxidant silymarin and skin cancer. Antioxid Redox Signal 4:655–663

Singh RP, Agarwal R (2005) Mechanisms and preclinical efficacy of silibinin in preventing skin cancer. Eur J Cancer 41:1969–1979

Stoner GD, Chen T, Kresty LA, Aziz RM, Reinemann T, Nines R (2006) Protection against esophageal cancer in rodents with lyophilized berries: potential mechanisms. Nutr Cancer 54:33–46

Strickland PT, Vitasa BC, West SK, Rosenthal FS, Emmett EA, Taylor HR (1989) Quantitative carcinogenesis in man: solar ultraviolet B dose dependence of skin cancer in Maryland watermen. J Natl Cancer Inst 81:1910–1913

Terui T, Tagami H (2000) Mediators of inflammation involved in UVB erythema. J Dermatol Sci 23(Suppl 1):S1–S5

The American Cancer Society. http://www.cancer.org/cancer/skincancerbasalandsquamouscell/index

Thomas-Ahner JM, Wulff BC, Tober KL, Kusewitt DF, Riggenbach JA, Oberyszyn TM (2007) Gender differences in UVB-induced skin carcinogenesis, inflammation, and DNA damage. Cancer Res 67:3468–3474

Ulrich C, Kanitakis J, Stockfleth E, Euvrard S (2008) Skin cancer in organ transplant recipients–where do we stand today? Am J Transplant 8:2192–2198

Vane JR, Mitchell JA, Appleton I, Tomlinson A, Bishop-Bailey D, Croxtall J et al (1994) Inducible isoforms of cyclooxygenase and nitric-oxide synthase in inflammation. Proc Natl Acad Sci USA 91:2046–2050

Ward PL, Koeppen H, Hurteau T, Schreiber H (1989) Tumor antigens defined by cloned immunological probes are highly polymorphic and are not detected on autologous normal cells. J Exp Med 170:217–232

Wei H, Zhang X, Wang Y, Lebwohl M (2002) Inhibition of ultraviolet light-induced oxidative events in the skin and internal organs of hairless mice by isoflavone genistein. Cancer Lett 185:21–29

Wilgus TA, Koki AT, Zweifel BS, Kusewitt DF, Rubal PA, Oberyszyn TM (2003a) Inhibition of cutaneous ultraviolet light B mediated inflammation and tumor formation with topical celecoxib treatment. Mol Carcinog 38:49–58

Wilgus TA, Koki AT, Zweifel BS, Rubal PA, Oberyszyn TM (2003b) Chemotherapeutic efficacy of topical celecoxib in a murine model of ultraviolet light B-induced skin cancer. Mol Carcinog 38:33–39

Wilgus TA, Ross MS, Parrett ML, Oberyszyn TM (2000) Topical application of a selective cyclooxygenase inhibitor suppresses UVB mediated cutaneous inflammation. Prostaglandins Other Lipid Mediat 62:367–384

Xue H, Aziz RM, Sun N, Cassady JM, Kamendulis LM, Xu Y et al (2001) Inhibition of cellular transformation by berry extracts. Carcinogenesis 22:351–356

Yamawaki M, Katiyar SK, Anderson CY, Tubesing KA, Mukhtar H, Elmets CA (1997) Genetic variation in low-dose UV-induced suppression of contact hypersensitivity and in the skin photocarcinogenesis response. J Invest Dermatol 109:716–721

Yu D, Berlin JA, Penning TM, Field J (2002) Reactive oxygen species generated by PAH o-quinones cause change-in-function mutations in p53. Chem Res Toxicol 15:832–842

Chapter 8
Chemopreventive Effects of Berries and Berry Components in the Rodent Esophagus

Claire M. Seguin, Li-Shu Wang, and Gary D. Stoner

Abstract Esophageal squamous cell carcinoma (ESCC) is the 7th leading cause of cancer death worldwide. Its etiology and late detection rate make it an important target for intensive studies in chemoprevention and treatment. The Fischer-344 rat model of esophageal squamous cell carcinoma has been used extensively to evaluate the ability of black raspberries (BRBs) and other berry types to inhibit esophageal tumorigenesis. In this model, tumors are induced by the nitrosamine carcinogen, *N*-nitrosomethylbenzylamine (NMBA). Dietary BRBs inhibit both the initiation and promotion/progression stages of esophageal tumorigenesis in the rat. They inhibit initiation events by influencing the metabolic activation and detoxification of NMBA, and promotion/progression events by reducing cell proliferation, inflammation, and angiogenesis and by stimulating apoptosis and differentiation. Genes associated with these cellular functions are positively modulated by BRBs. Biofractionation studies indicate that amongst the most active chemopreventive agents in BRBs are the anthocyanins. An anthocyanin-enriched fraction of BRBs was nearly as active as whole BRBs themselves in preventing esophageal tumorigenesis. However, the ellagitannins and other constituents in the fiber fraction of BRBs are also active and studies are underway to further identify these constituents. In a recent study, 7 different berry types, including the "exotic" berries (acai, noni and wolfberry [goji]), were compared for their ability to inhibit NMBA-tumorigenesis in the rat esophagus. All seven types were active, irrespective of their content of anthocyanins and ellagitannins. It appears that each berry type has unique constituents with cancer preventive potential.

Keywords Chemoprevention · Rodent · Esophagus · Cancer · Berries · Molecular biomarkers

---

G.D. Stoner (✉)
Department of Medicine, Medical College of Wisconsin, Milwaukee, WI 53226, USA
e-mail: gstoner@mcw.edu

G.D. Stoner, N.P. Seeram (eds.), *Berries and Cancer Prevention*,
DOI 10.1007/978-1-4419-7554-6_8, © Springer Science+Business Media, LLC 2011

1 Introduction

1.1 Esophageal Cancer

In 2009, there were approximately 545,000 new cases of esophageal cancer worldwide (DeMeester, 2009). This cancer exists in two principal forms with distinct etiological and pathological characteristics: squamous cell carcinoma (ESCC) and adenocarcinoma. Esophageal adenocarcinoma incidence is increasing rapidly in the Western world and has exceeded ESCC as the leading form of esophageal cancer in the United States (DeMeester, 2009). Worldwide, 90% of esophageal cancers are SCCs and 50% of ESCC occurs in China (Garcia et al., 2007). Both cancer types are usually detected at late stages of development and only 10–17% of treated patients survive more than 5 years (Ribeiro et al., 1997).

Epidemiological studies have identified multiple risk factors for human ESCC. These include tobacco use, alcohol consumption, and ingestion of salt-pickled, salt-cured and moldy foods (Wang et al., 2006; Stoner and Gupta, 2001). In addition, dietary deficiencies in certain vitamins (A, C, E, and riboflavin) and minerals (zinc, selenium, and iron) increase risk. High frequencies of ESCC are found in Iran, South Africa, Uruguay, France, Italy, Puerto Rico and parts of China, especially the *Shansi*, *Henana* and *Hopei* provinces (Stoner and Gupta, 2001). Studies in China indicate that N-nitroso compounds and their precursors (nitrates, nitrites, and secondary and tertiary amines) are present in contaminated and salt-preserved foods in the high risk provinces and are associated with the development of ESCC. Two nitrosamine carcinogens of potential importance for inducing human ESCC are *N*-nitrosomethylbenzylamine (NMBA) and *N*-nitrosomethylamylamine (NMAA), which have been identified in the gastric juices of Chinese subjects (Yang, 1992). Due to the association between lifestyle and dietary factors with risk for ESCC, prevention efforts addressing these factors are important for control of this disease (Stoner and Gupta, 2001).

1.2 Rat Model of Esophageal Squamous Cell Carcinoma

The Fisher 344 (F-344) rat has been used most extensively for investigations of esophageal carcinogenesis and chemoprevention (Stoner and Gupta, 2001; Stoner et al., 2007a). Our laboratory has used the F-344 rat to investigate the chemoprevention of ESCC by berries and berry components for more than 15 years (Stoner et al., 2007a). The rat model of ESCC involves the induction of tumors with NMBA, the most potent *N*-nitrosamine carcinogen for the rat esophagus (Stoner and Gupta, 2001; Stoner et al., 2007a).

1.2.1 Metabolism of NMBA

NMBA is a procarcinogen and must be metabolically activated to produce cancer (Stoner and Gupta, 2001; Stoner et al., 2007a). This activation occurs in the rat liver and esophagus. The first step in its metabolic activation is a cytochrome P450-mediated hydrolysis of the methylene carbon of NMBA producing an α–hydroxy derivative. This derivative spontaneously decomposes to methyldiazohydroxide and benzaldehyde. Methyldiazohydroxide then causes the formation of a highly electrophilic methylcarbonium ion which methylates guanine residues at the N^7 and O^6 positions. Although N^7-methylguanine is by far the most abundant adduct, it is very rapidly repaired and produces few, if any, mutations in esophageal DNA. In contrast, the O^6-methylguanine adduct is poorly repaired and produces single base mismatches in esophageal DNA. This leads to initiating GC→AT transition mutations in critical genes such as the *H-ras* oncogene which is mutated in nearly all NMBA-induced tumors in the rat esophagus (Stoner and Gupta, 2001; Stoner et al., 2007).

2 Chemoprevention of Esophageal Cancer in Rats

2.1 Chemoprevention Protocols

Bioassays of chemopreventive agents, including berries, in the F-344 rat have generally followed two protocols (Fig. 8.1). The complete protocol (Fig. 8.1a) consists of repeated subcutaneous injections of 0.25–0.50 mg NMBA/kg body weight once a week for 15 weeks to induce esophageal tumors. This protocol induces tumors in essentially 100% of treated rats within 20–25 weeks with a multiplicity of 4–8 tumors per rat (Stoner and Gupta, 2001; Stoner et al., 2007). In the complete protocol, chemopreventive agents including berry powder are added to the rat diet before, during, and after NMBA treatment to evaluate its ability to inhibit both the initiation and promotion/progression stages of esophageal carcinogenesis. The second protocol (Fig. 8.1b) simulates a post-initiation intervention. In this protocol, rats are injected with NMBA at 0.3 mg/kg b.w. 3 times per week for 5 weeks. This protocol also produces a 100% tumor incidence by week 25 with an average of 2–4 tumors per esophagus (Stoner and Gupta, 2001; Stoner et al., 2007). In the second protocol, berry powder is introduced into the diet about 1 week after the final injection of NMBA (week 6). At this time point, about 50–60% of the esophageal epithelium is hyperplastic and contains occasional foci of mild to moderate dysplasia. The post-initiation model is thought to be most relevant to the human situation because it mimics the strategy of using chemoprevention agents to inhibit the progression of dysplastic esophageal lesions in humans to SCC. In both protocols (1A and 1B), black raspberries (BRBs) reduced NMBA-induced esophageal tumorigenesis by 35–65% (Table 8.1) (Stoner and Gupta, 2001; Stoner et al., 2007).

The post-initiation protocol has been modified to model two other intervention schemes. In one scheme (Fig. 8.1c), dietary treatment with BRB powder was delayed until week 15 of the bioassay (i.e., 10 weeks after cessation of NMBA treatment). This models a condition in which premalignant dysplastic lesions are quite advanced before treatment with berries. BRB treatment reduced the tumor response

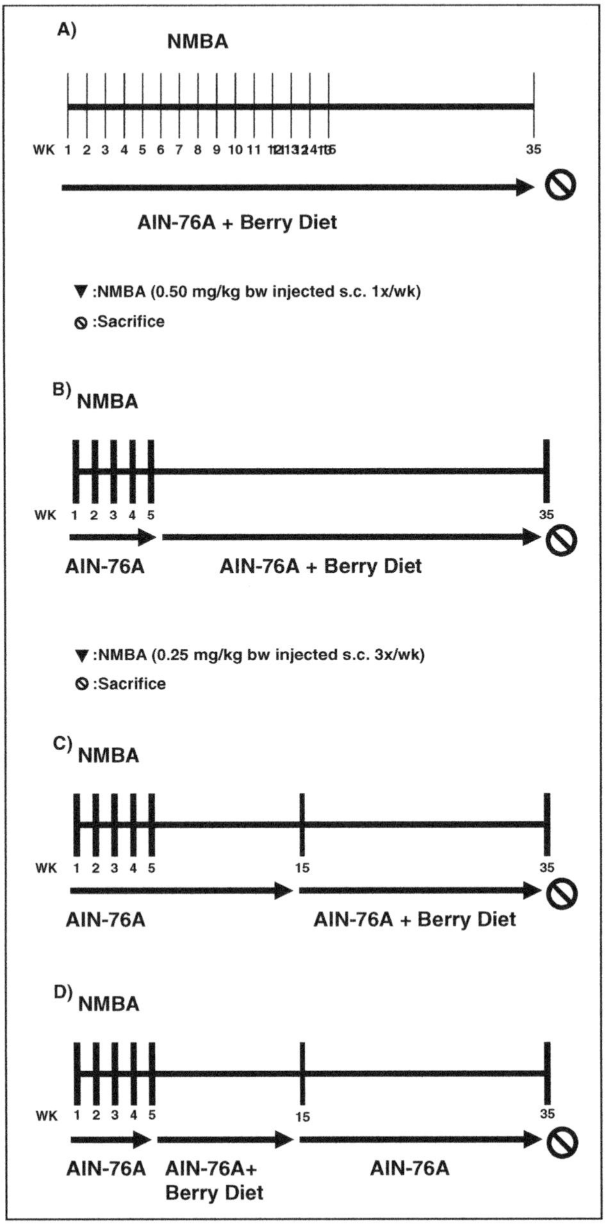

Fig. 8.1 Protocols for assessing the chemopreventive effects of berries in the NMBA model of rat esophageal carcinogenesis. **a** Complete protocol; **b**, post-initiation protocol; **c**, modified post-initiation protocol in which berries are added to the diet 10 weeks after NMBA treatment; **d**, modified post-initiation protocol in which berries are added to the diet immediately after NMBA treatment and then removed from the diet at 15 weeks

Table 8.1 Effects of dietary BRBs on NMBA-induced esophageal tumorigenesis using the complete and post-initiation protocols[a]

Diet administered	NMBA	Tumor incidence (%)	Multiplicity (± SE)
Complete protocol	0.25 mg/kg		
Week 25			
AIN-76A	–	0	0
AIN-76A	+	100	3.25 (0.31)
5% BRB	+	78	1.93 (0.40)[b]
10% BRB	+	92	1.61 (0.29)[b]
Post-initiation protocol	0.25 mg/kg		
Week 15			
AIN-76A	–	0	0
AIN-76A	+	50	75 (0.31)
5% BRB	+	25	0.12 (0.26)
10% BRB	+	12.5	0.13 (0.13)
Week 25			
AIN-76A	–	0	0
AIN-76A	+	86.6	1.40 (0.25)
5% BRB	+	40.0[b]	0.52 (0.19)[b]
10% BRB	+	46.7[b]	0.80 (0.30)[b]
Week 35			
AIN-76A	–	0	0
AIN-76A	+	92.9	2.00 (0.31)
5% BRB	+	53.3[b]	0.67 (0.19)[b]
10% BRB	+	80.0	1.53 (0.32)

[a]Data taken from Kresty et al. (2001).
[b]Statistically significant relative to NMBA controls ($P< 0.05$).

to NMBA by only 20–25% using this protocol, suggesting that advanced dysplastic lesions are more recalcitrant to berry effects than mildly dysplastic lesions. In the other scheme (Fig. 8.1d), BRB treatment began immediately after cessation of NMBA treatment and then the berries were removed from the diet at week 15 of the bioassay. Again, BRB treatment led to only a 25–30% reduction in the tumor response suggesting that premalignant lesions can re-emerge to progress to cancer after berry treatment has ceased.

It is important to note that most NMBA-induced tumors in the rat esophagus have the gross (Fig. 8.2a) and histologic (Fig. 8.2b) features of papillomas. Papillomas are the predominant tumors because they grow within the esophageal lumen and occlude the esophagus and tracheal airways before carcinomas have time to develop. One major difference between the rat model of ESCC and human ESCC is that there is no histological counterpart to the rat papilloma in the human disease. In contrast, preneoplastic lesions, including hyperplasia and epithelial dysplasia (Fig. 8.2b), in the rat esophagus closely mimic corresponding lesions in the human esophagus.

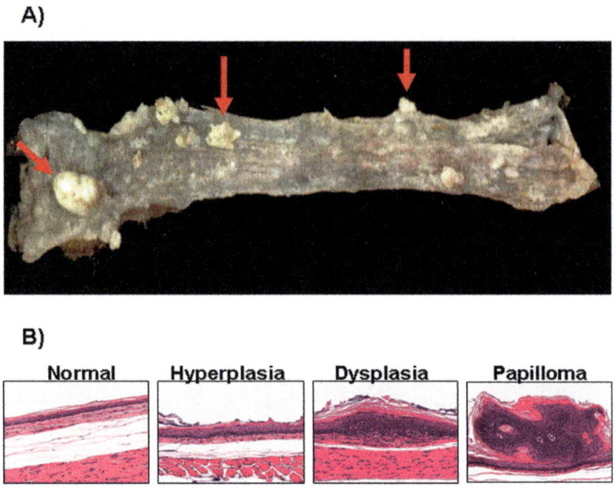

Fig. 8.2 Gross (**a**) and histological (**b**) appearance of NMBA-induced lesions in rat esophagus

Preneoplastic lesions, along with papillomas, are useful endpoints for evaluating the effects of berries and other chemopreventive agents on the multi-stage progression of esophageal cancer in rats.

2.2 Black Raspberries

Black raspberries (BRBs) have been used most extensively for chemoprevention studies in the rat esophagus (Stoner et al., 2007). The inclusion of BRBs or BRB components into the rat diet permits the localized absorption of these components into the esophagus on a consistent basis. This is very important because the chemopreventive anthocyanins and ellagitannins in BRBs are poorly absorbed into the blood stream and systemic delivery of these agents to the esophagus is minimal. In efforts to develop a "standardized" berry preparation, BRBs of the Jewel variety are purchased from a single Ohio farm on a yearly basis. The berries are grown on a specific region of the farm, picked mechanically when ripe, washed and stored frozen at –0°C. They are then shipped frozen to VanDrunen Farms (Momence, IL) to be freeze-dried and ground into a powder. The powder is stored frozen until use. BRB powders from different crop years have relatively constant concentrations (i.e., <25% degradation) of bio-active components when obtained as described. In addition, these components remain quite stable for at least 2 years when stored at –0°C (Stoner et al., 2007). The vitamins, especially vitamin C, are exceptions; they undergo considerable degradation in frozen berries before the berries are freeze-dried.

BRBs contain a wide range of bioactive phytochemicals, the most prominent of which are phenolic in nature as they have hydroxyl (OH^-) groups on aromatic rings.

Phytochemicals are non-nutritive constituents produced by secondary metabolism in plants. The bioactive phytochemicals in BRBs and other berry types fall into several structural and chemical classes including phenolic acids (hydroxycinnamic and hydroxybenzoic acids), flavonoids (anthocyanins, flavanols, and flavonols), condensed tannins (proanthocyanins), hydrolysable tannins (ellagitannins and gallotannins), stilbenoids, lignans, triterpenes, and sterols (Seeram, 2006). Amongst the most prevalent compounds in BRBs are the anthocyanins and ellagitannins which, collectively, are responsible for much of their antioxidant activity (Seeram, 2006). In addition to the anthocyanins and ellagitannins, BRBs contain many other constituents known to exhibit cancer-preventive effects including vitamins, such as A, C, E and folic acid, and minerals, such as calcium, selenium and zinc. They also contain appreciable levels of certain phytohormones such as beta-sitosterol, and low levels of carotenoids.

2.3 Berries Inhibit Initiating Events in NMBA-Treated Rat Esophagus

2.3.1 Effects on DNA Adduct Formation

Berries have long been known to influence the metabolism of NMBA. As indicated above, a result of NMBA metabolism is the formation of O^6-methylguanine (O^6-MeGua) adducts which cause single base mismatch mutations in DNA that are pro-tumorigenic (Stoner and Gupta, 2001; Stoner et al., 2007). O^6-MeGua adducts in esophageal DNA are quantified and used as biomarkers of the ability of berry components to inhibit the metabolic activation of NMBA. For example, treatment of F-344 rats with strawberry (STRW) powder at 5 or 10% of the diet for 2 weeks was found to significantly reduce O^6-MeGua adducts produced in esophageal DNA by a single injection of NMBA given on the last day of STRW treatment (Carlton et al., 2001). Using the same protocol, dietary BRBs were also found to reduce the formation of O^6-MeGua adducts produced by NMBA in the esophagus (Kresty et al., 2001). However, only the 5% BRB diet significantly inhibited adduct formation after an injection of 0.5 mg/kg body weight. The inability of 10% BRBs to inhibit adduct formation is an example of a lack of a dose-response effect with berry treatment. In the same study, ellagic acid significantly inhibited O^6-MeGua adduct formation when included in the diet at 0.04% (w/w).

2.3.2 Effects on Cytochrome P450 Enzymes

Expression studies have shown that the P-450 enzyme, *CYP2a2,* is markedly overexpressed in the rat esophagus during the first week of treatment with NMBA (Stoner et al., 2008a). However, when NMBA-treated rats were fed a diet containing 5% BRBs, *CYP2a2* expression in the esophagus returned to near-normal levels. These results suggest that *CYP2a2* may be important for the metabolic activation of NMBA and, potentially, for its ability to produce O^6-MeGua adducts in esophageal DNA. The consistent reduction in the formation of O^6-MeGua adducts in NMBA-treated esophagus by BRBs may well be due to their inhibitory effects on the expression of *CYP2a2*.

2.3.3 Potential Effects on H-ras Oncogene Activation

Inhibition of DNA adduct formation by berries might be expected to inhibit tumor initiation, in part, because one of the principal initiation events in rat esophageal carcinogenesis is mutational activation of the *H-ras* oncogene (Barch et al., 1991; Liston et al., 2001). Activation of this gene by NMBA is associated with GC$\rightarrow$AT transition mutations in the second base of codon 12. These mutations are consistent with the formation of O^6-MeGua adducts in DNA. Essentially, all NMBA-induced tumors in the rat esophagus display this *H-ras* mutation (Barch et al., 1991). Studies have shown that the relatively few early foci in NMBA-treated rat esophagus that possess *H-ras* mutations are the foci that progress to form papillomas (Liston et al., 2001). Therefore, if berries reduce *H-ras* activation in the esophagus by inhibiting the formation of O^6-MeGua adducts, this would likely reduce the number of NMBA-induced papillomas.

2.3.4 Effects on Gene Expression as Determined by DNA Microarray

Recent gene expression data further supports the ability of BRBs to prevent initiation events in NMBA-treated rat esophagus (Stoner et al., 2008). Six week-old F-344 rats were fed BRBs at 5% of the diet for a period of 3 weeks. During the third week of BRB administration, the rats received three subcutaneous injections of NMBA at 0.5 mg/kg body weight. Twenty four hours later, the rats were killed, esophagi removed, and the total RNA isolated for microarray analysis of 41,000 transcripts. Only 1 week of NMBA treatment led to either up-regulation or down-regulation of 2,261 genes more than $\geq$1.5-fold and BRBs modulated 462 of these genes to near normal levels of expression. The effects of berries on the expression of *CYP2a2* are mentioned above; if this enzyme is involved in NMBA activation, then its reduced expression by BRBs would influence initiation events. Several Phase II detoxifying enzymes, mostly glutathione-S-transferases (GSTs), were inhibited by NMBA-treatment and restored to higher than normal levels of expression by dietary BRBs. The importance of this with respect to NMBA detoxification is questionable however, because NMBA does not appear to be detoxified by a glutathione mechanism. Histopathological analysis of the esophagus of rats treated only three times with NMBA revealed marked changes in the epithelium including increased cell proliferation and apoptosis, and infiltration of inflammatory cells. Therefore, it was not surprising to observe that some of the 462 genes positively modulated by BRBs included genes involved in signal transduction, cell proliferation and cell cycle progression, apoptosis and cell death, response to stress and inflammation, cellular differentiation and morphogenesis, cell adhesion and motility, and angiogenesis (Table 8.2). Interestingly, several of the genes associated with signal transduction were genes that influence *ras* activity. Among these were *Apc1* and *Map2k3* whose dysregulation affects the activity of the *H-ras*1 protein. *Apc1* has transformative abilities and reduction of NMBA-induced upregulation of *Apc1* by BRBs would antagonize its pro-oncogenic abilities. The reader is referred to the article by Stoner et al. (2008) for a more extensive description of the effects of BRBs on the expression of genes in rat esophagus initiated by 1-week of treatment with NMBA.

2.4 Effects of BRBs on Preneoplastic Lesions and Papilloma Formation

The development of tumors in NMBA-treated rat esophagus is a multi-stage process in the order of normal epithelium > hyperplastic epithelium > foci of low- and high-grade dysplasia > papilloma > carcinoma. At the end of a standard chemoprevention bioassay using either the complete or post-initiation protocols, the epithelium of the esophagus will display all of these histologic features; however, as indicated above, there are likely to be few, if any, carcinomas. The effects of berry treatment on NMBA-treated rat esophagus can be seen by quantifying preneoplastic lesions microscopically and papillomas on the surface of the esophagus using a dissecting microscope. Kresty et al. (2001) showed that the percentage of hyperplastic esophageal epithelium that progresses to either low- or high-grade dysplasia is significantly reduced by the inclusion of BRBs in the diet of NMBA-treated rats. In the same study, however, BRB treatment did not reduce the amount of esophageal epithelium in the hyperplastic state. This finding suggests that BRBs are effective at preventing the progression of dysplastic lesions to papillomas, but not hyperplastic lesions to dysplasia. The molecular basis of these observations is currently under investigation.

The incidence (presence or absence) and multiplicity (number) of NMBA-induced tumors (papillomas) in the rat esophagus are also used as measures of the preventative effects of berries. Dietary BRB treatment has repeatedly reduced the incidence and multiplicity of NMBA-induced papillomas (>0.5 mm) in the rat esophagus (Stoner et al., 2007; Carlton et al., 2001; Kresty et al., 2001; Stoner et al., 2008) and the extent of inhibition is usually somewhat greater in the complete protocol (Fig. 8.1a) (about 55–70%) than in the post-initiation protocol (Fig. 8.1b) (about 45–60%). This is further evidence that the inhibition of initiation events in esophageal carcinogenesis is an important component of BRB effects. Interestingly, BRBs are about equally as effective at reducing incidence and multiplicity when included at either 5 or 10% of the diet. These results suggest that "more is not necessarily better" and most recent studies have used BRBs at 5% of the diet. At 2.5% of the diet, BRBs caused some reduction in tumor multiplicity in the complete protocol, but this was not significant (data not reported).

Table 8.2 Pathway and function clusters of genes and proteins dysregulated by NMBA and adjusted to near-normal levels by a 5% BRB diet in the rat esophagus[a]

Gene ontology/biological process/pathway	Gene symbol/protein symbol
Apoptosis/cell death	TUNEL
	Eif4g2_predicted, Grem1, Hmox1, Hip1, Hlf10, Mcl1, MGC72992, Miz1, Myd116, Pip5k1a_predicted, Prkg2, Rraga, Tgfa, Txn11
Angiogenesis	CD34
	VEGF-
	VEGF
	Anxa2, Cldn1, Fgfbp1, Tgfa, Ahnak, Klf5
Cell cycle/proliferation	Ki-67
	PCNA
	Bub1_predicted, Ccnc, Cdc42, Cops5, Eif4g2_predicted, H2afz, Kifap3_predicte, Klf10,LOC362587, Ndel1, Olfm3, Plk3, Ppp2ca, Prkar1a, Sh2d2a, Tgfa, Ube2c_predicted, Ywhah
Cell junction/adhesion/motility	*Apc1, Actn4, Actr2, Ambp, Anxa2, Arpc2_predicted, Cd44, Cdc42, Cldn1, Crk, Cttn, Dsc3_predicted, Kifap3_predicted, Lamb3, Msn, Ndel1, Ppp2r2a, PVR, Sdc1*
Cytoskeleton	*Actn4, Actr2, Anxa2, Arpc2_predicted, Bub1_predicted, Cdc42, Crk, Cttn, Gng12, Hip1, Kifap3_predicted, Krt20, Msn, MYO10, Ndel1, Pls3, Tubb6*
Differentiation	*Anxa2, Cd44, Cdc42, Cldn1, Fst, Grem1, Inhbb, Klf10, Lepr, Mcl1, Ndel1, Olfm3, Pcsk9, Prkar1a, Slc30a1, Tgfa, Ywhah*
Inflammation/stress response	*NOS2(iNOS), PTGS2(COX-2), JUN(c-Jun, AP1)*
	iNOS, COX-2, c-Jun
	COX-2, NF-κB, p50, CD45
	Adh6a_predicted, Akr1b8, Als2, Anxa2, Cyp2a2, Hmox1, Hspca, Map2k3, Mug1, Pcsk9, Ppp3ca, Pece, Phgdh
NMBA metabolism	*Cyp2a2, Taldo1*
Signal transduction	*Ambp, Ap3s1_predicted, Cacna2b, Cdc42, Cib2, Crk, Dusp5, Fst, Gabrd, Gng12, Grem1, Hmox1, Inhbb, Kifap3_predicted, Lamp2, Lepr, Lrba_predicted, Map2k3, Olfm3, Pmoc, Ppp2r2a, Ppp3ca, Prka1a, Prkg2, Rab1 Rbbp6, Rgs17_predicted, RragB, Sdc1, Sh2d2a, Spsb3_predicted, Tg, Tgfa, Tmed2, Tct1, Txnl1, Ube2c_predicted*

[a]Data taken from Stoner et al. (2008).

2.5 *Berries Inhibit Post-initiation Events in Rat Esophageal Carcinogenesis*

2.5.1 Effects on Genes Associated with Inflammation

Inflammation is an important component in the etiology of many cancers. The inflammatory response can create a pro-oncogenic microenvironment, in part, by producing DNA-damaging intracellular free radicals. The inflammation-associated enzyme, inducible nitric oxide synthase (iNOS), is overly expressed in many human cancers including esophageal squamous cell carcinoma (Tanaka et al., 1999). iNOS catalyzes the conversion of L-arginine to citrulline, a process that produces the free radical, nitric oxide (NO^+). Nitric oxide causes nitrosative stress, oxidative stress, and DNA damage. iNOS is elevated in NMBA-induced preneoplastic lesions and papillomas in the rat esophagus (Chen and Stoner, 2004), and this elevated expression is strongly inhibited by dietary BRBs. At 25 weeks of a post-initiation bioassay, a diet containing 5% BRBs was shown to inhibit the increase in iNOS mRNA expression in preneoplastic lesions by 95% and in papillomas by 60% (Chen et al., 2006). BRBs have also been shown to inhibit the inflammation-associated cyclooxygenase-2 (COX-2) enzyme and the level of prostaglandin E_2 in the esophagus of NMBA-treated rats (Chen et al., 2006). Because elevated levels of prostaglandins lead to enhanced cell proliferation, angiogenesis and metastasis, and reduced apoptosis and cell differentiation, reducing these levels may well be an important component of the chemopreventive effects of BRBs. Interestingly, the expression of inflammation-associated iNOS and COX-2 enzymes were not reduced when the rats were fed BRBs prior to treatment with NMBA (Stoner et al., 2008). This suggests that berry components are unable to affect inflammatory events associated with carcinogen administration; rather, they exert their inhibitory effects on these enzymes in the more advanced stages of tumor progression.

2.5.2 Effects on Genes Associated with Cell Proliferation and Cell Cycle Progression

BRBs have also been shown to reduce cell proliferation in the post-initiation protocol. Treatment of rats with NMBA increased the proliferating cell nuclear antigen (PCNA) labeling index (LI) in esophageal epithelium to 32.3%. Dietary administration of both 5 and 10% BRBs significantly reduced the LI to 22.7 and 25.7%, respectively (Kresty et al., 2001). This inhibition, however, was not related to the dietary concentration of berries. The gene *c-Jun* and its product c-Jun are increased significantly in the rat esophagus by NMBA treatment (Chen et al., 2006). c-Jun Protein is an important part of the activator protein (AP-1) complex, a major transcription factor involved in cell cycle and cell proliferation. c-Jun is typically up-regulated in transformed cell lines and human cancers and is often induced by the Ras family of oncogenes. BRBs were found to suppress the mRNA expression of c-Jun by 44% in esophageal papillomas and reduced protein expression by 36% relative to rats on control diet (Chen et al., 2006). The effects that BRBs have on PCNA levels and cell cycle proteins indicate that berries function, in part, by reducing cell proliferation in the rat esophagus after initiation with NMBA.

2.5.3 Effects on Genes Associated with Apoptosis and Cell Differentiation

In addition to their effects on cell proliferation, dietary BRBs have been shown to induce apoptosis in the esophagi of NMBA-treated rats. At week 25 of a bioassay, the esophagi of rats treated with NMBA only showed decreased levels of staining by TUNEL and these levels were enhanced by the 5% BRB diet (Wang et al., 2009, 2010a). The BCL2/Bax protein ratio is often used as an indicator of apoptotic signaling and the amount of induced-cell death. BRBs and an anthocyanin-enriched fraction of BRBs reduced this ratio in the esophagus of NMBA-treated rats further demonstrating their ability to stimulate apoptosis (Wang et al., 2009).

Microarray results indicated that BRBs also increase differentiation of cancer genes in NMBA-treated rat esophagus (Stoner et al., 2008). Eighteen genes associated with differentiation and morphogenesis that were dysregulated by NMBA treatment were brought back to near normal levels of expression by post-initiation treatment with BRBs (Table 8.2). Two notable genes were *Grem1* and the gene encoding the 14-3-3 family chaperone protein Ywhah. Grem1, which interacts with the Ywhah protein, encodes a secreted antagonist of the bone morphogenetic protein pathway which in turn plays a crucial role in regulating the balance between expansion and cell differentiation (Namkoong et al., 2006). In addition, Ywhah mediates signal transduction via activation of protein kinase C and calcium/calmodulin-dependent protein kinase II. Loss of the chaperone activity of Ywhah may also play a role in the oxidative signaling underlying oxidative damage. Another interesting gene is sciellin which encodes a precursor to the cornified envelope of terminally differentiated cells (Alibardi and Toni, 2007). Its down-regulation by NMBA could disrupt the normal differentiation program of esophageal squamous cells and promote cell transformation. These observations of differentiation-associated genes suggest that BRBs impede esophageal cell transformation.

2.5.4 Effects on Genes Associated with Angiogenesis

Angiogenesis, the formation of capillaries from pre-existing blood vessels, is essential for tumor growth and expansion because it enables general circulation and promotes metastasis. Solid tumors greater than 2 mm in diameter need capillaries for the delivery of oxygen and nutrients (Folkman, 1971). The angiogenic growth factor, vascular endothelial growth factor (VEGF), is highly specific mitogen for vascular endothelial cells and is considered the identifying angiogenesis factor during carcinogenesis. VEGF-C is known to be up-regulated in many human cancers including ESCC (Noguchi et al., 2002). At 25 weeks of a study using the post-initiation protocol, esophageal VEGF-C mRNA expression was significantly increased 2.38-fold in NMBA-treated rats given control diet. In contrast, in rats treated with NMBA plus a 5% BRB diet, the increase in VEGF mRNA expression was only 1.08-fold (Chen et al., 2006). The microvessel density (MVD) was also reduced in the esophagus of BRB-treated animals further demonstrating the ability of BRBs to reduce new blood vessel formation. Microarray analyses identified six genes associated with angiogenesis that were dysregulated in rat esophagus by NMBA treatment and re-regulated to normal levels of expression by BRBs (Table 8.2) (Stoner et al., 2008). These include *Klf5*, which was down-regulated by NMBA, and codes for a Kruppel-like zinc finger transcription factor that modulates cell proliferation, differentiation, cell cycle, apoptosis, and angiogenesis. Another gene is *Fgfbp1* which was up-regulated by NMBA and reduced to a near normal level of expression by BRBs. *Fgfbp1* codes for a secreted protein that enhances fibroblast growth factor activity and drives tumor angiogenesis (Kurtz et al., 2004). Collectively, these studies suggest that BRBs are capable of inhibiting the angiogenesis process.

3 Identification of Bioactive Agents in Berries for Prevention of Esophageal Cancer in Rats

We have used bioactivity-guided fractionation in attempts to identify the active chemopreventive constituents of black raspberries. Initially, freeze-dried BRB powder was extracted with organic solvents and water and the extract fractions tested for their ability to inhibit chemically-induced transformation of Syrian hamster embryo (SHE) cells (Xue et al., 2001). Of five extract fractions tested, an alcohol extract of BRBs was found to be the most effective in inhibiting cell transformation. These same extract fractions were evaluated by Huang et al. (2002) for their effects on transactivation of activated protein-1 (AP-1) and nuclear factor-κB (NF-κB) induced by the carcinogen, benzo(a)pyrene diol-epoxide (BPDE), in mouse epidermal cells. Again, the alcohol extract was found to be the most effective in down-regulating AP-1 and NF-κB activities, and its effect was mediated via inhibition of mitogen-activated protein kinase (MAPK) activation and inhibitory subunit κB phosphorylation, respectively. The alcohol extract was then fractionated by high-performance liquid chromatography to yield several bioactive subfractions which were tested individually for their ability to down-regulate AP-1 and NF-κB activities in mouse epidermal cells (Hecht et al., 2006). Interestingly, the major constituents of the most active subfractions were three of the four anthocyanins in BRBs: cyanidin-3-*O*-glucoside; cyanidin-3-*O*-rutinoside; and cyanidin 3-*O*-(2^G-xylosylrutinoside). These in vitro results suggested that the anthocyanins in BRBs are responsible for at least some of their chemopreventive activity.

In a follow-up study, these in vitro observations were extended to the rat model of esophageal SCC by determining if the anthocyanins in BRBs are among the most active chemopreventive constitutents in *vivo*. F-344 rats were fed diets containing either: (a) 5% whole BRB powder or (b) an anthocyanin-rich fraction (c) an alcohol/H_2O-soluble extract (d) an alcohol-insoluble (residue) fraction (e) a hexane extract, and (f) a sugar fraction of BRB powder before, during and after treatment with NMBA (Wang et al., 2009). The scheme for the preparation of these

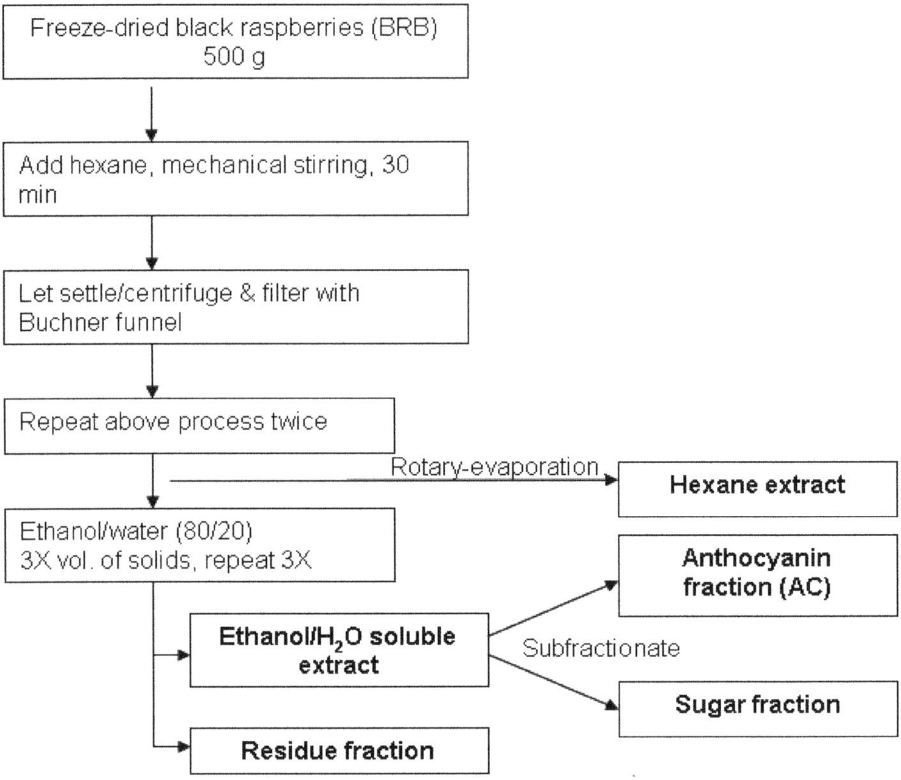

Fig. 8.3 Extraction scheme for isolation of extract and extract fractions from BRBs

different extracts/fractions is given in Fig. 8.3. The anthocyanin fraction and the alcohol/H_2O-soluble extract each contained the same amount of anthocyanins (~3.8 μmol/g diet) as were present in the diet containing 5% whole BRB powder. The residue fraction contained less than 0.02 μmol anthocyanins/g of diet, and the hexane extract and the sugar fraction had only trace quantities of anthocyanins. The results of these studies indicated that the anthocyanin treatments (diets a-c) were about equally effective in reducing NMBA tumorigenesis (multiplicity and size) in the esophagus, confirming that the anthocyanins in BRBs have chemopreventive potential.

Interestingly, the organic-insoluble (residue) fraction (d) was also effective. As expected, the hexane and sugar fractions were inactive, presumably because they contained only trace quantities of anthocyanins and other bioactives. Immunohistochemical and gene expression studies indicated that the anthocyanin-rich fraction and the residue fraction were equally as effective as whole 5% BRBs in re-regulating elevated protein levels of Ki-67, COX-2 and CD45 (leukocyte common antigen) in whole esophagus and in papillomas of NMBA-treated rats at the end of the study (Wang et al., 2009). Other biomarkers such as NF-κB and CD34 (a marker of angiogenesis) were reduced, and TUNEL (a marker of apoptosis) was increased in papillomas only.

A further investigation was undertaken in an attempt to identify the active component(s) in the residue fraction of BRBs. As indicated above, the residue fraction contained only 0.02 μmol of anthocyanins/g so its effectiveness in preventing esophageal cancer was not likely to be due to its content of anthocyanins. The residue fraction represents about 45% of whole BRB powder and likely contains cellulose, hemicelluloses, pectins, lignans, and protein. Chemical analysis of the residue indicated that it also contains ellagitannins (Wang et al., 2010). The ellagitannins are complex polyphenols in which the compound hexahydroxydiphenic acid forms diesters with sugars (Seeram, 2006). When hydrolyzed, the ellagitannins release ellagic acid which has chemopreventive activity in the rat esophagus (Mandal and Stoner, 1990). In a study in which the ellagic acid content of different fruits was measured, BRBs were found to have the highest content (1,500 μg/g of dry weight), STRWs were intermediate (630 μg/g of dry weight), and blueberries had among the lowest contents (<100 μg/g of dry weight) (Daniel et al., 1989). Given this information, we decided to evaluate the residue fractions of BRBs, STRWs and blueberries for their ability to prevent NMBA-tumorigenesis in the rat esophagus. On the basis of their contents of ellagitannins, we expected that the chemopreventive potential of the residue fractions of BRBs, STRWs and blueberries (BBs) would be in the order of BRB> STRW> BB. Surprisingly, the residue fraction of all three berry types was equally as effective as their whole berry equivalents at reducing papilloma incidence and multiplicity (Table 8.3) (Wang et al., 2010). These results suggest that the ellagitannins are not solely responsible for the chemopreventive effects of the residue fraction. Studies are currently underway in attempts to identify the role of the fiber itself in the prevention of esophageal carcinogenesis in the rat model.

4 Other Berry Types Also Prevent Esophageal Tumorigenesis in Rats

The expansion of efforts in berry research in the past 10 years has led to an increase in berry consumption by the public. One concern with BRBs is that they are more difficult to raise than most other berry types; thus, commercial production of these berries is relatively low. Moreover, they are usually not available for purchase several months each year. Given this, we decided to evaluate other berry types for their ability to prevent cancer using the rat esophageal SCC model. Two previous investigations in our laboratory showed that freeze-dried STRWs and blackberries exhibit chemopreventive potential in the rat esophagus, and both berry types were nearly as effective as BRBs (Carlton et al., 2001; Stoner et al., 2008). In a recent study, we compared the ability of four commonly consumed berries in the United States (strawberry, blueberry, red raspberry and black raspberry) and three "exotic" berry

Table 8.3 Effects of diets containing different amounts of ellagitannins (ET) derived from black raspberries (BRBs), strawberries (STRWs), and blueberries (BBs) on tumor number in NMBA-treated rat esophagus[a]

Gp[b]	1	2	3	4	5	6	7	8	9	10	11	12	13	14	15	16	17
NMBA	–	–	–	–	+	+	+	+	+	+	+	+	+	+	+	+	+
Residue or whole berry	–	Residue	Residue	Residue	–	Residue	Residue	Residue	Residue	Residue	Residue	Whole berry	Whole berry	Whole berry	Whole berry	Whole berry	Whole berry
Type of berry	–	BRB	STRW	BB	–	BRB	STRW	BB	BRB	STRW	BB	BRB	STRW	BB	BRB	STRW	BB
Average tumor number per rat[c,d]																	
Mean	–	–	–	–	10.2	5.5[e]	6.2[e]	4.9[e]	4.4[e]	5.2[e]	5.8[e]	5.7[e]	4.5[e]	5.4[e]	4.8[e]	5.2[e]	5.4[e]
SE	–	–	–	–	1.1	0.7	0.6	0.7	0.5	0.6	1.0	0.7	0.8	1.0	1.0	0.6	0.8

[a]Data taken from Wang et al. (2010).

[b]Animals in Groups 1–4 received s.c. injections of 0.2 mL of 20% DMSO, the vehicle for NMBA, once per week for 15 weeks. Animals in Groups 5–17 received s.c. injections of NMBA (0.3 mg/kg b.w.) in 0.2 mL of 20% DMSO, once per week for 15 weeks. The injections of vehicle or NMBA were started 2 weeks after initial administration of berry powders or residues to the diet.

[c]Animals in Groups 1 and 5 were fed AIN-76A diet only. All other groups were fed AIN-76A containing either residue or whole berry diets throughout the entire 30-week bioassay.

[d]$n = 15$ rats per groups

[e]significantly lower ($P < 0.05$) than rats treated with NMBA only (Group 1).

types (noni, goji and acai) to inhibit NMBA-induced tumors in the rat esophagus when administered in the diet using the post-initiation protocol (Stoner et al., 2010). We predicted that those berry types with higher levels of anthocyanins and ellagitannins might exhibit the strongest chemopreventive potential. A secondary goal of the study was to determine if we could identify inflammatory cytokines in the serum of carcinogen treated rats that might serve as indicators of the preventative effects of berries. Interestingly, at 5% of the diet, all seven berry types were about equally effective in reducing esophageal tumor incidence and multiplicity, but had no effect on tumor size (Table 8.4). In addition, all seven berry types were equally effective in reducing serum interleukin 5 (IL-5) and GRO/KC levels compared to the NMBA control group, suggesting that these two cytokines may be useful markers of the effects of chemopreventives on esophageal cancer development in this model.

This was the first study in which a "head-to-head" comparison was made between the ability of different berry types to influence chemically induced tumor development in an animal model system. It suggests that those berry types that contain relatively low levels of either anthocyanins or ellagitannins must have other constituents that are responsible for their chemopreventive effects. For example, the most active preventive agents in goji could well be their high content of carotenoids (Gross et al., 2006). Further studies are required to more fully evaluate the chemopreventive potential of black raspberries and of the other berry types, including berries that were not investigated in this study.

Table 8.4 Effect of different berry types on NMBA-induced esophageal tumors in F-344 rats when administered at 5% of the diet[a]

Gp	Diet	NMBA (0.3 mg/kg/inj)	Tumor incidence (%)	Tumor multiplicity (Mean ± SE)	Tumor size (mm^3) (Mean ± SE)
1	AIN-76A control diet	–	0	0	0
2	AIN-76A	+	95	2.15 ± 0.41	11.69 ± 5.07
3	AIN-76A + 5% BRBs	+	60[b]	1.07 ± 0.28[c]	7.50 ± 2.46
4	AIN-76A + 5% BBs	+	63[b]	1.00 ± 0.32[c]	9.21 ± 7.01
5	AIN-76A + 5% STRWs	+	75[b]	1.25 ± 0.32[c]	8.58 ± 3.46
6	AIN-76A + 5% RRBs (WGO2)	+	75[b]	1.19 ± 0.28[c]	6.72 ± 1.85
7	AIN-76A + 5% RRBs (Meeker)	+	63[b]	0.88 ± 0.27[c]	9.07 ± 3.86
8	AIN-76A + 5% noni	+	60[b]	1.10 ± 0.41[c]	7.93 ± 3.21
9	AIN-76A + 5% wolfberry	+	63[b]	0.94 ± 0.27[c]	5.73 ± 1.24
10	AIN-76A + 5% acai	+	75[b]	1.19 ± 0.25[c]	5.26 ± 2.15

BRBs, black raspberries; BBs, blueberries; STRWs, strawberries; RRBs, red raspberries.
[a]Data taken from Stoner et al.(2010).
[b]Significantly lower than Group 2 (NMBA only) as determined by χ^2 test ($P < 0.05$).
[c]Significantly lower than Group 2 (NMBA only) as determined by analysis of variance ($P < 0.05$).

References

Alibardi L, Toni M (2007) Characterization of keratins and associated proteins involved in the corneification of crocodilian epidermis. Tissue Cell 39:311–323

Barch DH, Jacoby RF, Brasitus TA et al (1991) Incidence of Harvey ras oncogene point mutations and their expression in methylbenzylnitrosamine-induced esophageal tumorigenesis. Carcinogenesis 12:2373–2377

Carlton PS, Kresty LA, Siglin JC et al (2001) Inhibition of *N*-nitrosomethylbenzylamine-induced tumorigenesis in the rat esophagus by dietary freeze-dried strawberries. Carcinogenesis 2: 441–446

Chen T, Hwang H, Rose ME et al (2006) Chemopreventive properties of black raspberries in *N*-nitrosomethylbenzylamine-induced rat esophageal tumorigenesis: down-regulation of COX-2, iNOS and c-Jun. Cancer Res 66:2853–2859

Chen T, Rose ME, Hwang H et al (2006) Black raspberries inhibit *N*-nitrosomethylbenzylamine-induced angiogenesis in rat esophagus parallel to the suppression of COX-2 and iNOS. Carcinogenesis 27:2301–2307

Chen T, Stoner GD (2004) Inducible nitric oxide synthase expression in *N*- nitrosomethylbenzylamine (NMBA)-induced rat esophageal tumorigenesis. Mol Carcinog 40:232–240

Daniel EM, Krupnick AD, Heur YH et al (1989) Extraction, stability, and quantitation of ellagic acid in various fruits and nuts. J Food Comp Anal 2:338–349

DeMeester SR (2009) Epidemiology and biology of esophageal cancer. Gastrointest Cancer Res 3:S2–S5

Folkman J (1971) Tumor angiogenesis: therapeutic implications. N Engl J Med 285:1182–1186

Garcia M, Jemal A, Ward EM et al (2007) Global cancer facts and figures 2007. American Cancer Society, Atlanta, GA

Gross PM, Zhang X, Zhang R (2006) Wolfberry: nature's bounty of nutrition and health, BookSurge Publishing, http://www.wolfberry.org

Hecht SS, Huang C, Stoner GD et al (2006) Identification of cyanidin glycosides as constituents of freeze-dried black raspberries which inhibit *anti*-benzo(a)pyrene-7,8-diol-9,10-epoxide induced NFkB and AP-1 activity. Carcinogenesis 27:1617–1626

Huang C, Huang Y, Li J et al (2002) Inhibition of BPDE-induced transactivation of AP-1 and NFkB by black raspberry extracts. Cancer Res 62:6857–6863

Kresty LA, Morse MA, Morgan C et al (2001) Chemoprevention of esophageal tumorigenesis by dietary administration of lyophilized black raspberries. Cancer Res 61:6112–6119

Kurtz A, Signer A, Cabal-Manzano RH et al (2004) Differential regulation of a fibroblast growth factor-binding protein during skin carcinogenesis and wound healing. Neoplasia 6:595–602

Liston BW, Gupta A, Nines R et al (2001) Incidence and effects of Ha-*ras* codon 12 G->A transition mutations in preneoplastic lesions induced by *N*-nitrosomethylbenzylamine (NMBA) in the rat esophagus. Mol Carcinog 32:1–8

Mandal S, Stoner GD (1990) Inhibition of N-nitrosobenzylmethylamine induced eosphageal tumorigenesis in rats by ellagic acid. Carcinogenesis 11:55–61

Namkoong H, Shin SM, Kim HK et al (2006) The bone morphogenetic protein antagonist gremlin 1 is overexpressed in human cancers and interacts with YWHAH protein. BMC Cancer 6:74

Noguchi T, Takeno S, Shibata T et al (2002) VEGF-C expression correlates with histological differentiation and metastasis in squamous cell carcinoma of the esophagus. Oncol Rep 9:995–999

Ribeiro U Jr, Posner MC, Safatle-Ribeiro AV et al (1997) Risk factors for squamous cell carcinoma of the oesophagus. Br J Surg 83:1174–1185

Seeram NP (2006) Berries. In: Heber D, Blackburn G, Go V, Milner J (eds) Nutritional oncology. Elsevier, Inc., Amsterdam

Stoner GD, Dombkowski AA, Reen RK et al (2008a) Carcinogen-altered genes in rat esophagus positively modulated to normal levels of expression by both black raspberries and phenylethyl isothiocyanate. Cancer Res 68:6460–6467

Stoner GD, Gupta A (2001) Etiology and chemoprevention of esophageal squamous cell carcinoma. Carcinogenesis 22:1737–1746

Stoner GD, Wang LS, Casto BC (2008b) Laboratory and clinical studies of cancer chemoprevention by antioxidants in berries. Carcinogenesis 29:1665–1674

Stoner GD, Wang LS, Chen T (2007a) Chemoprevention of esophageal squamous cell carcinoma. Toxicol Appl Pharmacol 224:337–349

Stoner GD, Wang LS, Seguin C et al (2010) Multiple berry types prevent N-nitrosomethylbenzylamine-induced esophageal cancer in rats. Pharm Res 27:1138–1145

Stoner GD, Wang LS, Zikri N et al (2007b) Cancer prevention with freeze-dried berries and berry components. Sem Cancer Biol 17:403–410

Tanaka H, Kijima H, Tokunaga T et al (1999) Frequent expression of inducible nitric oxide synthase in esophageal squamous cell carcinomas. Int J Oncol 14:1069–1073

Wang LS, Dombkowski AA, Rocha C et al (2010a) Effects of black raspberries on late events in N-nitrosomethylbenzylamine-induced rat esophageal carcinogenesis as determined by DNA microarray. Mol Carcinog (in press)

Wang LS, Hecht S, Carmella S et al (2009) Anthocyanins in black raspberries prevent esophageal tumors in rats. Cancer Prev Res 2(1):84–93. doi:10.1158/1940-6207.CPAR-08-0155

Wang LS, Hecht SS, Carmella SG et al (2010b) Berry ellagitannins may not be sufficient for prevention of tumors in the rodent esophagus. J Agric Food Chem 58:3992–3995

Wang Z, Tang L, Sun G et al (2006) Etiological study of esophageal squamous cell carcinoma in an endemic region: a population-based case control study in Huaian, China. BMC Cancer 6:287

Xue H, Aziz RM, Sun N et al (2001) Inhibition of cellular transformation by berry extracts. Carcinogenesis 22:351–361

Yang W (1992) Exposure level of N-nitrosamines in the gastric juice and its inhibition by vitamin C in high risk areas of esophageal cancer. Chin J Oncol 14:407–410

Chapter 9
Chemopreventive Effects of Berries and Berry Components in Animal Models: Prevention of Estrogen-Mediated Mammary Tumors in ACI Rats by Berries

Harini Aiyer, Srivani Ravoori, and Ramesh Gupta

Abstract Breast cancer is the most commonly diagnosed and the most prevalent cancer among women worldwide. There are several million women who could potentially benefit from prevention of both primary and recurring breast tumors. The female reproductive hormone 17ß-estradiol (E_2) has been implicated as a causative agent in breast cancer. ACI rats are susceptible to mammary adenocarcinomas induced by physiological levels of E_2, making it a preclinical model with a high applicability for clinical translation. We have shown that diets supplemented with blueberry or black raspberry (1, 2.5 and 5% w/w) show significant reduction in the latency, incidence, number, and volume of tumors in this animal model of E_2-mediated mammary tumorigenesis. Berry phytochemicals provide this protection by modulating E_2-metabolizing enzymes, preventing DNA damage, increasing DNA repair, reducing E_2-induced cell proliferation, lowering the levels of circulating prolactin, and by eliciting an anti-estrogenic effect. Further, upon conversion of effective rodent doses to human equivalents using allometry, it was found that a woman with an average caloric intake of 2,000 kcal/day may require only 1/2 to 1 cup of fresh or frozen berries to achieve significant protection against the risk posed by E_2. This dose can be effectively applied in a community setting to achieve primary prevention as well as in a clinical setting to prevent recurrence.

Keywords Hormonal breast cancer · ACI rat model · Prevention · Blueberry · Black raspberry · Ellagic acid allometric scaling

R. Gupta (✉)
James Graham Brown Cancer Center, University of Louisville, Louisville, KY 40202, USA; Department of Pharmacology and Toxicology, University of Louisville, Louisville, KY 40202, USA
e-mail: rcgupta@louisville.edu

Harini Aiyer and Srivani Ravoori contributed equally to this chapter.

G.D. Stoner, N.P. Seeram (eds.), *Berries and Cancer Prevention*,
DOI 10.1007/978-1-4419-7554-6_9,

1 Introduction

Breast cancer is the most prevalent cancer among women worldwide (Parkin et al., 2005; Parkin and Fernandez, 2006). According to the estimates provided by the International Agency for Research on Cancer (http://www-dep.iarc.fr/globocan/database.htm), the global incidence of cancer is estimated to be almost 11 million, and the mortality and prevalence figures are close to 7 and 25 million respectively (Parkin et al., 2005). Breast cancer is the most frequent cancer in women and contributes to 23% of all diagnosed cancers. Among the 1.15 million cases diagnosed globally, over 200,000 are in North America, which has the highest age-standardized incidence (122.9 per 100,000) (http://seer.cancer.gov/statfacts/html/breast.html#incidence-mortality). Generally, it is seen that the incidence of breast cancer is higher in developed countries than the developing nations, which is attributed to combined influence of differences in lifestyle, hereditary factors, and screening practices (Althuis et al., 2005). The mortality rate for breast cancer is the fifth highest ranking behind lung, stomach, liver, and colon cancers. The 5-year survival rate after diagnosis of a localized breast cancer is 98%. Due to such good prognosis, breast cancer ranks as the most prevalent cancer among all cancers (17.9%). Currently, there are over 2 million breast cancer survivors in the United States (ACS, 2007a, b). However, this survival rate varies with age, stage of tumor at diagnosis, race/ethnicity, and socioeconomic status of the patients (ACS, 2007a, b).

In developing countries such as Brazil, China, and India, there seems to be an increasing trend in the incidence of breast cancer. It is estimated that the number of new cancer cases globally will increase from 10 million in 2000 to 15 million in 2020 (Brown et al., 2006). The largest increase is expected to occur in developing countries, contributing to substantially more than 50% of the global cancer burden (http://www.who.int/mediacentre/news/releases/2003/pr27/en/). The improvements in the socio-economic conditions as well as changes to traditional food habits, reduced exercise, and the alarming increases in incidence of obesity among the populations in these countries is being cited as some reasons for this increasing trend (Porter, 2008). Further, the challenges in existing health care systems as well as poor screening practices further add to the cost of cancer.

1.1 Breast Cancer Risk Factors and Prevention

Epidemiological studies of breast cancer indicate at least two distinguishable causes. About 10% of all breast cancers diagnosed can be attributed to a familial or hereditary cause. The hereditary or familial breast cancer presents with germline mutations in certain genes that are passed on from one generation to another. Among these mutations, the most common are the BRCA 1 and BRCA 2 mutations. These high-penetrance genes are mutated in about 65% of all familial breast cancers diagnosed (Studzinski and Harrison, 2002). Somatic mutations in p53 gene involved in cell-cycle arrest are present in 50% of all cancers and about 15–30% of breast cancers. However, germline mutations in this gene are rare. More recently, mutations in the cell-cycle check point gene CHEK2 have been associated with familial breast cancer, but are not linked to BRCA 1 or BRCA 2 mutations (Vahteristo et al., 2002; Oldenburg et al., 2003; Thompson and Easton, 2004).

A great majority (90%) of breast cancer is considered sporadic since no single factor can be clearly attributed to causation and is thought to be caused by the interactions between multiple risk factors. Epidemiological studies have linked several risk factors to the etiology of breast cancer. These risk factors can be broadly classified into 3 categories:

1. Non-modifiable-risk factors such as age, gender, race/ethnicity, genetic polymorphisms, familial history, and previous breast history.
2. Modifiable- or lifestyle-risk factors that include diet, exercise, body weight, alcohol, and smoking.
3. Hormonal risk factors, including age at menarche and menopause, parity, breast feeding, and hormone-replacement therapy (HRT).

Prevention of breast cancer can be effectively achieved by targeting both the modifiable and hormonal risk factors listed above. The effect of 17ß-estradiol (E_2) as a complete carcinogen and the implications of berries as ideal chemopreventive agents in hormone-mediated breast cancer are discussed in detail further in this chapter. In terms of lifestyle factors that can be modified to achieve primary prevention, strategies include reduction of tobacco and alcohol consumption, higher dietary intake of fruits and vegetables, increase in activity levels, and control of the obesity epidemic (Hankinson et al., 2004; Warren et al., 2004).

Another key strategy of primary prevention, especially in certain high-risk women, has been the control of hormonal risk factors using anti-estrogen therapy. As noted previously, there are currently more than two million breast cancer survivors in the United States who are eligible for such an intervention (ACS, 2009). It must be stated that certain hormonal risk factors such as ages at menarche and menopause, parity, and breast feeding cannot be controlled. However, since these factors determine the cumulative exposure levels to the female reproductive hormone (E_2), anti-estrogen therapy typically targets women who have a high risk based on their circulating E_2 levels along with other risk factors such as inherited genetic mutations, family history, or previous breast disease (Amir et al., 2010). The conclusive finding that HRT significantly increases the risk of breast cancer has lead to discontinuation of HRT in many women, thus reducing their risks (Canfell et al., 2008; Parkin, 2009; Seradour et al., 2009).

As almost 70% of breast cancers diagnosed are estrogen receptor (ER)-positive, targeting this pathway with anti-estrogen therapy has been successfully used in the past three decades in both breast cancer treatment (as adjuvant therapy) (Jordan, 2008) and prevention (in high-risk women) (Powles, 2002; Virnig et al., 2010). Tamoxifen, a drug with over 10 million patient years of clinical data, is a selective-estrogen-receptor modulator (SERM). It acts as an ER-antagonist in the breast, while simultaneously acting as an ER-agonist in the bone and uterus. This selective modulation makes it a good choice for women who are at a high-risk for osteoporosis, either following menopause or after discontinuation of HRT. Currently, tamoxifen is the leading preventive therapy for breast cancer. However, treatment with tamoxifen involves numerous adverse effects, including increased incidence of endometrial cancer, cataracts, and thromboembolism (Cano and Hermenegildo, 2000; Morrow and Jordan, 2000). Although raloxifene, a second generation SERM and originally an osteoporosis-prevention drug, is equivalent to tamoxifen in prevention of invasive breast cancer with fewer adverse effects, thromboembolism, hot flashes, and leg cramps are still potential side effects (Cranney and Adachi, 2005; Jordan, 2006). In addition, raloxifene is poorly bioavailable and rapidly excreted, causing significantly reduced benefits in women with poor compliance (Jordan, 2006). Nevertheless, the search for better SERMs with fewer side effects is ongoing (Jordan, 2006). Another facet of anti-estrogen therapy is to stop the production of E_2. This is especially significant in post-menopausal women who convert androstenedione to estrone (E_1) via the enzyme aromatase, in the adipose and stromal tissue of the breast. E_1 is then converted to the more potent E_2 by the enzyme 17ß-hydroxysteroid dehydrogenase (17ßHSD). Aromatase inhibitors (AI) have proven extremely effective in this patient population and have provided better outcomes, without much of the side effects seen with the SERMs. Although these drugs are highly effective in the treatment and prevention of primary and recurrent breast cancer, respectively, they are associated with unpleasant side effects leading to reduced quality of life in breast cancer survivors as well as development of drug resistance. It is estimated that up to 50% of women with ER-positive breast cancer will fail to respond to or develop resistance to tamoxifen therapy (Clarke et al., 2001). No single approach can result in the complete prevention of breast cancer. For the best public health outcomes, a combination approach incorporating healthy-lifestyle modifications such as improved diet, exercise, and weight control regimens as well as regular screening, supported by anti-estrogen therapy where it is strongly implicated would be the most successful.

In this chapter, we will explain how estrogen acts as a complete carcinogen, introduce an animal model that can be used to study E_2-induced mammary tumors, and discuss the concept of why berries are ideal preventive agents in E_2-mediated mammary tumorigenesis. We further collate data from studies in this animal model conducted in our laboratory. Dietary berries show consistent reductions in mammary tumor incidence, latency, volume, and multiplicity. We will also briefly discuss the different mechanisms by which berries and berry polyphenols affect mammary tumorigenesis in vivo and in vitro and finally, the applicability and translatability of berry consumption to community as a whole, particularly highlighting the clinical settings.

1.2 Estrogen-Induced Mammary Tumors in ACI Rats

Of the risk factors associated with breast cancer, cumulative estrogen exposure has the highest positive correlation to incidence. This is corroborated by the following facts: (1) women with high serum levels of E_2 have a higher risk; (2) age at menarche and menopause, which are correlates of cumulative estrogen exposure determine risk; (3) removal of the ovary before or after breast cancer incidence results in a more positive outcome; (4) high levels of tissue E_2 are found in breast tumor biopsies, pointing to either accumulation or in-situ synthesis; and (5) treatment with anti-estrogens such as tamoxifen significantly reduces tumor recurrence (Liehr, 2001; Russo and Russo, 2004).

Animal models are indispensable to the study of breast cancer. Breast tumors undergo progression from the in-situ stage through invasive cancer to metastatic tumors (Clarke, 1996). Most animal models currently in use try to replicate this development from one stage to the other as closely as possible. The validity of most rodent tumor models has been derived based on the similarities, both histopathological and molecular, between tumors of rodent and human origin (Russo et al., 1990; Thompson and Singh, 2000). Although genetically engineered mouse models (transgenic and syngeneic) have illuminated to a large extent molecular mechanisms involved in breast tumorigenesis (Blackshear, 2001), their application in the treatment and prevention of sporadic human breast cancer is limited (Clarke, 1996; Kim et al., 2004). Also, explant models are less predictive of validity for translational research (Gutmann et al., 2006).

The use of chemical carcinogen-induced mammary tumors in rats as a preclinical model has been popular for the past 4 decades. Table 9.1 highlights the advantages and disadvantages of several carcinogen-induced mammary tumor models currently available. There is considerable heterogeneity in the incidence of mammary tumors in rats depending on the rat strain used, type of carcinogen, time and mode of carcinogen administration, etc. (Huggins et al., 1959, 1961; Thompson et al., 1992; Snyderwine et al., 1998; Shepel and Gould, 1999). Strikingly, the most common feature among all these models is that the disruption of the ovarian-endocrine axis by means of ovariectomy affects the ability of carcinogens to induce mammary tumors (Welsch, 1985; Shull et al., 1997; Thompson et al., 1998; Thordarson et al., 2001). This suggests the ovarian hormone dependence of mammary tumors (Blank et al., 2008). Further, increased circulating prolactin and pituitary hyperplasia is also seen in rats treated with any estrogenic compound (Dunning et al., 1947, 1953; Cutts and Noble, 1964; Holtzman et al., 1981; Mesia-Vela et al., 2008), suggesting that the pituitary-mammary axis also plays a crucial role in estrogen-induced mammary tumor development. The August-Copenhagen Irish-hooded (ACI) rat model initially described by Shull et al. (1997) using a 27 mg E_2-implant causes significant pituitary hyperplasia, leading to very high morbidity and mortality within a 6-month treatment period (Aiyer et al., 2008c). In order to refine the model, we reduced the dose of E_2 from 27 to 9 mg and the surface area of the implants from 3 to 1.2 cm (Ravoori et al., 2007). Although, there is still an increase in circulating prolactin levels, this improved model results in 100% mammary adenocarcinoma incidence without the associated pituitary hyperplasia-induced mortality. This model has been successfully used in several chemoprevention studies, including those involving berry intervention in our laboratory (Ravoori et al., 2008; Vadhanam et al., 2008; Gupta et al., 2009a, b; Ravoori et al., 2009; Aiyer and Gupta, 2010; Bansal et al., 2010; Vadhanam et al., 2010).

Table 9.1 Rat models of carcinogen-induced mammary tumors

Rat strain	Carcinogen	Age(d) at induction	Dose	Route	Incidence (%)	Latency (weeks)	Tumor type	Advantages	Disadvantages	References
SD	2-AAF	50	100 mg	PO	30	8	Carcinoma			Huggins et al. (1961)
	3-MC		100 mg	PO	100	7.3 ± 2	Carcinoma	A single dose of DMBA often induces 100% tumor incidence	DMBA is not a relevant human carcinogen	
	DMBA		20 mg	PO	100	6.1 ± 1	Carcinoma			
	DMBA	48	1 μM/gland	IM	100	10 ± 2	Adenocarcinoma (62%) Fibroadenoma (6%) Fibrosarcoma (28%)	A single NMU dose causes both in situ and invasive carcinoma	NMU tumors have an ovarian-independent phenotype	Cavalieri et al. (1991)
	DB[*a,l*]P				100	11± 1	Adenocarcinoma (83%) Fibroadenoma (0%) Fibrosarcoma (16%)	Both DMBA and NMU model have been extensively studied and documented	Genomic instability such as aneuploidy is rarely present	
	B[a]P				45	22 ± 1	Fibrosarcoma			
	NMU	50	50 mg/kg b.w	IP	100	8	In situ and invasive carcinoma		Harvey-ras mutations, commonly seen in DMBA- and NMU-induced tumors, are not present in humans	Thordarson et al. (2001)
	PhIP	43	75 mg/kg. b.w	PO- 10 doses	24	NR	Carcinoma			Snyderwine et al. (1998)

Table 9.1 (continued)

Rat strain	Carcinogen	Age(d) at induction	Dose	Route	Incidence (%)	Latency (weeks)	Tumor type	Advantages	Disadvantages	References
ACI	17ß-Estradiol	49	2 or 3 mg	SC-P	100	NR	In situ carcinoma	ACI rats do not develop spontaneous tumors Resistant to chemical-carcinogen-induced mammary tumors	Increased mortality due to pituitary adenoma	Li et al. (2002b)
		61–63	27 mg	SC-I	100	21 ± 3		ACI rats develop mammary adenocarcinomas in response to several types of estrogens	Tumors lack metastatic potential	Shull et al. (1997)
		36–49	9 mg	SC-I	100			Chromosomal instabilities observed in estrogen-induced tumors in ACI rats are often seen in humans as well	Relative dearth of both mechanistic and preventive studies	Ravoori et al. (2007), Aiyer and Gupta (2010)
	Estrone	30–40	8–11 mg	SC-P	86	43	Carcinoma (94.5%) Fibroadenoma (5.5%)			Cutts and Noble (1964)
	Ethynyl Estradiol	60–120	0.1 mg, 1 mg	SC-P	87	24	NR			Holtzman et al. (1981), Dunning and Curtis (1953)
	Diethyl Stilbesterol	60–120	2.3 mg	SC-P	47	21	Adenocarcinomas (> 95%)			

Abbreviations: 2-AAF, 2- alpha amino fluorine; 3-MC, 3- methylcholantherene; DMBA, 7, 12- Dimethylbenzanthracene; DB [a,l]P, Dibenzo [*a,l*] pyrene; B[*a*]P, Benzo [*a*] pyrene; NMU, N-nitroso-N-methylurea; PhIP, 2-amino-1-methyl-6-phenylimidazo[4,5-*b*]pyridine; SD, Sprague Dawley; ACI, August Copenhagen Irish-hooded; IP, Intraperitoneal; PO, Per Oral; SC-P, Subcutaneous Pellet; SC-I, Subcutaneous Implant; NR, Not Reported.

Several key points support the use of this animal model to study breast cancer prevention. First, estrogen is clearly and undisputedly associated with the etiology of the disease in humans. Second, estrogen-induced tumors in ACI rats exhibit chromosomal instabilities that are often seen in human breast cancer as well (Li et al., 2002a, 2004; Adamovic et al., 2007). Further, E_2– and DMBA-induced carcinogenesis involves genetically distinct mechanisms (Schaffer et al., 2006). Although these rats are susceptible to estrogen-induced prolactinomas, the loci that control the pituitary and mammary tumor susceptibilities are genetically distinct (Gould et al., 2004; Strecker et al., 2005; Schaffer et al., 2006). Recently, a genetically distinct strain of rats (ACI.COP-Ept2) that develop mammary tumors without any pituitary tumors have been developed (Kurz et al., 2008). In addition, the chromosomes that are affected in estrogen-induced carcinogenesis are homologous to those that are affected in humans (Adamovic et al., 2007). Finally, the mammary tissues show varying degrees of lobular and ductal epithelial hyperplasia, ductal carcinoma in situ, and tumors display molecular markers such as an overexpression of cyclin D1 and c-myc, similar to breast cancer pathology in humans (Weroha et al., 2006).

Although some intervention studies were done in the DES-induced mammary tumor model (Petrek et al., 1985; Holtzman, 1988), to date few studies have looked at the effect of preventive intervention in the estradiol-induced model. Of the few, recent studies by Bhat and coworkers (2003) indicate the effectiveness of dietary vitamin C and antioxidant butylated hydroxyl anisole, suggesting that antioxidants can prevent these tumors (Mense et al., 2009; Singh et al., 2009). Other studies include prevention using tamoxifen (Li et al., 2002b), phenobarbital (Mesia-Vela et al., 2006) and using α-napthaflavone, a CYP-inhibitor (Mense et al., 2009). Collectively, these facts make the ACI rat model an ideal preclinical model for exploring preventive intervention strategies that have a high applicability in the translational setting.

1.3 Berries in the Prevention of Estrogen-Mediated Mammary Tumorigenesis

Estrogen acts via 2 distinct pathways, both of which are equally important for its carcinogenic activity. In this section, we discuss the effect of berry extracts and phytochemicals on each of these distinct pathways to prevent mammary tumorigenesis. Figure 9.1 shows a simplified schematic diagram of E_2 action and the various stages at which berries affect E_2-mediated carcinogenesis.

First, estrogen causes genotoxicity via its metabolic pathway. E_2 is activated via hydroxylation at various positions by the phase I cytochrome P450 enzymes (Zhu and Conney, 1998). Of the different extra-hepatic P450s important in estrogen metabolism, CYP1A1 and 1B1 are present in the mammary tissue and produce 2- and 4- hydroxy metabolites, known as catechols, respectively (Zhu and Conney, 1998; Liehr, 2000). These data are further supported by numerous findings which

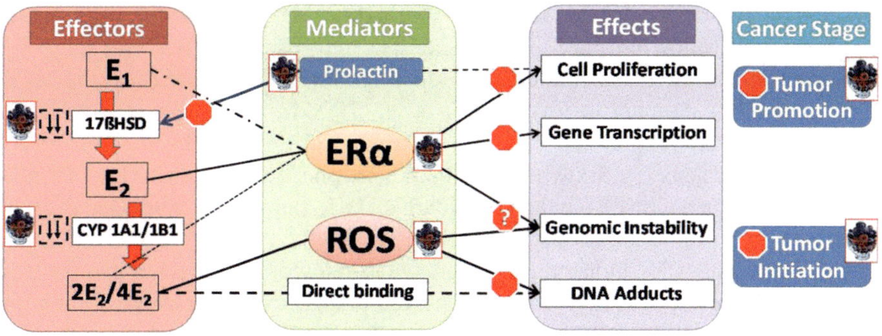

Fig. 9.1 A simplified schematic diagram of the effects of E_2 at different stages of mammary tumor devolpment and the role of berries in modulating the effects of E_2

were extensively reviewed by Liehr (2000, 2001) and can be summarized as follows. Pharmacological doses of estrogen induce renal-cell carcinomas in hamsters and mammary adenocarcinomas in ACI rats in the absence of other carcinogens (Li et al., 1983; Shull et al., 1997). E_2 by itself can induce chromosomal aberrations in cell culture similar to those seen in estrogen-induced tumors (Liehr, 2000; Li et al., 2002a). Catechol estrogens, which are active metabolites of E_2, can induce DNA damage causing both stable and unstable adducts (Cavalieri et al., 2000; Liehr, 2000). Further, enzymes that convert E_2 to its catechol metabolites, such as CYP1B1, are found in high levels in breast tumors, and microsomes from breast tumor tissues metabolize E_2 to potentially harmful catechols (Liehr and Ricci, 1996; Oyama et al., 2005). The hydroxylated metabolites are further either glucuronidated (by UDP-glucuronosyl transferase), methylated (by catechol-O-methyl transferase), or glutathione conjugated (by glutathione-S-transferase), by the phase II enzymes (Zhu and Conney, 1998). Polymorphisms that increase the metabolic activity of phase I enzymes, which activate and lower the activity of phase II enzymes, which detoxify E_2, are known to increase breast cancer risk (Thompson and Ambrosone, 2000). The oxidative stress induced by catechol-estrogen metabolites have been implicated in estrogen-induced carcinogenesis (Yager, 2000). Either E_2 alone or a combination of a strong oxidant (menadione) and weak estrogen (ethinyl estradiol) induce renal cell carcinomas and increase the levels of 8-iso-prostaglandin $F_{2\alpha}$, an oxidative-stress biomarker (Bhat et al., 2003). Further reports that catechol-estrogens can cause oxidative DNA damage in vitro in the presence of transition metal ions (Li et al., 1994; Hiraku et al., 2001; Aiyer et al., 2002; Srinivasan et al., 2002) designate a role for catechol-estrogens in inducing oxidative stress. Collectively, these facts provide evidence for the importance of estrogen metabolism in the causation of cancer.

In our in vitro studies, both ellagic acid (10 μM) and aqueous extracts of various berries (2%) were significantly effective in reducing 4-hydroxy etsradiol ($4E_2$)-induced oxidative DNA damage (Aiyer et al., 2008a, b). An important observation is that red-raspberry, which contains the highest concentration of ellagic acid among the various berries (blueberry, strawberry) tested, had the most significant reduction following pure ellagic acid. The red-raspberry diet also increased the expression of several hepatic DNA-repair genes, while decreasing the levels of baseline-DNA damage in vivo (Aiyer et al., 2008d). In another in vivo study, a mixed berry diet (containing an equal mixture of 5 different berries: blueberry, blackberry, red-raspberry, strawberry and black raspberry; 0.5% each) had a higher level of protection against E_2-induced oxidative DNA damage (8-oxodG) in the liver than the control diet or a blueberry-only diet (Aiyer et al., 2008b). These data again suggest reduction of E_2-induced DNA damage as one possible mechanism for their chemopreventive action. Previously, we showed that ellagic acid effectively inhibits the activation of benzo(a)pyrene (B(a)P) and subsequent DNA damage (Smith et al., 2001). A recent report by Singletary et al. (2007) shows similar mechanism of action by the blueberry-anthocyanidins and delphinidin in MCF-10F cells. Ellagic acid also inhibits DNA methyltransferase activity in MCF 7 cells, suggesting that it may have a role in epigenetic modification of the DNA (Paluszczak et al., 2010).

In a recent report, we showed that black raspberry, blueberry and ellagic acid diets significantly reverse the E_2-induced changes in the mRNA expression of several enzymes involved in E_2-metabolism in the mammary tissue of the ACI rat (Aiyer and Gupta, 2010). E_2-treatment in ACI rats significantly up-regulates the mammary tissue expression of 17ßHSD, which converts E_1 to E_2 and of CYP1A1, a mixed function oxygenase that can convert E_2 to both $2E_2$ and $4E_2$ (Cribb et al., 2006). The black raspberry and blueberry diet significantly offset E_2-induced up-regulation of both 17ßHSD and CYP1A1 during the early phase of E_2-mediated mammary carcinogenesis (Aiyer and Gupta, 2010). These berries also reduce the CYP1B1 expression compared with both untreated and E_2-treated rats. Ellagic acid does not affect CYP1A1 expression, but down-regulates CYP1B1 in a manner similar to berries. Studies suggest that ellagic acid decreases the activity of CYP1A1 (Ahn et al., 1996) without altering its expression (Aiyer and Gupta, 2010). Thus, berry phytochemicals may significantly reverse the tumor initiating effects of E_2 by affecting the in situ synthesis and phase I metabolism of E_2 and by reducing the DNA damage caused by its genotoxic catechol-estrogen metabolites (Fig. 9.1).

The other important pathway crucial for estrogen carcinogenicity is its role as a growth factor via steroid receptor signaling. The 2 types of estrogen receptors, ERα and ERß, have been extensively studied. Of these, ERα is considered a diagnostic marker and an indicator of response to anti-estrogen therapy in breast cancer (Clarke et al., 2001; Balfe et al., 2004). E_2 is proliferative primarily through its action on ERα, which is also required for normal development and differentiation of the mammary gland (Dickson and Stancel, 2000). Therapy for breast cancer targets this pathway using antiestrogens or SERMs (Sims et al., 2007). There is clear evidence to suggest that berry phytochemicals are potent antiestrogenic agents and interact with the ERα pathway. The chemical structure of both anthocyanins and ellagic acid is similar to estradiol (Fig. 9.2). This similarity suggests a potential for SERM-like activity of these phytochemicals. In fact, both ellagic acid and berry anthocyanins show potent anti-estrogenic activities (Schmitt and Stopper, 2001; Papoutsi et al., 2005; Larrosa et al., 2006). Other evidence for their anti-estrogenic

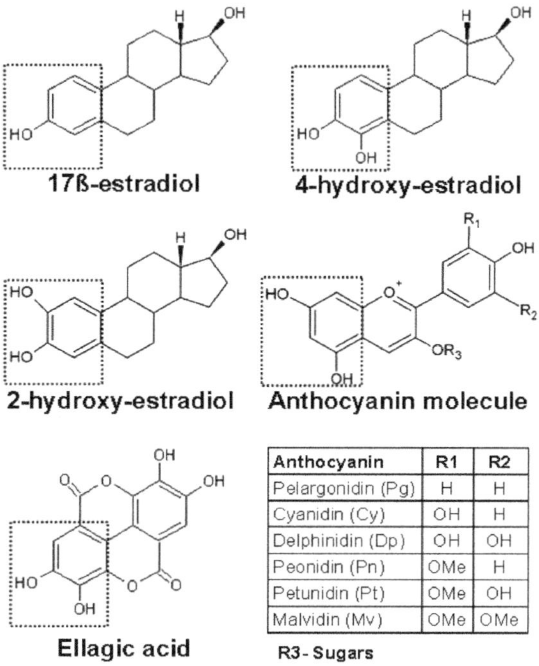

Anthocyanin	R1	R2
Pelargonidin (Pg)	H	H
Cyanidin (Cy)	OH	H
Delphinidin (Dp)	OH	OH
Peonidin (Pn)	OMe	H
Petunidin (Pt)	OMe	OH
Malvidin (Mv)	OMe	OMe

Fig. 9.2 Chemical Structures of 17β-estradiol, its metabolites and berry phytochemicals. The structural similarities that may be responsible for possible estrogen-receptor binding of the various chemicals are highlighted. Table of different functional groups in the anthocyanin molecule adapted from (Wu and Prior, 2005)

effect comes from our studies. As noted earlier in the chapter, E_2-treatment in ACI rats induces ER-mediated increase in pituitary proliferation (Lyle et al., 1984; Chen et al., 2009). Rats fed diets supplemented with black raspberry, blueberry, and ellagic acid experienced significant reduction in pituitary weight (Aiyer and Gupta, 2010), pituitary prolactinoma-induced mortality (Aiyer et al., 2008c), and circulating prolactin levels. Prolactin levels measured in the serum of E_2-treated rats (Table 9.2) were attenuated by both blueberry (34.3%; $p = 0.03$) and black raspberry (27.2%; $p = 0.07$). Further, all dietary interventions significantly offset the overexpression of 17ßHSD, a gene known to be controlled by prolactin, at 6 weeks after E_2-treatment (Aiyer and Gupta, 2010). Another key evidence for the

Table 9.2 Serum prolactin levels of rats fed the blueberry and black raspberry diets 3 weeks after E_2 administration

Implant	Diet	Mean ± SD	*p*-value
Sham	Control diet (AIN-93 M)	213.9 ± 146.9	
	5% Blueberry	212.3 ± 97.85	
	5% Black raspberry	395.3 ± 186.5	
E_2	Control diet (AIN-93 M)	733.4 ± 203.6	
	5% Blueberry	482 ± 159.3	0.0307
	5% Black raspberry	533.7 ± 173	0.0666

anti-estrogenic activity of berry phytochemicals is their effect on the uterus and ovaries. Compared with sham treatment, the combined wet weight of the ovary and uterus increased significantly in animals treated with 27 mg E_2 for 24 weeks (620 $\pm$ 80 mg vs. 870 $\pm$ 50; $p<0.01$). This increase in tissue weight was significantly reduced after dietary intervention (blueberry diet: 650 $\pm$ 18; black raspberry diet: 600 $\pm$ 77; ellagic acid diet: 650 $\pm$ 42 mg; $p<0.05$). These results are similar in trend, but not in magnitude, to tamoxifen treatment (Li et al., 2002b; S. Li, personal communication). Together, these findings suggest that both berries and ellagic acid at the concentrations tested may act as antiestrogens, but at a much lower capacity compared to tamoxifen. Further studies are required to confirm the SERM effects of these dietary agents in the bone, neurological, and cardiovascular tissues.

The antiproliferative activity of anthocyanins and ellagic acid as well as berry extracts has been shown in vitro using breast cancer cell lines (Seeram et al., 2006; Boivin et al., 2007; Adams et al., 2010; Fernandes et al., 2010; Nguyen et al., 2010). In the ACI rat model, a short-term study to test the effect of blueberry and black raspberry diets revealed significant antiproliferative activity. Estrogen treatment for 3 weeks increased the proliferation of mammary tissue by fivefold ($p<0.0001$), as assessed by deep positivity for PCNA (Fig. 9.3). A significant reduction in the proliferation of mammary tissue was observed in rats fed the 5% blueberry (66% reduction; $p<0.0003$) and 5% black raspberry diet (32% reduction; $p<0.0071$). For blueberry, this trend held even after 12 weeks of E_2-treatment, even at a 2.5% dose (Aiyer et al., 2008a).

In another study, pooled RNA samples (3–4 rats/group) from mammary tissues of tumor endpoint were subjected to microarray analyses using Genechip rat genome 230 2.0 array (Affymetrix, Inc.), containing probe sets to measure over 30,000 transcripts. Mammary tissue from estrogen-treated rats revealed dysregulation of over 700 genes involved in cancer pathways. Of these genes, about 150 were restored to near-normal levels by berry diets. Key genes modulated include genes associated with cell proliferation, cell-cycle regulation, and signal transduction (data not shown). Similar observation was made by Stoner and colleagues (2008) where the black raspberry diet restored about 462 genes dysregulated by NMBA treatment of rat esophagus involving phase I and II enzymes, oncogenes, tumor suppressor genes and genes involved in apoptosis, cell cycling and angiogenesis.

1.4 Prevention of Mammary Tumorigenesis by Dietary Berries

In several studies conducted in our laboratory, dietary intervention with black raspberry, blueberry, and ellagic acid has shown consistent reductions in E_2-induced mammary tumor indices in ACI rats (Aiyer et al., 2008c; Ravoori et al., 2008, 2009; Aiyer and Gupta, 2010; Aiyer et al., 2010). Compared with an unsupplemented diet, black raspberry supplementation at 1% (w/w) caused a 19% reduction in tumor incidence at 26 weeks (Fig. 9.4a), 44% reduction in tumor volume (Fig. 9.4d), and a 43% reduction in tumor multiplicity (Fig. 9.4e). There was a linear dose response at

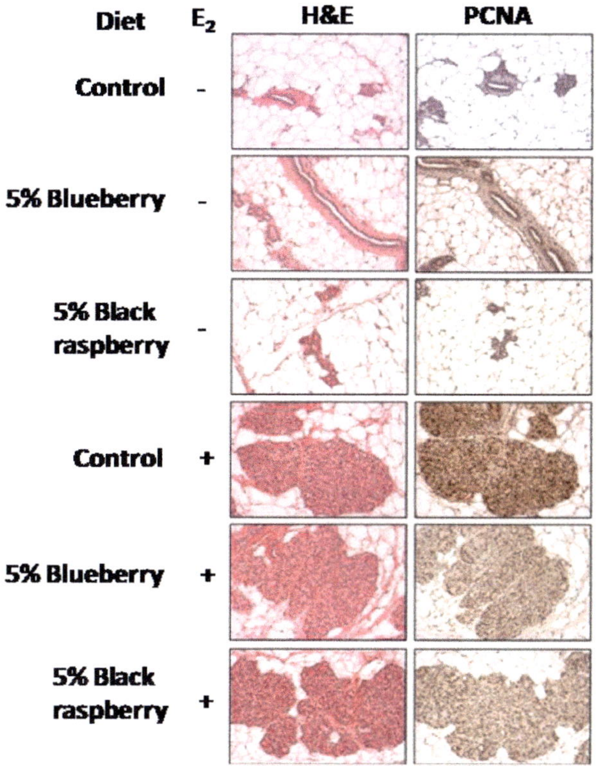

Fig. 9.3 Anti-proliferative effects of blueberry and black raspberry diets. Mammary tissue sections were analysed for proliferation by immunohistochemistry using a biotinylated PCNA monoclonal antibody. Streptavidin-peroxidase was used to generate signal and visualized using 3,3′-diaminobenzidine. Slides were counter-stained with hematoxylin and observed using light microscope

2.5% dose in most of the tumor indices – a 13% reduction in incidence, 67% reduction in volume, and 51% reduction in multiplicity. Although 2.5% blueberry was more effective in reducing tumor incidence at 26 weeks (69%; Fig. 9.4b), it was less effective in reducing tumor volume and multiplicity, with 59 and 38% reductions, respectively. Blueberry at 1% dose was only marginally effective in reducing tumor volume (41%), but not other indices. Ellagic acid supplementation at 400 ppm also reduced tumor incidence (19%), volume (65%), and multiplicity (41%) (Fig. 9.4 c–e). The inconsistency seen between reduction in tumor incidence and tumor volume/multiplicity can be explained by the time lag in the measurement of these two indices. Tumor incidence was measured in live animals based on palpation. The tumor incidence was considered 100% when all E_2-treated animals in the unsupplemented diet control group presented with palpable mammary tumors (Fig. 9.4a–c). However, the tumor volume and multiplicity (Fig. 9.4d–e) were measured after six more weeks of E_2 treatment when the animals were euthanized.

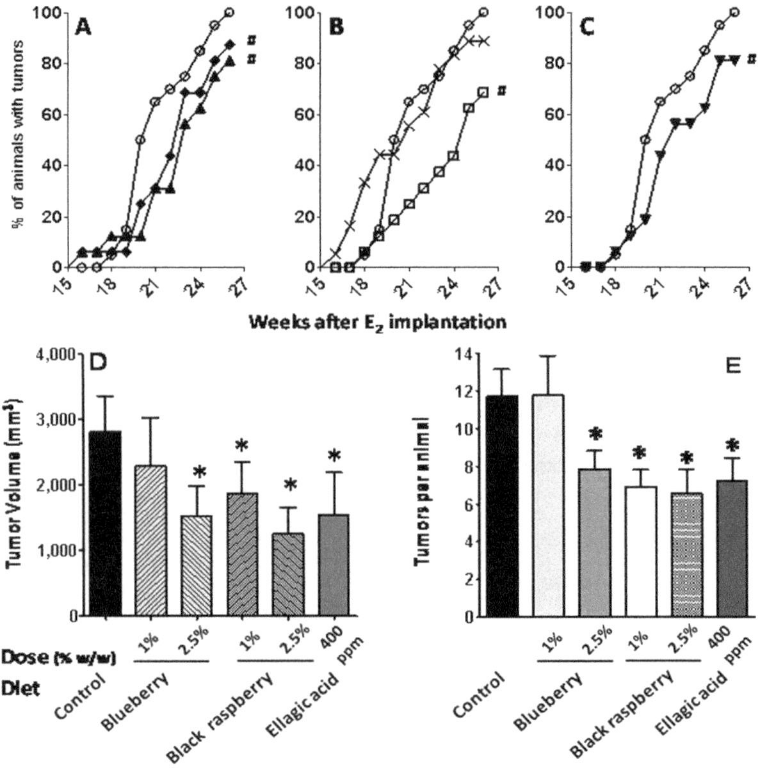

Fig. 9.4 Comparison of tumor indices in berry- or acid – fed animals. Tumor incidence (%) among animals fed control diet (**a–c**) and either black raspberry (**b**) or ellagic acid (**c**) diets. The tumor incidence is calculated based on the number animals per group with palpable tumors and measured until 26 weeks after implantation with 9 mg E_2. In animals fed control diet 100% tumor incidence occurred at 26 weeks. The animals supplemented with black raspberry at both doses 1 and 2.5% (**a**), blueberry at 2.5% (**b**), and 400 ppm ellagic acid (**c**) had significantly less tumor incidence (log rank test, $p < 0.005$; denoted by #) at 26 weeks; 1% blueberry did not differ significantly from the control (**b**). Tumor volume (**d**) and multiplicity (**e**) among animals fed control or supplemented diets. Data presented is mean ± SE and significant differences are marked by an asterisk

More recent studies with berries supplemented at a dose of 5% in the diet showed no significant differences in body weight gain or diet intake, suggesting no toxicity of a higher dose of the berries in the diet. Tumor palpation from 14 weeks till termination revealed a tumor latency of 84 days in control group. A clear dose response for the berry diets was observed with regard to tumor latency. The 5% blueberry and black raspberry diets delayed the appearance of first tumor by 24 and 39 days ($P = 0.04$), respectively, compared to 18 and 20 days, with a 2.5% dose (and not significant). Although, there was a significant reduction in tumor volume by blueberry (50% reduction) and black raspberry (42.5% reduction) diets, a clear dose-response could not be demonstrated. However, at the higher dose of 5%, blueberry appears to elicit more protection than black raspberry (Ravoori et al., 2009, 2010). Similar reductions were observed with the tumor multiplicity as well, for both diets. The most significant finding is the high effectiveness of black raspberry in delaying the incidence of first tumor by up to 5 weeks (Ravoori et al., 2009).

1.5 Correlation Between Chemopreventive Potential and Anthocyanin Profiles of Blueberry and Black Raspberry

The concentration of total phenolics in black raspberry and blueberry were 17.2 and 4.3 mg/g dry weight, respectively (Fig. 9.5a). The black raspberry diet at each dose (1–5%) provided typically has a much higher total phenolic and anthocyanin content than the blueberry diet (Table 9.2). However, when the anthocyanin spectrum is measured, blueberry has a wider spectrum of anthocyanins but in lower quantities, while black raspberry contains predominantly one anthocyanin but in much higher amounts (Fig. 9.5b). Black raspberry contains almost exclusively cyanidin glycosides (97.4%), while blueberry contains five major anthocyanins: glycosides of cyanidin (7.7%); delphinidin (31.2%); peonidin (18.6%); petunidin (8.8%); and malvidin (33.8%) (Fig. 9.5b). This diverse spectrum of anthocyanins might explain the higher protection of a 5% blueberry diet in reducing tumor volume compared to a 5% black raspberry diet as noted previously. A recent report shows that delphinidin is more cytotoxic than cyanidin to ER+ MCF7 cells, whereas cyanidin reduced the levels of ER itself (Fernandes et al., 2010). In our studies (Ravoori S, Kausar H, Gupta RC, unpublished data), MCF-7 cells treated with delphinidin, cyanidin, malvidin, petunidin, and peonidin either individually or as a mixture showed antiproliferative effects in the following order: mixture > delphinidin > malvidin > peonidin > cyanidin > petunidin. This is clearly indicative of the synergistic effects of the anthocyanidins when present as a mixture, but also that delphinidin is a more potent antagonist of breast cancer cell proliferation than cyanidin. Delphinidin

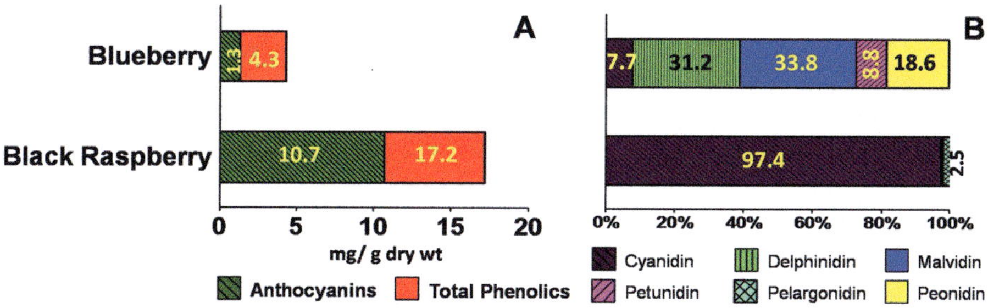

Fig. 9.5 **a** The total phenolics and anthocyanin contents of black raspberry and blueberry used in our rodent studies were measured by generating HPLC fingerprints of phenolics-enriched extracts of indicated berries (Aiyer et al., 2008a) Extracts were analyzed using a Premier C18 reversed phase column with UV detection at 250 nm. **b** Anthocyanin spectrum interpreted from data derived from Wada and Ou (2002) and Wu et al. (2006)

has also been shown to interact with the EGFR pathway and cause apoptosis in breast cancer cells via the mitogen-activated protein kinase pathway (Afaq et al., 2008). This effect is supported by our in vivo data where blueberry diet, regardless of the dose, consistently showed a higher inhibition of cell proliferation during early stages of E_2-treatment than the black raspberry diet (Fig. 9.1a) (Aiyer et al., 2008a). Collectively, these data suggest that despite twofold and eightfold lower contents of total phenolics and anthocyanins, respectively in blueberry than in black raspberry, the former elicits higher antiproliferation of estrogen-treated mammary tissue than the latter. This can be attributed to the presence of a wider spectrum of anthocyanins and their possible synergistic effects.

1.6 Translation to Community and Clinical Nutrition

In order to establish the translational relevance of our studies, we calculated the human equivalent for berry intakes in rodent studies using allometric calculations. Allometric scaling involves using either body weight or caloric consumption data to extrapolate rodent doses to human equivalent (Schneider et al., 2004; Reagan-Shaw et al., 2008; Hao et al., 2009). We used the latter approach as we believe that a scaling based on caloric intake is more appropriate for translational purpose as these berries were provided via the dietary route. Box 9.1 shows the basic methods of calculation and a comparison between the two approaches for a 1% (w/w) dose. Human equivalent dose values of berry consumption for 1, 2.5 and 5% berry diets is calculated based on caloric intake and tabulated (Table 9.3). The allometric scaling calculations show that an average pre-menopausal woman with a 2,000 kcal/day caloric intake needs a minimum of 1 cup of fresh/frozen berries every day to significantly reduce the carcinogenic effects of circulating E_2. Not only is this meaningful, but is also easily achievable and highly translatable. Berries can be incorporated in the diet in the fresh, frozen or dried forms. As berries are already a part of the American culinary repertoire, the adaptation of these doses for a community nutrition setting can be easily adapted.

The time from diagnosis of neoplastic disease until the time of treatment varies for most cancer types. Based on data obtained from Kentucky Cancer Registry during the period of 1995–2005, our preliminary analyses have revealed that nearly 25% of breast cancer patients undergo a 3 week waiting period since the time of diagnosis before any treatment is administered (Groves and Gupta, 2009). This “lead time” between diagnosis and treatment provides a novel window of opportunity for the clinical trial of nutritional supplements such as berries (Groves and Gupta, 2009). The diversity of phytochemicals in berries provides additive and/or synergistic activity and could potentially target multiple processes in estrogen-mediated carcinogenesis favorably. Identification of specific molecular markers modulated by the berry phytochemicals will enable higher translatability. In effect, patients diagnosed with breast cancer could be provided with berry supplements during this waiting period and the effect of these supplements on biomarkers in both the tumor

Table 9.3 Total phenolic, anthocyanin and ellagic acid content of berry diets used in rodent studies and recommended human equivalents for berry consumption based on allometric calculations

		Control diet	Blueberry diet			Black raspberry diet			Ellagic acid diet
	Units	AIN-93M	1%	2.5%	5%	1%	2.5%	5%	400 ppm
Total ellagic acid[a]	ppm	–	<1	<2.5	< 5.0	20	50	100	400
Total anthocyanins[b]	mg/g dry wt	–	13	32.5	65	107	267.5	535	–
Total phenolics[c]	mg/g dry wt	–	43	107.5	215	172	430	860	400
Average feed intake (mean ± SD)[d]	g/rat/day	9.35 ± 0.7	10.02 ± 0.85	9.84± 0.65	9.53 ± 0.3	9.41 ± 1.0	9.63 ± 1.0	10.0 ± 0.6	9.58 ± 0.75
Berry intake based on feed consumption[e] (∼10 g/rat/day)[d]	mg	–	100	250	500	100	250	500	NA
Berry consumed based on caloric intake (1 g feed = 4 kcal)[f]	mg/kcal/day	–	2.5	6.25	12.5	2.5	6.25	12.5	0.01
Allometric scaling to human consumption (2,000 kcal/day)[g]	g dried berry powder	–	5	12.5	25	5	12.5	25	0.02
Common conversion for dried berries[h]	Tbsp/d	–	0.5	1.25	2.5	0.5	1.25	2.5	NA
Common conversion for fresh berries[i]	Cups/d	–	0.4	1	2	0.4	1	2	–

Abbreviations: BB, Blueberry; BRB, Black raspberry; EA, Ellagic acid; NA, Not applicable.

[a,b,c]The equivalent content of ellagic acid and total anthocyanins in the blueberry and black raspberry diets when supplemented at 1, 2.5 and 5% (w/w) are derived from previously published reports (Daniel et al., 1989; Wu et al., 2006; Aiyer et al., 2008b).

[d]Feed intake of the rats consuming different diets was measured for a period of 5 days. It was assessed by subtracting the unused diet after 5 days from the initial known amount provided per cage, then dividing that by the number of rats in the cage and is represented as g/rat/day. This measurement was performed periodically throughout the study and averaged for performing the allometric scaling calculations. Supplementation with berries did not significantly alter the feed intake. Data presented is the mean ± SD of 13 individual measurements over a period of 30 weeks during the course of the study.

[e]Average diet intake in ACI rats was estimated to be10 g/rat/day for ease of calculations.

[f]Based on information in Harlan-Teklad product literature available at (www.harlan.com).

[g]Allometric scaling calculations based on caloric demand are explained further in Materials and Methods.

[h,i]Approximate measures based on food exchange lists for diabetics provided by the American Dietetic Association at http://www.eatright.org/ada/files/Fruits.pdf. 1 g dried berries = 10 g fresh berries.

as well as the adjacent normal tissue could be assessed. Further, there are nearly two million breast cancer survivors who have undergone chemotherapy following breast conserving surgery after their diagnosis that essentially receive no form of intervention whatsoever. This area of research remains largely unexplored and could be effectively utilized to study the effect of nutritional supplementation on biomarkers of breast tumors. The outcome from such studies, with berries for example, can therefore benefit breast cancer survivors who are at a higher risk for secondary cancers.

In summary, combined data from an animal model of breast cancer that is highly relevant to the human scenario suggests that berries at doses as low as 1% powder (w/w) can elicit significant reductions in E_2-mediated tumor indices. The primary mechanisms by which dietary berries prevent mammary tumors include modulation of E_2-metabolizing enzymes, reduction in DNA damage, decreased circulating prolactin levels, antiestrogenic, and antiproliferative actions. Translation of the rodent doses to human equivalents using allometric scaling reveals that an average woman needs approximately only a cup of fresh/frozen berries daily to achieve significant protection from the risk posed by high circulating E_2-levels. The case for the use of berries in breast cancer prevention is strong because berries have been used for centuries without any reported adverse side effects (other than allergic reactions in some), they are a part of the Western culinary tradition, their tolerability studies are positive, their protective nutrients are bioavailable (Stoner et al., 2005), and they show anti-estrogenic, antioxidant, anti-inflammatory, anti-angiogenic and pro-apoptotic activities that will be beneficial in breast cancer prevention. It is also evident that simple and effective nutritional intervention strategies using berries can be developed to be tested in a clinical research setting either prior to or as adjuvant to the traditional treatment(s) to benefit breast cancer patients and in survivors who receive no prophylactic treatment prior to the recurrence of cancer.

Box 9.1 Methods of allometric scaling conversions for extrapolating rodent intakes of berry diets into human equivalents

Calculation based on body surface area for 1% (w/w) dose

Average feed intake/rat/day- 10 g
Berry dose/rat/day @1% (w/w) supplement- 100 mg
Average body weight of female ACI rat- 200 g[1] (0.2 kg)
Intake of dried berries (mg/kg body weight) @ 1% = 100 mg/0.2 kg = 500 mg

Human Equivalent Dose (mg/kg) = Animal dose (mg/kg) × (Animal K_m [6 for rats]/Human K_m [37 for 60 kg adult])[2] where K_m *factor* is the body weight (kg) divided by body surface area (m^2)

HED for berries @ 1% dose = 500 mg × (6/37) = 81 mg (equivalent of 0.8 g of fresh berries).

1. The average weight of each group over the entire study period rounded to the nearest hundred g for ease of calculations.
2. The allometric scaling based on body weight was done as described in (Reagan-Shaw et al., 2008).

Calculation based on caloric intake for a 1% (w/w) dose

Average feed intake/rat/day- 10 g
Berry dose/rat/day @1% (w/w) supplement = 1% of 10 g = 100 mg
Average calories consumed/rat/day 40 kcal[3] (based on 4 kcal/g diet)
Dose of berries (mg/kg body weight) @ 1% = 100 mg/40 kcal = 2.5 mg
Average caloric intake for a 60 kg human 2,000 kcal

Human Equivalent Dose (mg dried berries/day) = 2.5 mg × 2,000 kcal = 5,000 mg or 5 g

3. The allometric scaling calculations based on caloric demand were done as described (Hao et al., 2009 and Schneider et al., 2004).

Acknowledgment The authors would like to acknowledge Dr. Manicka V. Vadhanam for support during the initial studies using the ACI rat model in the laboratory. This research was supported by NIH grants CA-118114, CA-90892, and CA-92758 and Agnes Brown Duggan Endowment. Dr. Harini S. Aiyer was a graduate student of Dr. Ramesh Gupta when she conducted a large part of the berry intervention studies described here. Dr. Ramesh Gupta holds the Agnes Brown Duggan Chair in Oncological Research.

References

ACS (2007a) Breast cancer facts and figures-2007. American Cancer Society, Atlanta, GA

ACS (2007b) Cancer facts and figures-2007. American Cancer Society, Atlanta, GA

ACS (2009) Cancer Facts and Figures-2009. American Cancer Society, Atlanta, GA

Adamovic T, Roshani L, Chen L, Schaffer BS, Helou K, Levan G, Olsson B, Shull JD (2007) Nonrandom pattern of chromosome aberrations in 17beta-estradiol-induced rat mammary tumors: indications of distinct pathways for tumor development. Genes Chromosomes Cancer 46:459–469

Adams LS, Zhang Y, Seeram NP, Heber D, Chen S (2010) Pomegranate ellagitannin-derived compounds exhibit antiproliferative and antiaromatase activity in breast cancer cells in vitro. Cancer Prev Res (Phila Pa) 3:108–113

Afaq F, Zaman N, Khan N, Syed DN, Sarfaraz S, Zaid MA, Mukhtar H (2008) Inhibition of epidermal growth factor receptor signaling pathway by delphinidin, an anthocyanidin in pigmented fruits and vegetables. Int J Cancer 123:1508–1515

Ahn D, Putt D, Kresty L, Stoner GD, Fromm D, Hollenberg PF (1996) The effects of dietary ellagic acid on rat hepatic and esophageal mucosal cytochromes P450 and phase II enzymes. Carcinogenesis 17:821–828

Aiyer HS, Gupta RC (2010) Berries and ellagic acid prevent estrogen-induced mammary tumorigenesis by modulating enzymes of estrogen metabolism. Cancer Prev Res (Phila) 3: 727–737

Aiyer HS, Kichambare S, Gupta RC (2008b) Prevention of oxidative DNA damage by bioactive berry components. Nutr Cancer 60(Suppl 1):36–42

Aiyer HS, Li Y, Liu QH, Reuter N, Martin RC (2010) Dietary freeze-dried black raspberry's effect on cellular antioxidant status during reflux-induced esophagitis in rats. Nutrition, in press

Aiyer H, Ravoori S, Schultz D, Gupta RC (2008a) The effect of dietary berries and ellagic acid on cell proliferation, estrogen-metabolizing enzymes and tumor indices in an estrogen-induced rat mammary tumor model. Proceedings of the International Conference on New Developments in Drug Discovery from Natural Products and Traditional Medicines.

Aiyer HS, Srinivasan C, Gupta RC (2008c) Dietary berries and ellagic acid diminish estrogen-mediated mammary tumorigenesis in ACI rats. Nutr Cancer 60:227–234

Aiyer HS, Vadhanam MV, Gupta RC (2002) Efficacy of cancer chemopreventive agents in protecting against oxidative DNA damage from Cu^{2+}-mediated activation of 4-hydroxy estradiol. Am Assoc Cancer Res 43:1146

Aiyer HS, Vadhanam MV, Stoyanova R, Caprio GD, Clapper ML, Gupta RC (2008d) Dietary berries and ellagic acid prevent oxidative DNA damage and modulate expression of DNA repair genes. Int J Mol Sci 9:327–341

Althuis MD, Dozier JM, Anderson WF, Devesa SS, Brinton LA (2005) Global trends in breast cancer incidence and mortality 1973–1997. Int J Epidemiol 34:405–412

Amir E, Freedman OC, Seruga B, Evans DG (2010) Assessing women at high risk of breast cancer: a review of risk assessment models. J Natl Cancer Inst 102:680–691

Balfe PJ, McCann AH, Welch HM, Kerin MJ (2004) Estrogen receptor beta and breast cancer. Eur J Surg Oncol 30:1043–1050

Bansal S, Kausar H, Aqil F, Vadhanam M, Gupta R (2010) Polymeric implants enhance bioavailability of curcumin by providing a continous ("24/7") delivery system. Proc Am Assoc Cancer Res 51:Abst 1880

Bhat HK, Calaf G, Hei TK, Loya T, Vadgama JV (2003) Critical role of oxidative stress in estrogen-induced carcinogenesis. Proc Natl Acad Sci USA 100:3913–3918

Blackshear PE (2001) Genetically engineered rodent models of mammary gland carcinogenesis: an overview. Toxicol Pathol 29:105–116

Blank EW, Wong PY, Lakshmanaswamy R, Guzman R, Nandi S (2008) Both ovarian hormones estrogen and progesterone are necessary for hormonal mammary carcinogenesis in ovariectomized ACI rats. Proc Natl Acad Sci USA 105:3527–3532

Boivin D, Blanchette M, Barrette S, Moghrabi A, Beliveau R (2007) Inhibition of cancer cell proliferation and suppression of TNF-induced activation of NFkappaB by edible berry juice. Anticancer Res 27:937–948

Brown ML, Goldie S, Draisma G, Harford J, Lipscomb J (2006) Health service interventions for cancer control in developing countries. In: Jamison DT, Breman JG, Measham AR, Alleyne G, Claeson M, Evans DB, Jha P, Mills A, Musgrove P (eds) Disease control in developing countries. Oxford University Press, New York, NY, pp 569–589

Canfell K, Banks E, Moa AM, Beral V (2008) Decrease in breast cancer incidence following a rapid fall in use of hormone replacement therapy in Australia. Med J Aust 188:641–644

Cano A, Hermenegildo C (2000) The endometrial effects of SERMs. Hum Reprod Update 6: 244–254

Cavalieri E, Frenkel K, Liehr JG, Rogan E, Roy D (2000) Estrogens as endogenous genotoxic agents – DNA adducts and mutations. J Natl Cancer Inst Monogr 27:75–93

Cavalieri EL, Higginbotham S, Ramakrishna NV, Devanesan PD, Todorovic R, Rogan EG, Salmasi S (1991) Comparative dose-response tumorigenicity studies of dibenzo[alpha,l]pyrene versus

7,12-dimethylbenz[alpha]anthracene, benzo[alpha]pyrene and two dibenzo[alpha,l]pyrene dihydrodiols in mouse skin and rat mammary gland. Carcinogenesis 12: 1939–1944
Chen S, Bangaru ML, Sneade L, Dunckley JA, Ben-Jonathan N, Kansra S (2009) Epidermal growth factor receptor cross-talks with ligand-occupied estrogen receptor-alpha to modulate both lactotroph proliferation and prolactin gene expression. Am J Physiol Endocrinol Metab 297:E331–E339
Clarke R (1996) Animal models of breast cancer: their diversity and role in biomedical research. Breast Cancer Res Treat 39:1–6
Clarke R, Leonessa F, Welch JN, Skaar TC (2001) Cellular and molecular pharmacology of antiestrogen action and resistance. Pharmacol Rev 53:25–71
Cranney A, Adachi JD (2005) Benefit-risk assessment of raloxifene in postmenopausal osteoporosis. Drug Saf 28:721–730
Cribb AE, Knight MJ, Dryer D, Guernsey J, Hender K, Tesch M, Saleh TM (2006) Role of polymorphic human cytochrome P450 enzymes in estrone oxidation. Cancer Epidemiol Biomarkers Prev 15:551–558
Cutts JH, Noble RL (1964) Estrone-induced Mammary Tumors in the RAT. I. Induction and behavior of tumors. Cancer Res 24:1116–1123
Daniel EM, Krupnick AS, Heur Y, Blinzler JA, Nims RW, Stoner GD (1989) Extraction, stability and quantitation of ellagic acid in various fruits and nuts. J Food Compost Anal 2:338–349
Dickson RB, Stancel GM (2000) Estrogen receptor-mediated processes in normal and cancer cells. J Natl Cancer Inst Monogr 27:135–145
Dunning WF, Curtis MR, Segaloff A (1947) Strain differences in response to diethylstilbesterol and the induction of mammary gland and bladder cancer in the rat. Cancer Res 7: 511–521
Dunning WF, Curtis MR, Segaloff A (1953) Strain differences in response to estrone and the induction of mammary gland, adrenal, and bladder cancer in rats. Cancer Res 13:147–152
Fernandes I, Faria A, Azevedo J, Soares S, Calhau C, De Freitas V, Mateus N (2010) Influence of anthocyanins, derivative pigments and other catechol and pyrogallol-type phenolics on breast cancer cell proliferation. J Agric Food Chem 58:3785–3792
Gould KA, Tochacek M, Schaffer BS, Reindl TM, Murrin CR, Lachel CM, VanderWoude EA, Pennington KL, Flood LA, Bynote KK, Meza JL, Newton MA, Shull JD (2004) Genetic determination of susceptibility to estrogen-induced mammary cancer in the ACI rat: mapping of Emca1 and Emca2 to chromosomes 5 and 18. Genetics 168:2113–2125
Groves FD, Gupta RC (2009) Lead time between diagnosis and treatment of cancer in Kentucky. Soc Epidemiol Res 42:Abst 203
Gupta RC, Bansal SS, Aqil F, Cao P, Jeyabalan J, Russell GK, Ravoori S, Vadhanam MV (2009a) A novel concept in delivering chemopreventive compounds. Proc Am Assoc Cancer Res 50: Abst 944
Gupta RC, Jeyabalan J, Aqil F, Vadhanam MV, Schultz DJ, Ravoori S (2009b) Potent chemoprotective activity of Apiaceae spices. NCI Translational Science Meeting
Gutmann DH, Hunter-Schaedle K, Shannon KM (2006) Harnessing preclinical mouse models to inform human clinical cancer trials. J Clin Invest 116:847–852
Hankinson SE, Colditz GA, Willett WC (2004) Towards an integrated model for breast cancer etiology: the lifelong interplay of genes, lifestyle, and hormones. Breast Cancer Res 6: 213–218
Hao J, Zhang B, Liu B, Lee M, Hao X, Reuhl KR, Chen X, Yang CS (2009) Effect of alpha-tocopherol, N-acetylcysteine and omeprazole on esophageal adenocarcinoma formation in a rat surgical model. Int J Cancer 124:1270–1275
Hiraku Y, Yamashita N, Nishiguchi M, Kawanishi S (2001) Catechol estrogens induce oxidative DNA damage and estradiol enhances cell proliferation. Int J Cancer 92:333–337
Holtzman S (1988) Retinyl acetate inhibits estrogen-induced mammary carcinogenesis in female ACI rats. Carcinogenesis 9:305–307

Holtzman S, Stone JP, Shellabarger CJ (1981) Synergism of estrogens and X-rays in mammary carcinogenesis in female ACI rats. J Natl Cancer Inst 67:455–459
Huggins C, Briziarelli G, Sutton H Jr (1959) Rapid induction of mammary carcinoma in the rat and the influence of hormones on the tumors. J Exp Med 109:25–42
Huggins C, Grand LC, Brillantes FP (1961) Mammary cancer induced by a single feeding of polymucular hydrocarbons, and its suppression. Nature 189:204–207
Jordan VC (2006) Optimising endocrine approaches for the chemoprevention of breast cancer beyond the study of tamoxifen and raloxifene (STAR) trial. Eur J Cancer 42:2909–2913
Jordan VC (2008) Tamoxifen: catalyst for the change to targeted therapy. Eur J Cancer 44:30–38
Kim JB, O'Hare MJ, Stein R (2004) Models of breast cancer: is merging human and animal models the future? Breast Cancer Res 6:22–30
Kurz SG, Hansen KK, McLaughlin MT, Shivaswamy V, Schaffer BS, Gould KA, McComb RD, Meza JL, Shull JD (2008) Tissue-specific actions of the Ept1, Ept2, Ept6, and Ept9 genetic determinants of responsiveness to estrogens in the female rat. Endocrinology 149: 3850–3859
Larrosa M, Gonzalez-Sarrias A, Garcia-Conesa MT, Tomas-Barberan FA, Espin JC (2006) Urolithins, ellagic acid-derived metabolites produced by human colonic microflora, exhibit estrogenic and antiestrogenic activities. J Agric Food Chem 54:1611–1620
Li JJ, Li SA, Klicka JK, Parsons JA, Lam LK (1983) Relative carcinogenic activity of various synthetic and natural estrogens in the Syrian hamster kidney. Cancer Res 43: 5200–5204
Li JJ, Papa D, Davis MF, Weroha SJ, Aldaz CM, El-Bayoumy K, Ballenger J, Tawfik O, Li SA (2002a) Ploidy differences between hormone- and chemical carcinogen-induced rat mammary neoplasms: comparison to invasive human ductal breast cancer. Mol Carcinog 33:56–65
Li Y, Trush MA, Yager JD (1994) DNA damage caused by reactive oxygen species originating from a copper-dependent oxidation of the 2-hydroxy catechol of estradiol. Carcinogenesis 15: 1421–1427
Li JJ, Weroha SJ, Lingle WL, Papa D, Salisbury JL, Li SA (2004) Estrogen mediates Aurora-A overexpression, centrosome amplification, chromosomal instability, and breast cancer in female ACI rats. Proc Natl Acad Sci USA 101:18123–18128
Li SA, Weroha SJ, Tawfik O, Li JJ (2002b) Prevention of solely estrogen-induced mammary tumors in female aci rats by tamoxifen: evidence for estrogen receptor mediation. J Endocrinol 175:297–305
Liehr JG (2000) Is estradiol a genotoxic mutagenic carcinogen? Endocr Rev 21:40–54
Liehr JG (2001) Genotoxicity of the steroidal oestrogens oestrone and oestradiol: possible mechanism of uterine and mammary cancer development. Hum Reprod Update 7:273–281
Liehr JG, Ricci MJ (1996) 4-Hydroxylation of estrogens as marker of human mammary tumors. Proc Natl Acad Sci USA 93:3294–3296
Lyle SF, Wright K, Collins DC (1984) Comparative effects of tamoxifen and bromocriptine on prolactin and pituitary weight in estradiol-treated male rats. Cancer 53:1473–1477
Mense SM, Singh B, Remotti F, Liu X, Bhat HK (2009) Vitamin C and alpha-naphthoflavone prevent estrogen-induced mammary tumors and decrease oxidative stress in female ACI rats. Carcinogenesis 30:1202–1208
Mesia-Vela S, Sanchez RI, Reuhl KR, Conney AH, Kauffman FC (2006) Phenobarbital treatment inhibits the formation of estradiol-dependent mammary tumors in the August-Copenhagen Irish rat. J Pharmacol Exp Ther 317:590–597
Mesia-Vela S, Sanchez RI, Roberts KG, Reuhl KR, Conney AH, Kauffman FC (2008) Dietary clofibrate stimulates the formation and size of estradiol-induced breast tumors in female August-Copenhagen Irish (ACI) rats. Toxicology 246:63–72
Morrow M, Jordan VC (2000) Tamoxifen for the prevention of breast cancer in the high-risk woman. Ann Surg Oncol 7:67–71
Nguyen V, Tang J, Oroudjev E, Lee CJ, Marasigan C, Wilson L, Ayoub G (2010) Cytotoxic effects of bilberry extract on MCF7-GFP-tubulin breast cancer cells. J Med Food 13:278–285

Oldenburg RA, Kroeze-Jansema K, Kraan J, Morreau H, Klijn JG, Hoogerbrugge N, Ligtenberg MJ, van Asperen CJ, Vasen HF, Meijers C, Meijers-Heijboer H, de Bock TH, Cornelisse CJ, Devilee P (2003) The CHEK2*1100delC variant acts as a breast cancer risk modifier in non-BRCA1/BRCA2 multiple-case families. Cancer Res 63:8153–8157
Oyama T, Morita M, Isse T, Kagawa N, Nakata S, So T, Mizukami M, Ichiki Y, Ono K, Sugaya M, Uramoto H, Yoshimatsu T, Hanagiri T, Sugio K, Kawamoto T, Yasumoto K (2005) Immunohistochemical evaluation of cytochrome P450 (CYP) and p53 in breast cancer. Front Biosci 10:1156–1161
Paluszczak J, Krajka-Kuzniak V, Baer-Dubowska W (2010) The effect of dietary polyphenols on the epigenetic regulation of gene expression in MCF7 breast cancer cells. Toxicol Lett 192: 119–125
Papoutsi Z, Kassi E, Tsiapara A, Fokialakis N, Chrousos GP, Moutsatsou P (2005) Evaluation of estrogenic/antiestrogenic activity of ellagic acid via the estrogen receptor subtypes ERalpha and ERbeta. J Agric Food Chem 53:7715–7720
Parkin DM (2009) Is the recent fall in incidence of post-menopausal breast cancer in UK related to changes in use of hormone replacement therapy? Eur J Cancer 45:1649–1653
Parkin DM, Bray F, Ferlay J, Pisani P (2005) Global cancer statistics, 2002. Ca Cancer J Clin 55:74–108
Parkin DM, Fernandez LM (2006) Use of statistics to assess the global burden of breast cancer. Breast J 12(Suppl 1):S70–S80
Petrek JA, Sandberg WA, Cole MN, Silberman MS, Collins DC (1985) The inhibitory effect of caffeine on hormone-induced rat breast cancer. Cancer 56:1977–1981
Porter P (2008) "Westernizing" women's risks? Breast cancer in lower-income countries. N Engl J Med 358:213–216
Powles TJ (2002) Anti-oestrogenic prevention of breast cancer–the make or break point. Nat Rev Cancer 2:787–794
Ravoori S, Aqil F, Gupta RC (2009) Prevention of breast cancers in rat model by berries and potential mechanisms. Am Assoc Cancer Res 50:Abst 931
Ravoori S, Kausar H, Aqil F, Gupta RC (2010) Distinct molecular targets of blueberry and black raspberry in breast cancer prevention. Proc Am Assoc Cancer Res 51:Abst 1887
Ravoori S, Vadhanam M, Kausar H, Moktar A, Vuppalapati P, Schultz D, Gupta R (2008) Effect of select berries on estrogen-induced mammary tissue proliferation. Proc Am Assoc Cancer Res 49:Abst 3821
Ravoori S, Vadhanam MV, Sahoo S, Srinivasan C, Gupta RC (2007) Mammary tumor induction in ACI rats exposed to low levels of 17beta-estradiol. Int J Oncol 31:113–120
Reagan-Shaw S, Nihal M, Ahmad N (2008) Dose translation from animal to human studies revisited. FASEB J 22:659–661
Russo J, Gusterson BA, Rogers AE, Russo IH, Wellings SR, van Zwieten MJ (1990) Comparative study of human and rat mammary tumorigenesis. Lab Invest 62:244–278
Russo J, Russo IH (2004) Genotoxicity of steroidal estrogens. Trends Endocrinol Metab 15: 211–214
Schaffer BS, Lachel CM, Pennington KL, Murrin CR, Strecker TE, Tochacek M, Gould KA, Meza JL, McComb RD, Shull JD (2006) Genetic bases of estrogen-induced tumorigenesis in the rat: mapping of loci controlling susceptibility to mammary cancer in a Brown Norway x ACI intercross. Cancer Res 66:7793–7800
Schmitt E, Stopper H (2001) Estrogenic activity of naturally occurring anthocyanidins. Nutr Cancer 41:145–149
Schneider K, Oltmanns J, Hassauer M (2004) Allometric principles for interspecies extrapolation in toxicological risk assessment – empirical investigations. Regul Toxicol Pharmacol 39: 334–347
Seeram NP, Adams LS, Zhang Y, Lee R, Sand D, Scheuller HS, Heber D (2006) Blackberry, black raspberry, blueberry, cranberry, red raspberry, and strawberry extracts inhibit growth and stimulate apoptosis of human cancer cells in vitro. J Agric Food Chem 54:9329–9339

Seradour B, Allemand H, Weill A, Ricordeau P (2009) Changes by age in breast cancer incidence, mammography screening and hormone therapy use in France from 2000 to 2006. Bull Cancer 96:E1–E6

Shepel LA, Gould MN (1999) The genetic components of susceptibility to breast cancer in the rat. Prog Exp Tumor Res 35:158–169

Shull JD, Spady TJ, Snyder MC, Johansson SL, Pennington KL (1997) Ovary-intact, but not ovariectomized female ACI rats treated with 17beta-estradiol rapidly develop mammary carcinoma. Carcinogenesis 18:1595–1601

Sims AH, Howell A, Howell SJ, Clarke RB (2007) Origins of breast cancer subtypes and therapeutic implications. Nat Clin Pract Oncol 4:516–525

Singh B, Mense SM, Remotti F, Liu X, Bhat HK (2009) Antioxidant butylated hydroxyanisole inhibits estrogen-induced breast carcinogenesis in female ACI rats. J Biochem Mol Toxicol 23:202–211

Singletary KW, Jung KJ, Giusti M (2007) Anthocyanin-rich grape extract blocks breast cell DNA damage. J Med Food 10:244–251

Smith WA, Freeman JW, Gupta RC (2001) Effect of chemopreventive agents on DNA adduction induced by the potent mammary carcinogen dibenzo[a,l]pyrene in the human breast cells MCF-7. Mutat Res 480-481:97–108

Snyderwine EG, Thorgeirsson UP, Venugopal M, Roberts-Thomson SJ (1998) Mammary gland carcinogenicity of 2-amino-1-methyl-6-phenylimidazo[4,5-b]pyridine in Sprague-Dawley rats on high- and low-fat diets. Nutr Cancer 31:160–167

Srinivasan P, Vadhanam MV, Arif JM, Gupta RC (2002) A rapid screening assay for antioxidant potential of natural and synthetic agents in vitro. Int J Oncol 20:983–986

Stoner GD, Sardo C, Apseloff G, Mullet D, Wargo W, Pound V, Singh A, Sanders J, Aziz R, Casto B, Sun X (2005) Pharmacokinetics of anthocyanins and ellagic acid in healthy volunteers fed freeze-dried black raspberries daily for 7 days. J Clin Pharmacol 45:1153–1164

Stoner GD, Dombkowski AA, Reen RK, Cukovic D, Salagrama S, Wang LS, Lechner JF (2008) Carcinogen-altered genes in rat esophagus positively modulated to normal levels of expression by both black raspberries and phenylethyl isothiocyanate. Cancer Res 68:6460–6467

Strecker TE, Spady TJ, Schaffer BS, Gould KA, Kaufman AE, Shen F, McLaughlin MT, Pennington KL, Meza JL, Shull JD (2005) Genetic bases of estrogen-induced pituitary tumorigenesis: identification of genetic loci determining estrogen-induced pituitary growth in reciprocal crosses between the ACI and Copenhagen rat strains. Genetics 169: 2189–2197

Studzinski G, Harrison L (2002) Genetic Basis for the Emergence and Progression of Breast Cancer. In: Donegan WL, Spratt JS (eds) Cancer of the Breast. Saunders, Philadelphia, PA, pp 169–179

Thompson HJ, Adlakha H, Singh M (1992) Effect of carcinogen dose and age at administration on induction of mammary carcinogenesis by 1-methyl-1-nitrosourea. Carcinogenesis 13: 1535–1539

Thompson PA, Ambrosone C (2000) Molecular epidemiology of genetic polymorphisms in estrogen metabolizing enzymes in human breast cancer. J Natl Cancer Inst Monogr 125–134

Thompson D, Easton D (2004) The genetic epidemiology of breast cancer genes. J Mammary Gland Biol Neoplasia 9:221–236

Thompson HJ, McGinley J, Rothhammer K, Singh M (1998) Ovarian hormone dependence of pre-malignant and malignant mammary gland lesions induced in pre-pubertal rats by 1-methyl-1-nitrosourea. Carcinogenesis 19:383–386

Thompson HJ, Singh M (2000) Rat models of premalignant breast disease. J Mammary Gland Biol Neoplasia 5:409–420

Thordarson G, Lee AV, McCarty M, Van Horn K, Chu O, Chou YC, Yang J, Guzman RC, Nandi S, Talamantes F (2001) Growth and characterization of N-methyl-N-nitrosourea-induced mammary tumors in intact and ovariectomized rats. Carcinogenesis 22:2039–2047

Vadhanam M, Aqil F, Bansal S, Cao P, Jeyabalan J, Ravoori S, Gupta R (2010) Controlled-release systemic delivery of chemopreventive agents – An update. Proc Am Assoc Cancer Res 51: Abst 5673
Vadhanam M, Ravoori S, Aqil F, Gupta R (2008) Ellagic acid administered by a novel, sustained drug-delivery system inhibits estrogen-induced mammary carcinogenicity. Proc Am Assoc Cancer Res 49:Abst 3835
Vahteristo P, Bartkova J, Eerola H, Syrjakoski K, Ojala S, Kilpivaara O, Tamminen A, Kononen J, Aittomaki K, Heikkila P, Holli K, Blomqvist C, Bartek J, Kallioniemi OP, Nevanlinna H (2002) A CHEK2 genetic variant contributing to a substantial fraction of familial breast cancer. Am J Hum Genet 71:432–438
Virnig BA, Tuttle TM, Shamliyan T, Kane RL (2010) Ductal carcinoma in situ of the breast: a systematic review of incidence, treatment, and outcomes. J Natl Cancer Inst 102:170–178
Wada L, Ou B (2002) Antioxidant activity and phenolic content of Oregon caneberries. J Agric Food Chem 50:3495–3500
Warren R, Harvie M, Howell A (2004) Strategies for managing breast cancer risk after the menopause. Treat Endocrinol 3:289–307
Welsch CW (1985) Host factors affecting the growth of carcinogen-induced rat mammary carcinomas: a review and tribute to Charles Brenton Huggins. Cancer Res 45:3415–3443
Weroha SJ, Li SA, Tawfik O, Li JJ (2006) Overexpression of cyclins D1 and D3 during estrogen-induced breast oncogenesis in female ACI rats. Carcinogenesis 27:491–498
Wu X, Beecher GR, Holden JM, Haytowitz DB, Gebhardt SE, Prior RL (2006) Concentrations of anthocyanins in common foods in the United States and estimation of normal consumption. J Agric Food Chem 54:4069–4075
Wu X, Prior RL (2005) Systematic identification and characterization of anthocyanins by HPLC-ESI-MS/MS in common foods in the United States: fruits and berries. J Agric Food Chem 53:2589–2599
Yager JD (2000) Endogenous estrogens as carcinogens through metabolic activation. J Natl Cancer Inst Monogr 27:67–73
Zhu BT, Conney AH (1998) Functional role of estrogen metabolism in target cells: review and perspectives. Carcinogenesis 19:1–27

Chapter 10
Inhibition of Oral Cancer in Animal Models by Black Raspberries and Berry Components

Bruce C. Casto, Thomas J. Knobloch, and Christopher M. Weghorst

Abstract It is estimated that there will be 35,720 cases and 7,600 deaths resulting from oral cancer in the United States this year. Even more common worldwide, oral cancer is the 6th most prevalent cancer internationally, the majority of which are squamous cell carcinomas that have been etiologically linked to carcinogens in tobacco. Current surgical and adjuvant therapies remain only modestly effective and are often associated with significant physical and physiological side effects. Therefore, alternative or complementary intervention strategies, such as oral cancer chemoprevention, should be developed and tested in appropriate preclinical animal models of experimental oral carcinogenesis. The best characterized model of chemically-induced oral cancer, the hamster cheek pouch, has been employed to evaluate the ability of dietary lyophilized black raspberries (LBR) to inhibit oral tumors. Tumors induced by DMBA were significantly inhibited by the administration of dietary LBR. A discussion of berry components and inhibition of oral cancers in hamsters, rats, and mice is included. These data show that administration of berries or berry components effectively inhibit chemically-induced tumor formation in several comparative animal models of experimental oral carcinogenesis.

Keywords Oral cancer · Black raspberries · Berries · DMBA · Chemoprevention · Nutraceutical · Animal model · Preclinical · Food-based · Cancer prevention · Dietary · Hamster cheek pouch

Abbreviations

4NQO	4-Nitroquinoline-1-oxide
CCB	Complete Chemoprevention Bioassay
DMBA	7,12-dimethylbenz(a)anthracene
DMSO	Dimethylsulfoxide

B.C. Casto (✉)
Division of Environmental Health Sciences, College of Public Health, The Ohio State University, Columbus, OH 43210, USA
e-mail: casto.44@osu.edu

G.D. Stoner, N.P. Seeram (eds.), *Berries and Cancer Prevention*,
DOI 10.1007/978-1-4419-7554-6_10,

HCP	Hamster cheek pouch
IUPAC	International Union of Pure and Applied Chemists
LBR	Lyophilized black raspberries
PCB	Post-initiation Chemoprevention Bioassay
OSCC	Oral squamous cell carcinoma
AP-1	Activator protein 1
Bcl2	B-cell leukemia/lymphoma 2 gene (rodent homolog)
Cdkn2a	Cyclin-dependent kinase inhibitor 2A gene (rodent homolog)
Egfr	Epidermal growth factor receptor (rodent homolog)
Erbb2	v-erb-b2 erythroblastic leukemia viral oncogene homolog 2, neuro/glioblastoma derived oncogene (rodent homolog)
Hras1	Harvey rat sarcoma virus oncogene 1 (rodent homolog)
NFκB	Nuclear factor of kappa light polypeptide gene enhancer in B-cells protein
Pcna	Proliferating cell nuclear antigen gene (rodent homolog)
Trp53	Transformation related protein 53 gene (rodent homolog)

1 Oral Cancer as a Site for Chemoprevention

1.1 Oral Cancer

Oral cancer represents approximately 2.4% of the total cancers that will occur in the United States this year with an estimated 35,720 cases and 7,600 deaths (American Cancer Society, 2009). Even more common internationally, oral cancer is the 6th most prevalent cancer in the world (Mignogna et al., 2004; Parkin et al., 2005). The majority (90%) of these cancers are oral squamous cell carcinomas (OSCCs), which have been etiologically linked to the individual's exposure to known carcinogens, mainly in tobacco and alcohol (American Cancer Society, 2009). The overall prognosis for patients is poor, with a 5-year survival rate ranging from 54 to 65% (American Cancer Society, 2009). Present therapies for OSCC patients typically involve surgical resection (stages I and II), in combination with radiation (stages III and IV), and with chemotherapy for high risk patients with nodal involvement or metastases. In addition to the physical disfiguration associated with surgical procedures, there are significant complications following radiation therapy (tissue necrosis, fibrosis, atrophy, and xerostomia). Tumor recurrence is also a problem for oral cancer patients, as nearly 20% will exhibit locoregional recurrence within 18 months post-surgery, and an additional 22–42% of patients will present with a second primary tumor 5–8 years after their initial tumor diagnosis (Cooper et al., 1989; Leon et al., 1999). Unfortunately, despite important advances in OSCC treatment over the past 30 years, overall survival rates have remained relatively unchanged (American Cancer Society, 2009). Since current therapeutic protocols remain modestly effective and physically damaging, it is appropriate that alternative or complementary strategies, such as chemoprevention, be developed and tested in applicable preclinical model systems. These preclinical studies can be translated into early stage clinical investigations and potentially into standard of care practices.

1.2 Oral Cancer and Chemoprevention

The oral cavity is ideally suited for preclinical and clinical chemoprevention studies for several reasons. First, the anatomical location allows for rapid and largely non-intrusive accessibility to the tissue at risk. Second, chemopreventive agents can be accurately and directly administered to affected areas. Third, tissues can be readily biopsied, lesions accurately measured, and photo documentation acquired. Fourth, high risk populations primarily associated with coupled tobacco use and alcohol consumption are easily identified and readily available. Fifth, it has been proposed that the oral cavity may serve as a reliable surrogate for determining genetic and epigenetic changes that occur in other respiratory tissues due to cigarette smoking (Bhutani et al., 2008; Sidransky, 2008). One of the attractive characteristics of chemoprevention strategies is the extended window of opportunity during which intervention can begin and the desired outcomes obtained. Since the multistep process of cancer development involves the accumulation of critical genetic insults over a 10–20 year period of time and includes numerous molecular pathways, there are many points at which chemopreventive agents can intervene in disease progression. This may have special relevance to past smokers who remain at higher risk for oral cancer (Spira et al., 2004) and former OSCC patients who are free of disease after local therapy yet remain at high risk for both recurrent and second primary tumors. In these individuals, an important paradigm in cancer chemoprevention must be to inhibit the progression of premalignant lesions, such as oral dysplasias, into malignant OSCC.

1.3 Berry-Based Chemoprevention

Numerous epidemiological studies have shown a strong correlation between frequent consumption of fresh fruits and vegetables and a decreased risk of oral cancer (Pavia et al., 2006; Freedman et al., 2008). In support of these data, several preclinical studies in human cell cultures and animal models have been conducted that demonstrate the remarkable chemopreventive activity of two berry fruits, namely black raspberries and strawberries, that inhibit both human oral cancer cell growth in vitro (Han et al., 2005) and development of chemically-induced aerodigestive tract tumors in the oral cavity, esophagus, and colon in vivo (Carlton et al., 2001; Kresty et al., 2001; Casto et al., 2002; Harris et al., 2002). These studies in cell culture and animal models have employed lyophilized powders or extracts of ripe fruits containing a complex mixture of bioactive berry components. One major group of compounds present in these berry preparations is the anthocyanins of which the daily intake in humans is estimated to be 180–215 mg (Kühnau, 1976;

Hertog et al., 1993). Epidemiological evidence suggests that diets rich in anthocyanins (often indicated by blue, red, and purple colored fruits and vegetables) reduce the overall risk of cancer, especially in the esophagus, breast and colon (Colditz et al., 1985; Adlercreutz, 1998; Almendingen, Hofstad, and Vatn, 2004; Wang et al., 2009). There is also substantial laboratory evidence that anthocyanins and anthocyanin-rich extracts inhibit cell growth of various human and animal tumor cells in culture and demonstrate chemopreventive activity in animal models of colon, mammary, and skin cancer (Cooke et al., 2005; Fimognari et al., 2008). In addition to the diverse family of anthocyanins, there are numerous other phenolic compounds in berries that have demonstrated striking antioxidant and growth inhibitory activity in cell culture and remarkable chemopreventive activity in animal models of cancer (Wang and Lin, 2000; Stoner and Casto, 2004; Nichenametla et al., 2006; Stoner, 2009). These additional food-based chemopreventive compounds include the phenolic acids (caffeic, chlorogenic, ellagic, ferulic, gallic, p-coumaric, p-hydroxybenzoic, protocatechuic, and vanillic acids), the flavonols (isorhamntin, kaempferol, mycetrin, and quercetin), flavan-3-ols (catechins), and complex polyphenols (lignans, ellagitannin, and gallotannin). A review of the pharmacologic and chemopreventive activity of berries and individual berry components can be found in book chapters "Chemoprevention of Oral Carcinogenesis" by Tanaka (1995), "Chemoprevention by Fruit Phenolics" by Stoner and Casto (2004), "Berries" by Seeram (2006), and "Laboratory and Clinical Studies of Cancer Chemoprevention by Antioxidants in Berries" by Stoner et al. (2008).

2 Animal Models of Chemically-Induced Oral Cancer

The most commonly used animal models for chemically-induced oral cancer research are the hamster cheek pouch and the rat or mouse tongue/palate using the chemical carcinogens DMBA (IUPAC: 7,12-dimethylbenz(a)anthracene) or 4NQO (IUPAC: 4-nitro-1-oxidoquinolin-1-ium), respectively. Each model has its own advantages and disadvantages, but the sequence of events that characterize the development of oral carcinogenesis is represented in each.

2.1 *Hamster Oral Carcinogenesis Model*

The hamster cheek pouch (HCP) has been used since 1954 as a model for oral cavity cancer (Salley, 1954). This well-established model has been used to follow the early development of oral cancers (Polverini and Solt, 1988; Gimenez-Conti et al., 1990; Conti, 1991; Sacks et al., 1991) to identify and characterize some of the genetic alterations occurring early and late in the progression of OSCC (Solt and Shklar, 1982; Moroco et al., 1990; Shklar, 1999; Balasenthil et al., 2000), and for over 30 years, to investigate the effectiveness of selected food components as anti-cancer agents (Meng and Shyu, 1990; Tanaka, 1995; Balasubramanian and Govindasamy,

1996; Shklar and Schwartz, 1996; Li et al., 2002; Bhuvaneswari et al., 2004; Miller et al., 2004). Most experimental data in the HCP model have been accumulated using a prototypic polycyclic hydrocarbon (DMBA) that can be derived from a direct coal liquefaction process (Mahlum et al., 1984) and is metabolized by the same CYP1B1 enzyme (Buters et al., 1999) that is heavily involved in the biological processing of polycyclic hydrocarbons found in tobacco smoke (Thier et al., 2002). To more closely simulate tobacco smoke exposure, Schwartz et al. (2004) have described a hamster tongue assay using the even more potent tobacco smoke carcinogen, dibenzo(a,l)pyrene (Hecht, 2002; Mahadevan et al., 2005).

The HCP carcinogenesis model mimics many of the morphologic and physiologic characteristics that are seen in human OSCCs (Gimenez-Conti and Slaga, 1993; Schwartz et al., 2004; Vairaktaris et al., 2008) (Fig. 10.1). Similar molecular events are present in both human and hamster OSCC which may serve as viable biomarkers. As with human oral cancer, some tumors that develop in the HCP begin as verrucae or papillomas that become malignant and invasive, while other tumors evolve from relatively flat dysplastic lesions comparable to leukoplakias in human oral mucosa (Salley, 1957; Shklar, 1972; Conti, 1991). Chemically-induced HCP tumors exhibit many of the same genetic events that are present in human OSCC. These may include early *Hras1* mutations (Husain et al., 1989; Kwong et al., 1992), amplification and over-expression of *Erbb2* and *Egfr* (Wong and Biswas, 1987; Husain et al., 1989; Shin et al.,1990), and alterations in the *Trp53* (p53) and *Cdkn2a* (p16) tumor suppressor genes (Chang et al., 1996; Gimenez-Conti et al., 1996; Li et al., 2008). It has been estimated that greater than 75% of oral cancers are related to use of tobacco products. Since up to 40–50% of oral cancers are located in the buccal mucosa (Asian populations) and 40–50% are found on the tongue (US and European populations) (Warnakulasuriya, 2009), Schwartz et al. (2000) developed a hamster model using both the buccal mucosa and the lateral border of the tongue as sites of carcinogen application. Using DMBA at the two distinct anatomical sites resulted in differences in corresponding tumor aggressiveness, differentiation, invasiveness, and *Pcna*, *Trp53* and *Bcl2* expression.

2.2 Rat and Mouse Oral Carcinogenesis Models

Wallenuis and Lekholm (1973) first described the induction of oral dysplasia and tumors on the rat palate and other oral surfaces following several applications of 0.5% 4NQO. Since that time, several investigations have been published in which variations of this model have been used to produce palatal and tongue tumors in rats and mice that mimic the series of events that occur during oral cancer development in the human oral cavity (Nauta et al., 1995; Ribeiro et al., 2004; Vered et al., 2005; Kanojia and Vaidya, 2006; Vitale-Cross et al., 2009). 4NQO is a synthetic, water-soluble carcinogen that can be administered either by direct application or given in drinking water at typical levels of 20, 50, or 100 ppm. It has been described as a UV mimetic, since the kinetics of 4NQO-induced DNA repair resemble the

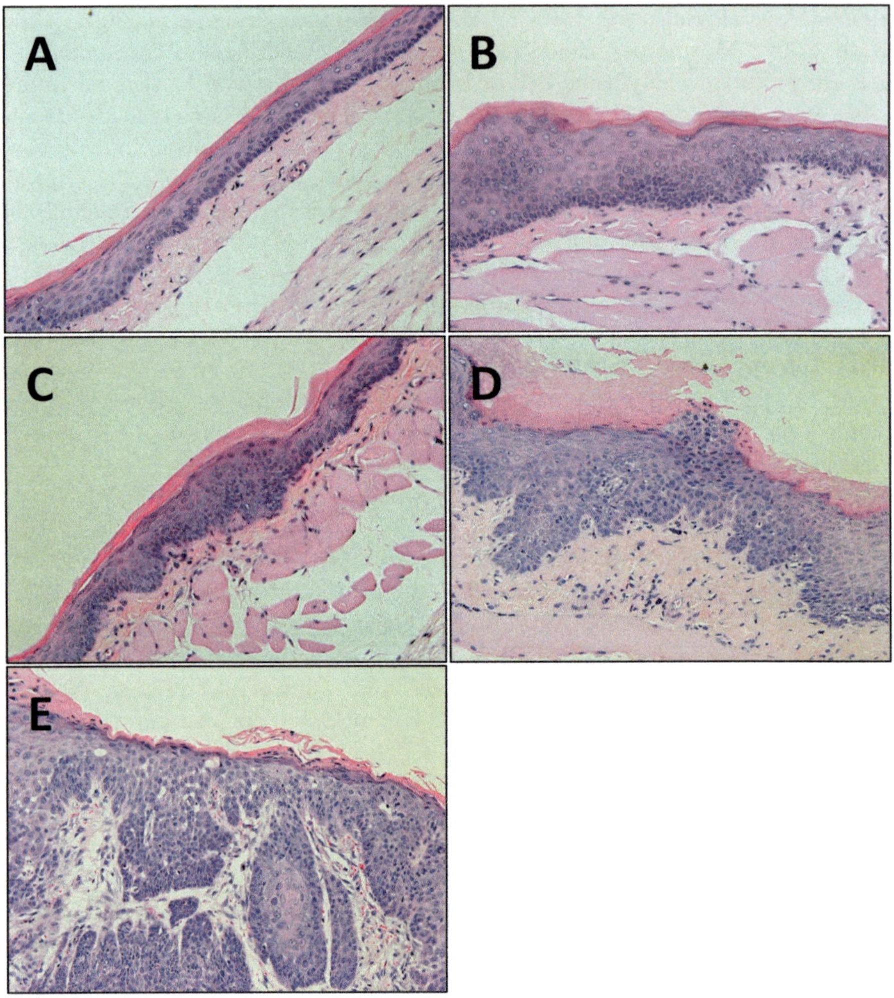

Fig. 10.1 DMBA-induced hamster cheek pouch oral carcinogenesis. Hamster cheek pouches were painted 3× per week with 0.2% DMBA in DMSO and collected 6 weeks after carcinogen exposure. At the time of collection, pouches were flattened onto biopsy sponges, placed into tissue cassettes, and fixed in 10% neutral buffered formalin overnight at room temperature. Tissue samples were embedded in paraffin blocks, 4 μm sectioned, stained with hematoxylin & eosin, and microscopically examined at 20× magnification. (**a**) Normal epithelium; (**b**) Low-grade (mild) dysplasia, characterized by basilar crowding, hyperplasia, cellular disorganization, and maturational disturbances not extending more than one-third of the epithelial thickness with little interruption of the keratin layer; (**c**) High-grade (severe) dysplasia, included the above "mild" parameters and extending beyond one-half of the epithelial thickness, but not affecting the entirety of the epithelium. Additional features included frequent mitotic figures, cellular pleomorphism, nuclear atypia, and some early disturbance of the keratin layer; (**d**) *Carcinoma-in-situ*, presented as a full thickness epithelial changes with an expansion of multiple layers of cells into the suprabasal and intermediate layers, and with disturbance of the keratin layer, but without penetration of the basement membrane, (**e**) Oral squamous cell carcinoma, characterized by cellular and nuclear pleomorphism, mitotic figures, and invasion of the underlying lamina propria as islands, nests, and cords of atypical epithelium

rates of UV-induced DNA damage repair. Unlike polycyclic hydrocarbons that are metabolized via cytochrome P450 mechanisms, 4NQO is processed by NADH to 4-hydroxyaminoquinoline 1-oxide (Arima et al., 2006) which subsequently forms 8-oxo-7-hydrodeoxyguanosine DNA adducts. In contrast to the adducts formed with polycyclic hydrocarbons, 4NQO DNA adducts are quickly repaired over a relatively short period (Stich et al., 1972). Tumors on the rat tongue or palate develop after multiple dosing (Wong and Wilson, 1983) over an experimental period of 20–32 weeks and the yield of tumors is limited. However, Dayan et al. (1997) found that the time-to-tumor could be considerably shortened if the submandibular and sublingual glands in rats were excised and the parotid ducts were ligated. Under these modified conditions, 0.001% 4NQO in the drinking water yielded tongue lesions in as little as 7 weeks, whereas the sham-operated control rats required up to 22 weeks to present the same type of oral lesions.

A mouse model for chemically-induced oral carcinogenesis was first described by Fujino et al. (1965) in which 4NQO was applied by daily brushing, eventually resulting in the formation of OSCCs. Steidler and Reade (1984) demonstrated an increased incidence of dysplasias and OSCCs in mouse palates after 50 weeks as the application of 4NQO was extended from 2 to 16 weeks. Reviews and thorough observations on the 4NQO-mouse oral cancer model have been presented in detail by Hawkins et al. (1994), Kim et al. (2002), Schoop et al. (2009), Vitale-Cross et al. (2009).

3 Prevention of Oral Cancer by Black Raspberries

Based on studies demonstrating the successful inhibition of aerodigestive tract cancers using dietary black raspberries in rat esophagus and colon (Kresty et al., 2001; Harris et al., 2002), it was hypothesized that cells progressing towards cancer in the oral cavity would also be targets for inhibition by black raspberries. Black raspberries *(Rubus occidentalis)* are attractive as a cancer preventive agent due to the presence of numerous compounds with demonstrated chemopreventive activity, including vitamins C and E, folic acid, calcium, selenium, β-sitosterol, ellagic and ferulic acids, and quercetin (Stoner, 2009). Black raspberries also contain significant amounts of ellagitannins and fiber in the form of lignin and cellulose. Ellagitannins from raspberries have been shown to inhibit phorbol ester-induced DNA synthesis and polyamine synthesis via decreased ornithine decarboxylase activity (Clifford and Scalbert, 2000). The biopolymers lignin and cellulose have also been reported to reduce the number of premalignant lesions in F344 rats (Nigro et al., 1979) and inhibit colon tumors in Sprague-Dawley rats (Serraino and Thompson, 1992). When compared to other plant products, berries also display marked antioxidant activity (Wang et al., 1996; Kahkone'n et al., 1999), a common feature of many food-based chemopreventives (Stoner et al., 2008). Evidence that berries, or their derivative compounds, could be effective against oral cancer was demonstrated by several studies that established individual components of berries as effective inhibitors of cell growth and cell transformation in vitro and successful suppressors of oral cavity lesions in experimental animal models (Suda et al., 1986; Balasubramanian and Govindasamy, 1996; Ohnishi et al., 1997; Xue et al., 2001; Han et al., 2005; Balakrishnan et al., 2008). Subsequently, a series of food-based experiments with black raspberries using a Complete Chemoprevention Bioassay (CCB) were conducted by Casto et al. (2002) during which the black raspberries were present before, during, and after chemical carcinogen induction of oral lesions.

3.1 Complete Chemoprevention Bioassay with Dietary Administration of Black Raspberries

In the CCB, 3–4 week-old male Syrian Golden hamsters (*Mesocricetus auratus*) weighing 50–60 g, were obtained from the Charles River Laboratories (Wilmington, MA) and given either a control AIN-76A diet (Dyets, Inc.; Bethlehem, PA) or a modified AIN-76A diet containing lyophilized black raspberry powder (LBR) at 5 and 10% concentrations (Casto et al., 2002). After 2 weeks of animal habituation, cheek pouch surfaces were treated 3× per week for 8 weeks with 0.2% DMBA in DMSO. Water and AIN-76A diets (±LBR) were given ad libitum and animals were weighed biweekly during the 12 week carcinogen and LBR dietary intervention. All experimental conditions were in accordance with NIH guidelines (Guide for the Care and Use of Laboratory Animals, 1996) and with protocols approved by The Ohio State University Institutional Animal Care and Use Committee.

Fresh black raspberries were supplied from a single source (Dale Stokes Berry Farm; Wilmington, OH) and shipped frozen to Van Drunen Farms (Momence, IL) for freeze-drying. Detailed characteristics of the LBR powder composition were determined by Covance Laboratories (Madison, WI) and have been presented previously (Kresty et al., 2001; Casto et al., 2002). Carcinogen application was performed using a No.4 camel hair brush and a modification of methods initially described by Morris (1961). Tumors in the DMBA-only control group reached 5–10 mm in greatest length approximately 12 weeks after beginning carcinogen exposure. Following CO_2 euthanasia (AVMA Panel on Euthanasia, 2001), the HCP tumors were measured, harvested, and processed for evaluation. After tumor removal, the HCPs were sectioned and either fixed in 10% neutral buffered formalin overnight at room temperature for histochemistry or frozen in liquid nitrogen for subsequent gene expression analysis.

The number of oral tumors in LBR-exposed HCPs was reduced from 48 in 15 animals receiving control AIN-76A diet to 27 in 14 animals given 5% LBR in the diet and to 39 in animals receiving 10% LBR in the diet (Casto et al., 2002). Whereas there was a significant 40% reduction in tumor multiplicity in the animals receiving 5% LBR, the 19% reduction in animals receiving 10% LBR in the diet did not reach significance. The tumor incidence between the control and LBR supplemented diet groups was not significantly altered. The greater reduction in tumor multiplicity with 5% LBR vs. 10% LBR administration are similar to data generated in the rat esophagus by Kresty et al. (2001) in that 5% dietary LBR was more effective than 10% LBR in inhibiting esophageal tumors (38% vs. 31% reduction). It has been hypothesized that while both dietary LBR concentrations decrease tumor multiplicity, the dose-response anomaly may be associated with the complex nutraceutical composition of this food-based intervention strategy. Whole black raspberries contain powerful antioxidants and tumor inhibitory agents, some of which have been characterized; however, an abundance of additional phenolics, micronutrients, phytosterols, and competing compounds are also present that may interact in the tumor microenvironment to interfere with tumor inhibition as the concentration of LBR in the diet increases.

A part of the tumor inhibitory activity exhibited by LBR in the oral cavity can be attributed to a reduction in carcinogen-initiated DNA damage. For example, hamsters administered 5% dietary LBR for 2 weeks prior to DMBA exposure demonstrated a 28.5% decrease in DNA adducts at 24 h and a 54.7% reduction in total DNA adducts at 48 hours after carcinogen exposure (Casto et al., 2002). However, the mechanisms of LBR-mediated inhibition of tumor formation appear to extend beyond the ability to suppress chemically-induced DNA-damaging initiation events. Both Carlton et al. (2001) with strawberries and Kresty et al. (2001) with LBR demonstrated a significant reduction in esophageal tumors when the berries were added after tumor initiation. These studies indicate that berry components affected not only early lesional induction (initiation), but also the subsequent stages of tumor development (promotion/progression).

4 Prevention of Oral Cancer by Berry Components

Chemoprevention using lyophilized whole berry powders or berry extracts that contain a complex mixture of components is striking in both cell cultures and animal models of oral cancer. However, it remains unclear what specific bioactive food components in berries are responsible for these remarkable growth inhibitory and anti-tumorigenic responses. Many of the same bioactive compounds are present in black raspberries and strawberries, although there are distinctive profiles in both the type and number of anthocyanins between the different berries. In addition to the inhibition of oral and aerodigestive tract cancers by dietary LBR powders in the animal models described above, various isolated or enriched berry components have been shown to be effective for suppressing oral cancer development in both HCP and rat tongue experimental animal models. It has been demonstrated that there are bioactive compounds and micronutrients in berries that modulate gene expression patterns in key regulatory pathways in both hamster and rat models that correlate with oral cancer chemopreventive activities (Shklar, 1998). These unique berry-responsive gene expression profiles are transcriptional biomarkers of exposure and may further represent surrogate endpoints of chemopreventive potential in preclinical animal studies. Validation of the berry-mediated transcriptional biomarker profiles is fundamental to translating the animal model data into future food-based human oral cancer prevention trials.

Evidence that components of berries may have chemopreventive potential originates from the findings that berry extracts inhibit the growth of human cancer cells in vitro (Meyers et al., 2003; Han et al., 2005; Olsson et al., 2006; Seeram et al., 2006;

Nadova et al., 2007), demonstrate antimicrobial activity (Nohynek et al., 2006), and reduce obesity by inhibiting enzymes associated with digestion of starch, protein, and fat (McDougall and Stewart, 2005). Berry extracts also inhibit key transcriptional modulators of cellular proliferation, stress responsiveness, inflammation, and apoptosis, including AP-1 and NF-κB (Wang et al., 2005) in cultured cells. In the following sections, a short list of previously studied berry components known to exhibit chemopreventive activity in animal models of oral cancer is presented.

4.1 Quercetin

Quercetin (IUPAC: 2-(3,4-dihydroxyphenyl)-3,5,7-trihydroxychromen-4-one), a flavonol found in black raspberries and strawberries at concentrations ranging from 0.65 to 1.03 mg/100 g wet weight, has been shown to inhibit both DMBA-induced papillomas (41% decrease) and oral tumors (37% decrease) in the HCP when given in the diet at a 2% concentration (Balasubramanian and Govindasamy, 1996). Makita et al. (1996) evaluated quercetin in the 4NQO rat tongue model using two bioassay protocols. First, rats received diets with 500 ppm quercetin beginning 1 week prior to, and 1 week after, 8 weeks of treatment with 4NQO (20 ppm) in the drinking water. Second, rats were treated for 8 weeks with 4NQO and 1 week later received the quercetin diet through 22 weeks. In the first bioassay, the incidence of hyperplasias was reduced from 100 to 69%, dysplasias from 87 to 50%, papillomas 27 to 6%, and OSCCs from 60 to 13%. In the second bioassay, dietary administration of quercetin 1 week after cessation of 4NQO exposure resulted in the decreased incidence of hyperplasia from 100 to 67%, dysplasia from 87 to 80%, papillomas from 27 to 7%, and OSCCs from 60 to 7%. These data demonstrated that the oral cancer chemopreventive activities of dietary quercetin are effective both when given during carcinogen exposure and after such contact is discontinued. Oral cancer prevention by quercetin during both a "complete" and "post-initiation" type of chemical carcinogenesis protocol demonstrates the potential of this chemopreventive agent to act at several intervention points along the extended multistep process of oral squamous cell carcinoma development.

4.2 Ferulic Acid

Ferulic acid (FA; 4-hydroxy-3-methoxycinnamic acid; IUPAC: (E)-3-(4-hydroxy-3-methoxy-phenyl)prop-2-enoic acid) is a major phenolic acid in berries ranging in concentration in black raspberries from 17 to 32 mg/100 g of berry powder. Ferulic acid has been shown to inhibit growth of both premalignant and malignant human oral cells in vitro with blockage at the G_2/M interface in cells with increases in cyclin B1 (CCNB1) and cyclin-dependent kinase 1 (CDK1/CDC2) proteins (Han et al., 2005). Using the HCP model, Balakrishnan et al. (2008) showed that FA completely inhibited development of malignant tumors when given orally at

40 mg/kg of body weight beginning 1 week before carcinogen exposure and continuing on days alternate to DMBA painting (3× per week) for 14 weeks. Microscopic examination revealed that oral FA administration reduced the appearance of dysplasias from severe to mild and reduced hyperplasia from severe to moderate. Accompanying the striking inhibition of tumor formation, Phase II liver enzyme activities increased in FA administered hamsters relative to DMBA-only exposed animals and demonstrated levels comparable to healthy control animals.

Previously, Tanaka et al. (1993) showed that dietary FA (500 ppm) was effective in reducing the incidence of hyperplasias, dysplasias, papillomas, and carcinomas in the rat tongue oral cancer model. One week after receiving the FA diet, 4NQO (20 ppm) was delivered in the drinking water for 5 weeks and lesions were assessed at 7 weeks. Mori et al. (1999) demonstrated a significant reduction in the incidence of rat tongue carcinomas and severe dysplasias when FA was given in the diet at 500 ppm after 5 weeks of 4NQO exposure, indicating that FA was also an effective chemopreventive when administered after tumor initiation.

4.3 β-carotene

β-carotene (IUPAC: 1,3,3-trimethyl-2-[(1E,3E,5E,7E,9E,11E,13E,15E,17E)-3,7,12,16-tetramethyl-18-(2,6,6-trimethylcyclohexen-1-yl)octadeca-1,3,5,7,9,11,13,15,17-nonaenyl]cyclohexene) is one of a number of antioxidants found in strawberries and black raspberries, ranging in concentration from 7 to 12 μg/100 g whole berries. Suda, Schwartz and Shklar (1986) demonstrated the inhibition of initiation of DMBA-induced tumors in the HCP model following topical application of β-carotene. Furthermore, it was established that β-carotene administration after DMBA exposure and during benzoyl peroxide application (post-initiation) resulted in inhibition of the promotion phase of tumor development. Schwartz and Shklar (1988) later reported that twice weekly injections of β-carotene (250 μg) into the tumor-bearing HCPs for 4 weeks would also induce regression of established tumors. Schwartz et al. (1989) then administered oral β-carotene and observed an inhibition of HCP tumors and suggested a mechanism associated with the release of tumor necrosis factor alpha (TNF-α) in conjunction with an inflammatory response consisting of cytotoxic lymphocytes, macrophages, and histiocytes into areas of dysplasia, carcinoma-in-situ, and early tumor development. Tanaka et al. (1994), using the rat tongue model, demonstrated the inhibition of oral tumors when β-carotene (500 ppm) was administered 1 week before, during, and 1 week after 8 weeks of 4NQO exposure (20 ppm) or when given beginning 1 week after the final carcinogen exposure. The incidence of papillomas was reduced from 17 to 12% and the incidence of carcinomas from 54 to 18% when β-carotene was administered during the initiation period. When β-carotene was given post-initiation, the incidence of papillomas did not significantly change; however, the incidence of carcinomas was reduced from 54 to 24% compared to control animals. β-carotene significantly reduced the appearance of dysplasias when received during the initiation period, but not when administered post-initiation. Accompanying the reductions in tumor incidence was a significant decrease in markers of cell proliferation. Shklar (1998) has extensively discussed three of the major mechanisms whereby antioxidants such as β-carotene direct their cancer preventive effects, including the production of immune cytokines, stimulation of tumor suppressor genes, and inhibition of angiogenesis.

4.4 Protocatechuic Acid

Protocatechuic acid (PCA; IUPAC: 3,4-dihydroxybenzoic acid) is a major metabolite of cyanidin-3-glucoside (CyG) (Nurmi et al., 2009), one of the anthocyanins found in strawberries at concentrations ranging from 1.66 to 5.30 μg/g of whole berries (Hernanz et al., 2007). The CyG parental compound has been shown to be a scavenger for reactive oxygen species in cell cultures, decreased UV or 12-O-tetradecanoylphorbol-13-acetate (TPA) transactivation of AP-1 and NF-κB in JB6 cells, inhibit expression of COX-2 and TNF-α, repress promotion of skin tumors in mice, and inhibit in vitro transformation of JB6 cells by TPA (Ding et al., 2006). Dietary administration of blood orange juice containing 71 mg of CyG to human volunteers resulted in serum concentrations of only 1.9 nmol/L of CyG after 30 min, but 492 nmol/L of PCA after 2 h, and accounted for approximately 73% of the total intake of CyG (Vitaglione et al., 2007). The authors suggested that the observed antioxidant activity in plasma following anthocyanin ingestion might be largely related to PCA activity. Similarly, Koli et al. (2010) found that following 8 weeks of a dietary intervention including 160 g/day of berries (bilberries, lingonberries, black currants, and chokeberries), there were significant increases in the plasma concentration of PCA and quercetin. These studies demonstrate that PCA and other phenolic acids become bioavailable when subjects are administered a diet enriched with berries.

Ohnishi et al. (1997) demonstrated the efficacy of PCA-mediated oral cancer inhibition in HCPs that had been exposed to DMBA. Dietary administration of PCA (200 ppm) followed the last DMBA exposure and continued for 17 weeks. Delivery of PCA in the diet did not affect the incidence or multiplicity of papillomas or carcinomas in the HCP. However, when tumor volume was considered, the mean tumor burden was significantly reduced by 65% from 655 mm^3 in DMBA-only controls to 231 mm^3 in hamsters receiving dietary PCA. In addition, there were significant reductions in the total number of dysplastic lesions in the PCA administered HCPs.

The inhibitory effect of PCA on oral tumor progression was further described by Suzuki et al. (2003) who exposed rats to 20 ppm 4NQO (initiation) followed by four cycles of 2-week treatments with 4NQO and water (progression). After 12 weeks of 4NQO exposure, rats were administered diets supplemented with PCA (2,000 ppm) for the remainder of the study. Rats exposed to only 4NQO presented with a 16% incidence of tongue papillomas at 32 weeks with no observed carcinomas. In rats exposed to 4NQO followed by cyclic treatment with 4NQO, there was a 32% incidence of papillomas and a 47% incidence of carcinomas. In each case, these incidences were reduced to a level of 10% following administration of PCA in the diet. Furthermore, in rats receiving dietary PCA, the incidence of papillary hyperplasia was reduced from 100 to 25% and severe dysplasia reduced from 87 to 25%.

5 Summary and Discussion

The major risk factor for oral cancer is the combinatorial use of tobacco and alcoholic beverages, which may account for approximately 75% of all oral cancers in the United States (Mashberg et al., 1993). Additional and independent risk factors for oral cancer include poor nutrition and exposure to viruses such as the Epstein Barr virus (EBV) (Lanier et al., 1991; Shamaa et al. 2008) and human papillomavirus (HPV) (Greer et al., 1990; Woods et al., 1993; Gillison and Shah, 2001; Dahlgren et al., 2004; Campisi et al., 2007). Despite advances over the past 3 decades in detection, surgical intervention, and adjuvant treatment, the survival rates for oral cancer patients have not significantly changed for those cases that have spread beyond the mucosa. Thus, chemoprevention strategies in conjunction with tobacco and alcohol cessation programs offer an alternate/complementary tactic for averting primary disease and recurrent or second primary oral malignancies (Hong et al., 2000). Whole berries, their simple derivatives, and individual bioactive components have been shown to modulate cancer-associated processes in vitro and to inhibit in vivo development of oral tumors in well-established animal models when administered before, during, or after initiation by chemical carcinogens. When coupled with the overwhelming epidemiologic data associating dietary fruit and vegetable consumption with decreased cancer risks, these findings provide powerful evidence for the value of whole foods and their derivatives in the inhibition of oral cancer. The robust and expanding knowledge base of food-based intervention studies that have been systematically examined in appropriate preclinical experimental animal models of oral carcinogenesis is the cornerstone of subsequent human clinical trials. It is through structured in vitro cell culture experiments that transition into preclinical animal model surrogates, and ultimately, translate into clinical trials and standard of care practices.

References

Adlercreutz H (1998) Epidemiology of phytoestrogens. Baillieres Clin Endocrinol Metab 12: 605–623

Almendingen K, Hofstad B, Vatn MH (2004) Dietary habits and growth and recurrence of colorectal adenomas: results from a three-year endoscopic follow-up study. Nutr Cancer 49:131–138

American Cancer Society 2009 Cancer Facts & Figures 2009. American Cancer Society, Atlanta, GA

AVMA Panel on Euthanasia (2001) 2000 Report of the AVMA panel on Euthanasia. J Am Vet Med Assoc 218:669–696

Arima Y, Nishigori C, Takeuchi T, Oka S, Morimoto K, Utani A, Miyachi Y (2006) 4-Nitroquinoline 1-oxide forms 8-hydroxydeoxyguanosine in human fibroblasts through reactive oxygen species. Toxicol Sciences 91:382–392
Balakrishnan S, Menon VP, Manoharan S (2008) Ferulic acid inhibits 7, 12-dimethylbenz[a]anthracene-induced hamster buccal pouch carcinogenesis. J Med Food 11:693–700
Balasenthil S, Saroja M, Ramachandran CR, Nagini S (2000) Of humans and hamsters: comparative analysis of lipid peroxidation, glutathione and glutathione dependent enzymes during oral carcinogenesis. Br J Oral Maxillofac Surg 38:267–270
Balasubramanian S, Govindasamy S (1996) Inhibitory effect of dietary flavonol quercetin on 7, 12-dimethylbenz[a]anthracene-induced hamster buccal pouch carcinogenesis. Carcinogenesis 17:877–879
Bhutani M, Pathak AK, Fan YH, Liu DD, Lee JJ, Tang H, Kurie JM, Morice RC, Kim ES, Hong WK, Mao L (2008) Oral epithelium as a surrogate tissue for assessing smoking-induced molecular alterations in the lungs. Cancer Prev Res 1:39–44
Bhuvaneswari V, Velmurugan B, Nagini S (2004) Dose-response effect of tomato paste on 7, 12-dimethylbenz[a]anthracene-induced hamster buccal pouch carcinogenesis. J Exp Clin Cancer Res 23:241–249
Buters JT, Sakai S, Richter T, Pineau T, Alexander DL, Savas U, Doehmer J, Ward JM, Jefcoate CR, Gonzalez FJ (1999) Cytochrome P450 CYP1B1 determines susceptibility to 7, 12-dimethylbenz[a]anthracene-induced lymphomas. Proc Natl Acad Sci USA 96:1977–1982
Campisi G, Panzarella V, Giuliani M, Lajolo C, Di Fede O, Falaschini S, Di Liberto C, Scully C, Lo Muzio L (2007) Human papillomavirus: its identity and controversial role in oral oncogenesis, premalignant and malignant lesions (review). Int J Oncol 30:813–823
Carlton PS, Kresty LA, Siglin JC, Morse MA, Lu J, Morgan C, Stoner GD (2001) Inhibition of N-nitrosomethylbenzylamine-induced tumorigenesis in the rat esophagus by dietary freeze-dried strawberries. Carcinogenesis 22:441–446
Casto BC, Kresty LA, Kraly CL, Pearl DK, Knobloch TJ, Schut HA, Stoner GD, Mallery SR, Weghorst CM (2002) Chemoprevention of oral cancer by black raspberries. Anticancer Res 22:4005–4016
Chang KW, Lin S-C, Koos S, Pather K, Solt D (1996) P53 and H-ras mutations in chemically induced buccal pouch carcinomas. Carcinogenesis 17:595–600
Clifford MN, Scalbert A (2000) Ellagitannins-nature, occurrence and dietary burden. J Sci Food Agric 80:1118–1125
Colditz GA, Branch LG, Lipnick RJ, Willett WC, Rosner B, Posner BM, Hennekens CH (1985) Increased green and yellow vegetable intake and lowered cancer deaths in an elderly population. Am J Clin Nutr 41:32–36
Conti CJ (1991) Animal models in the study of the premalignant process. Cancer Bull 43:499–503
Cooke D, Steward WP, Gescher AJ, Marczylo T (2005) Anthocyanins from fruits and vegetables–does bright colour signal cancer chemopreventive activity? Eur J Cancer 41:1931–1940
Cooper JS, Pajak TF, Rubin P, Tupchong L, Brady LW, Leibel SA, Laramore GE, Marcial VA, Davis LW, Cox JD (1989) Second malignancies in patients who have head and neck cancer: incidence, effect on survival and implications based on the ROTG experience. Int J Radiat Oncol Biol Phys 17:449–456
Dahlgren L, Dahlstrand HM, Lindquist D, Högmo A, Björnestål L, Lindholm J, Lundberg B, Dalianis T, Munck-Wikland E (2004) Human papillomavirus is more common in base of tongue than in mobile tongue cancer and is a favorable prognostic factor in base of tongue cancer patients. Int J Cancer 112:1015–1019
Dayan D, Hirshberg A, Kaplan I, Rotem N, Bodner L (1997) Experimental tongue cancer in desalivated rats. Oral Oncol 33:105–109
Ding M, Feng R, Wang SY, Bowman L, Lu Y, Qian Y, Castranova V, Jiang BH, Shi X (2006) Cyanidin-3-glucoside, a natural product derived from blackberry, exhibits chemopreventive and chemotherapeutic activity. J Biol Chem 281:17359–17368

Fimognari C, Lenzi M, Hrelia P (2008) Chemoprevention of cancer by isothiocyanates and anthocyanins: mechanisms of action and structure-activity relationship. Curr Med Chem 15:440–447

Freedman ND, Park Y, Subar AF, Hollenbeck AR, Leitzmann MF, Schatzkin A, Abnet CC (2008) Fruit and vegetable intake and head and neck cancer risk in a large united states prospective cohort study. Int J Cancer 122:2330–2336

Fujino H, Chino T, Imai T (1965) Experimental production of labial and lingual carcinoma by local application of 4-nitroquinoline N-oxide. J Natl Cancer Inst 35:907–918

Gillison ML, Shah KV (2001) Human papillomavirus-associated head and neck squamous cell carcinoma: mounting evidence for an etiologic role for human papillomavirus in a subset of head and neck cancers. Curr Opin Oncol 13:183–188

Gimenez-Conti IB, Shin DM, Bianchi AB, Roop DR, Hong WK, Conti CJ, Slaga TJ (1990) Changes in keratin expression during 7,12-dimethylbenz(a)anthracene induced hamster cheek pouch carcinogenesis. Cancer Res 50:4441–4445

Gimenez-Conti IB, LaBate M, Liu F, Osterndorff E (1996) P53 alterations in chemically induced hamster cheek-pouch lesions. Molec Carcinogenesis 16:197–202

Gimenez-Conti IB, Slaga TJ (1993) The hamster cheek pouch carcinogenesis model. J Cell Biochem Suppl 17F:83–90

Greer RO, Douglas JM, Breese P (1990) Evaluation of oral and laryngeal specimens for human papillomavirus (HPV) DNA by dot blot hybridization. J Oral Pathol Med 19:35–38

Han C, Ding H, Casto B, Stoner GD, D'Ambrosio SM (2005) Inhibition of the growth of premalignant and malignant human oral cell lines by extracts and components of black raspberries. Nutr Cancer 51:207–217

Harris GK, Gupta A, Nines RG, Kresty LA, Habib SG, Frankel WL, LaPerle K, Gallaher DD, Schwartz SJ, Stoner GD (2002) Effects of lyophilized black raspberries on azoxymethane-induced colon cancer and 8-hydroxy-2'-deoxyguanosine levels in the Fischer 344 rat. Nutr Cancer 40:125–133

Hawkins BL, Heniford BW, Ackermann DM, Leonberger M, Martinez SA, Hendler FJ (1994) 4NQO carcinogenesis: a mouse model of oral cavity squamous cell carcinoma. Head Neck 16:424–432

Hecht SS (2002) Tobacco smoke carcinogens and breast cancer. Environ Mol Mutagen 39: 119–126

Hernanz D, Recamales AF, Meléndez-Martínez AJ, González-Miret ML, Heredia FJ (2007) Assessment of the differences in the phenolic composition of five strawberry cultivars (*Fragaria x ananassa Duch.*) grown in two different soilless systems. J Agric Food Chem 55: 1846–1852

Hertog MG, Hollman PC, Katan MB, Kromhout D (1993) Intake of potentially anticarcinogenic flavonoids and their determinants in adults in the netherlands. Nutr Cancer 20:21–29

Hong WK, Spitz MR, Lippman SM (2000) Cancer chemoprevention in the 21st century: genetics, risk modeling, and molecular targets. J Clin Oncol 18(Suppl):9S–18S

Husain Z, Fei Y, Roy S, Solt DB, Polverini PJ, Biswas DK (1989) Cooperative interaction of c-Ha-ras and c-erbB genes in chemically induced hamster buccal pouch carcinogenesis. Proc Soc Natl Acad Sci USA 86:1264–1268

Institute of Laboratory Animal Resources, Commission on Life Sciences, National Research Council (1996) Guide for the care and use of laboratory animals. National Academy Press, Washington, DC

Kahkone'n MP, Hopia AI, Vuorela HJ, Rauha JP, Pihlaja K, Kujala TS, Heinonen M (1999) Antioxidant activity of plant extracts containing phenolic compounds. J Agric Food Chem 47:3954–3962

Kanojia D, Vaidya MM (2006) 4-nitroquinoline-1-oxide induced experimental oral carcinogenesis. Oral Oncol 42:655–667

Kim TW, Chen Q, Shen X, Regezi JA, Ramos DM, Tanaka H, Jordan RC, Kramer RH (2002) Oral mucosal carcinogenesis in SENCAR mice. Anticancer Res 22:2733–2740

Koli R, Erlund I, Jula A, Marniemi J, Mattila P, Alfthan G (2010) Bioavailability of Various Polyphenols from a Diet Containing Moderate Amounts of Berries (dagger). J Agric Food Chem 58:3927–3932
Kresty LA, Morse MA, Morgan C, Carlton PS, Lu J, Gupta A, Blackwood M, Stoner GD (2001) Chemoprevention of esophageal tumorigenesis by dietary administration of lyophilized black raspberries. Cancer Res 61:6112–6119
Kühnau J (1976) The flavonoids. A class of semi-essential food components: their role in human nutrition. World Rev Nutr Diet 24:117–191
Kwong YY, Husain A, Biswas DK (1992) c-Ha-ras gene mutation and activation precede pathological changes in DMBA-induced in vivo carcinogenesis. Oncogene 7:1481–1489
Lanier AP, Clift SR, Bornkamm G, Henle W, Goepfert H, Raab-Traub N (1991) Epstein-Barr virus and malignant lymphoepithelial lesions of the salivary gland. Arctic Med Res 50: 55–61
Leon X, Quer M, Diez S, Orus C, Lopez-Pousa A, Burgues J (1999) Second neoplasm in patients with head and neck cancer. Head Neck 21:204–210
Li J, Warner B, Casto BC, Knobloch TJ, Weghorst CM (2008) Tumor suppressor p16(INK4A)/Cdkn2a alterations in 7,12-dimethylbenz(a)anthracene (DMBA)-induced hamster cheek pouch tumors. Mol Carcinogenesis 47:733–738
Li N, Chen X, Liao J, Yang G, Wang S, Josephson Y, Han C, Chen J, Huang MT, Yang CS (2002) Inhibition of 7,12-dimethylbenz[a]anthracene (DMBA)-induced oral carcinogenesis in hamsters by tea and curcumin. Carcinogenesis 23:1307–1313
Mahadevan B, Luch A, Bravo CF, Atkin J, Steppan LB, Pereira C, Kerkvliet NI, Baird WM (2005) Dibenzo[a,l]pyrene induced DNA adduct formation in lung tissue in vivo. Cancer Lett 227: 25–32
Mahlum DD, Wright CW, Chess EK, Wilson BW (1984) Fractionation of skin tumor-initiating activity in coal liquids. Cancer Res 44:5176–5181
Makita H, Tanaka T, Fujitsuka H, Tatematsu N, Satoh K, Hara A, Mori H (1996) Chemoprevention of 4-nitroquinoline 1-oxide-induced rat oral carcinogenesis by the dietary flavonoids chalcone, 2-hydroxychalcone, and quercetin. Cancer Res 56:4904–4909
Mashberg A, Boffetta P, Winkelman R, Garfinkel L (1993) Tobacco smoking, alcohol drinking and cancer of the oral cavity and oropharynx among US veterans. Cancer 72:1369–1375
McDougall GJ, Stewart D (2005) The inhibitory effects of berry polyphenols on digestive enzymes. Biofactors 23:189–195
Meng C, Shyu KW (1990) Inhibition of experimental carcinogenesis by painting with garlic extract. Nutr Cancer 14:207–217
Meyers KJ, Watkins CB, Pritts MP, Liu RH (2003) Antioxidant and antiproliferative activities of strawberries. J Agric Food Chem 51:6887–6892
Mignogna MD, Fedele S, Lo Russo L (2004) The World Cancer Report and the burden of oral cancer. Eur J Cancer Prev 13:139–142
Miller EG, Porter JL, Binnie WH, Guo IY, Hasegawa S (2004) Further studies on the anticancer activity of citrus limonoids. J Agric Food Chem 52:4908–4912
Mori H, Kawabata K, Yoshimi N, Tanaka T, Murakami T, Okada T, Murai H (1999) Chemopreventive effects of ferulic acid on oral and rice germ on large bowel carcinogenesis. Anticancer Res 19:3775–3778
Moroco JR, Solt DB, Polverini PJ (1990) Sequential loss of suppressor genes for three specific functions during in vivo carcinogenesis. Lab Invest 63:298–306
Morris AL (1961) Factors influencing experimental carcinogenesis in the hamster cheek pouch. J Dental Res 40:3–15
Nadova S, Miadokova E, Cipak L (2007) Flavonoids potentiate the efficacy of cytarabine through modulation of drug-induced apoptosis. Neoplasma 54:202–206
Nauta JM, Roodenburg JL, Nikkels PG, Witjes MJ, Vermey A (1995) Comparison of epithelial dysplasia – the 4NQO rat palate model and human oral mucosa. Int J Oral Maxillofac Surg 24:53–58

Nichenametla SN, Taruscio TG, Barney DL, Exon JH (2006) A review of the effects and mechanisms of polyphenolics in cancer. Crit Rev Food Sci Nutr 46:161–183
Nigro ND, Bull AW, Klopfer BA, Pak MS, Campbell RL (1979) Effect of dietary fiber on azoxymethane-induced intestinal carcinogenesis in rats. J Natl Cancer Inst 62:1097–1102
Nohynek LJ, Alakomi HL, Kahkonen MP, Heinonen M, Helander IM, Oksman-Caldentey KM, Puupponen-Pimia RH (2006) Berry phenolics: antimicrobial properties and mechanisms of action against severe human pathogens. Nutr Cancer 54:18–32
Nurmi T, Mursu J, Heinonen M, Nurmi A, Hiltunen R, Voutilainen S (2009) Metabolism of Berry Anthocyanins to Phenolic Acids in Humans. J Agric Food Chem 57:2274–2281
Ohnishi M, Yoshimi N, Kawamori T, Ino N, Hirose Y, Tanaka T, Yamahara J, Miyata H, Mori H (1997) Inhibitory effects of dietary protocatechuic acid and costunolide on 7,12-dimethylbenz[a]anthracene-induced hamster cheek pouch carcinogenesis. Jpn J Cancer Res 88:111–119
Olsson ME, Andersson CS, Oredsson S, Berglund RH, Gustavsson KE (2006) Antioxidant levels and inhibition of cancer cell proliferation in vitro by extracts from organically and conventionally cultivated strawberries. J Agric Food Chem 54:1248–1255
Parkin DM, Bray F, Ferlay J, Pisani P (2005) Global cancer statistics, 2002. CA Cancer J Clin 55:74–108
Pavia M, Pileggi C, Nobile CG, Angelillo IF (2006) Association between fruit and vegetable consumption and oral cancer: a meta-analysis of observational studies. Am J Clin Nutr 83:1126–1134
Polverini PJ, Solt DB (1988) Expression of the angiogenic phenotype by a subpopulation of keratinocytes derived from 7,12 dimethylbenz(a)anthracene-initiated hamster buccal pouch epithelium. Carcinogenesis 9:117–122
Ribeiro DA, Fávero Salvadori DM, da Silva RN, Ribeiro Darros B, Alencar Marques ME (2004) Genomic instability in non-neoplastic oral mucosa cells can predict risk during 4-nitroquinoline 1-oxide-induced rat tongue carcinogenesis. Oral Oncol 40:910–915
Sacks PG, Hong WK, Hittelman WN (1991) In vitro studies of the premalignant process: initial culture of oral premalignant lesions. Cancer Bull 43:485–489
Salley JJ (1954) Experimental carcinogenesis in the cheek pouch of the Syrian hamster. J Dent Res 33:253–262
Salley JJ (1957) Histologic changes in the hamster cheek pouch during early hydrocarbon carcinogenesis. J Dent Res 36:48–55
Schoop RA, Noteborn MH, Baatenburg de Jong RJ (2009) A mouse model for oral squamous cell carcinoma. J Mol Histol 40:177–181
Schwartz J, Baker V, Larios E, Desai D, Amin S (2004) Inhibition of experimental tobacco carcinogen induced head and neck carcinogenesis. Oral Oncol 40:611–623
Schwartz J, Shklar G (1988) Regression of experimental oral carcinomas by local injection of beta-carotene and canthaxanthin. Nutr Cancer 11:35–40
Schwartz JL, Gu X, Kittles RA, Baptiste A, Shklar G (2000) Experimental oral carcinoma of the tongue and buccal mucosa: possible biologic markers linked to cancers at two anatomic sites. Oral Oncol 36:225–235
Schwartz JL, Sloane D, Shklar G (1989) Prevention and inhibition of oral cancer in the hamster buccal pouch model associated with carotenoid immune enhancement. Tumour Biol 10: 297–309
Seeram NP, Adams LS, Zhang Y, Lee R, Sand D, Scheuller HS, Heber D (2006) Blackberry, black raspberry, blueberry, cranberry, red raspberry, and strawberry extracts inhibit growth and stimulate apoptosis of human cancer cells in vitro. J Agric Food Chem 54:9329–9339
Seeram NP (2006) Chapter 37, berries. In: Heber D, Blackburn G, Go V, Milner J (eds) Nutritional oncology, Elsevier, Amsterdam, pp 615–628
Serraino M, Thompson LU (1992) Flaxseed supplementation and early markers of colon carcinogenesis. Cancer Lett 63:159–165

Shamaa AA, Zyada MM, Wagner M, Awad SS, Osman MM, Azeem AA (2008) The significance of Epstein Barr Virus (EBV) & DNA Topoisomerase II alpha (DNA-Topo II alpha) immunoreactivity in normal oral mucosa, Oral Epithelial Dysplasia (OED) and Oral Squamous Cell Carcinoma (OSCC). Diagn Pathol 3:45

Shin DM, Gimenez IB, Lee JS, Nishioka K, Wargovich MJ, Thacher S, Lotan R, Slaga TJ, Hong WK (1990) Expression of epidermal growth factor receptor, polyamine levels, ornithine decarboxylase activity, micronuclei, and transglutaminase i in a 7,12-dimethylbenz(a)anthracene induced hamster buccal pouch carcinogenesis model. Cancer Res 50:2505–2510

Shklar G, Schwartz JL (1996) Vitamin e inhibits experimental carcinogenesis and tumour angiogenesis. Eur J Cancer B Oral Oncol 32B:114–119

Shklar G (1998) Mechanisms of cancer inhibition by anti-oxidant nutrients. Oral Oncol 34:24–29

Shklar G (1972) Experimental oral pathology in the Syrian hamster. Prog Exp Tumor Res 16: 518–538

Shklar G (1999) Development of experimental oral carcinogenesis and its impact on current oral cancer research. J Dent Res 78:1768–1772

Sidransky D (2008) The oral cavity as a molecular mirror of lung carcinogenesis. Cancer Prev Res 1:12–14

Solt DB, Shklar G (1982) Rapid induction of gamma-glutamyl transpeptidase-rich intraepithelial clones in 7,12-DMBA-treated hamster buccal pouch. Cancer Res 42:285–291

Spira A, Beane J, Shah V, Liu G, Schembri F, Yang X, Palma J, Brody JS (2004) Effects of cigarette smoke on the human airway epithelial cell transcriptome. Proc Natl Acad Sci USA 101: 10143–10148

Steidler NE, Reade PC (1984) Experimental induction of oral squamous cell carcinomas in mice with 4-nitroquinolone-1-oxide. Oral Surg Oral Med Oral Pathol Oral Radiol Endod 57:524–531

Stich HF, Hammerberg O, Casto BC (1972) The combined effect of chemical mutagen and virus on DNA repair, chromosome aberrations, and neoplastic transformation. Can J Genet Cytol 14:911–917

Stoner GD, Casto BC (2004) Chemoprevention by fruit phenolic compounds. In: Kelloff GJ, Hawk ET, Sigman CC (eds) Cancer chemoprevention chapter 29, volume I: promising cancer chemoprevention agents, Humana Press, Inc., Totowa NJ, pp 419–435

Stoner GD, Wang LS, Casto BC (2008) Laboratory and clinical studies of cancer chemoprevention by antioxidants in berries. Carcinogenesis 29:1665–1674

Stoner GD (2009) Foodstuffs for preventing cancer: the preclinical and clinical development of berries. Cancer Prev Res 2:187–194

Stoner GD, Dombkowski AA, Reen RK, Cukovic D, Salagrama S, Wang LS, Lechner JF (2008) Carcinogen-altered genes in rat esophagus positively modulated to normal levels of expression by both black raspberries and phenylethyl isothiocyanate. Cancer Res 68:6460–6467

Suda D, Schwartz J, Shklar G (1986) Inhibition of experimental oral carcinogenesis by topical beta carotene. Carcinogenesis 7:711–715

Suzuki R, Kohno H, Sugie S, Tanaka T (2003) Dietary protocatechuic acid during the progression phase exerts chemopreventive effects on chemically induced rat tongue carcinogenesis. Asian Pac J Cancer Prev 4:319–326

Tanaka T, Kojima T, Kawamori T, Wang A, Suzui M, Okamoto K, Mori H (1993) Inhibition of 4-nitroquinoline-1-oxide-induced rat tongue carcinogenesis by the naturally occurring plant phenolics caffeic, ellagic, chlorogenic and ferulic acids. Carcinogenesis 14:1321–1325

Tanaka T, Makita H, Ohnishi M, Hirose Y, Wang A, Mori H, Satoh K, Hara A, Ogawa H (1994) Chemoprevention of 4-nitroquinoline 1-oxide-induced oral carcinogenesis by dietary curcumin and hesperidin: comparison with the protective effect of beta-carotene. Cancer Res 54: 4653–4659

Tanaka T (1995) Chemoprevention of oral carcinogenesis: review. Eur J Cancer B Oral Oncol 31B:3–15

Thier R, Brüning T, Roos PH, Bolt HM (2002) Cytochrome P450 1B1, a new keystone in gene-environment interactions related to human head and neck cancer? Arch Toxicol 76:249–256

Vairaktaris E, Spyridonidou S, Papakosta V, Vylliotis A, Lazaris A, Perrea D, Yapijakis C, Patsouris E (2008) The hamster model of sequential oral oncogenesis. Oral Oncol 44:315–324

Vered M, Yarom N, Dayan D (2005) 4NQO oral carcinogenesis: animal models, molecular markers and future expectations. Oral Oncol 41:337–339

Vitaglione P, Donnarumma G, Napolitano A, Galvano F, Gallo A, Scalfi L, Fogliano V (2007) Protocatechuic acid is the major human metabolite of cyanidin-glucosides. J Nutr 137: 2043–2048

Vitale-Cross L, Czerninski R, Amornphimoltham P, Patel V, Molinolo AA, Gutkind JS (2009) Chemical carcinogenesis models for evaluating molecular-targeted prevention and treatment of oral cancer. Cancer Prev Res 2:419–422

Wallenius K, Lekholm U (1973) Oral cancer in rats induced by the water-soluble carcinogen 4-nitroqhinoline N-oxide. Odontol Rev 24:39–48

Wang H, Cao G, Prior RL (1996) Total antioxidant capacity of fruits. J Agric Food Chem 44: 701–705

Wang LS, Hecht SS, Carmella SG, Yu N, Larue B, Henry C, McIntyre C, Rocha C, Lechner JF, Stoner GD (2009) Anthocyanins in black raspberries prevent esophageal tumors in rats. Cancer Prev Res 2:84–93

Wang SY, Lin HS (2000) Antioxidant activity in fruits and leaves of blackberry, raspberry, and strawberry varies with cultivar and developmental stage. J Agric Food Chem 48:140–146

Wang SY, Feng R, Lu Y, Bowman L, Ding M (2005) Inhibitory effect on activator protein-1, nuclear factor-kappaB, and cell transformation by extracts of strawberries (*Fragaria x ananassa Duch.*). J Agric Food Chem 53:4187–4193

Warnakulasuriya S (2009) Global epidemiology of oral and oropharyngeal cancer. Oral Oncol 45:309–316

Wong PN, Wilson DF (1983) 4 Nitroquinoline 1-oxide-induced carcinogenesis in the rat palate. J Oral Pathol 12:375–384

Wong DTW, Biswas DK (1987) Expression of c-erbb proto-oncogene during dimethylbenzanthracene induced tumorigenesis in hamster cheek pouch. Oncogene 2:67–72

Woods KV, Shillitoe EJ, Spitz MR (1993) Analysis of human papillomavirus DNA in oral squamous cell carcinomas. J Oral Pathol Med 22:101–108

Xue H, Aziz RM, Sun N, Cassady JM, Kamendulis LM, Xu Y, Stoner GD, Klaunig JE (2001) Inhibition of cellular transformation by berry extracts. Carcinogenesis 22:351–356

Chapter 11
Prevention of Cancer with Pomegranate and Pomegranate Anthocyanins

Vaqar Mustafa Adhami, Naghma Khan, and Hasan Mukhtar

Abstract The fruit of the pomegranate tree (*Punica granatum* L.) has recently attracted attention based on anecdotal evidence and studies suggesting that it possesses antioxidant, anti-inflammatory and anti-cancer properties. The pomegranate (literally translated as seeded apple) plant is a shrub that commonly grows 6–15 ft tall. The fruit is a berry (globose) that is 2–3 inches in diameter and reddish when fully mature. It is filled with crunchy and juicy seeds that are eaten and used for extracting the juice. However, industrial preparations use the whole fruit for juice extraction. Antioxidant activity of flavonoids extracted from pomegranate fermented juice showed strong activity close to that of green tea and significantly higher than that of red wine. Preclinical laboratory studies have suggested that pomegranate and its constituents possess cancer preventive properties against skin, prostate, breast, colon, and lung cancers. Epidemiological, clinical, and case-control studies have not been conducted for pomegranate; however, a phase II clinical trial was recently conducted in patients with rising prostate specific antigen (PSA), a clinical marker for prostate cancer. Pomegranate juice given to men with rising PSA following surgery or radiation offered positive and beneficially significant effects on PSA parameters, suggesting a potential of pomegranate derived products for prevention of human prostate cancer. This chapter will focus on the laboratory and some clinical evidence on the cancer preventive properties of the pomegranate.

Keywords Pomegranate · Chemoprevention · Cancer · Anthocyanins

1 Pomegranates: An overview

The pomegranate fruit has an ancient history and is mentioned in many Holy Scriptures such as the Torah, the Bible, and the Quran (Langley, 2000; Longtin, 2003). For centuries, the fruit has been revered in Greek mythology,

H. Mukhtar (✉)
Department of Dermatology, University of Wisconsin, Madison, WI 53706, USA
e-mail: hmukhtar@wisc.edu

G.D. Stoner, N.P. Seeram (eds.), *Berries and Cancer Prevention*,
DOI 10.1007/978-1-4419-7554-6_11,

Christianity, Judaism, Islam, Buddhism and Hinduism (Longtin, 2003; Jurenka, 2008). Sculptured representations of the fruit are found on the ancient monuments of Egypt and the Assyrian ruins. The tree is native to the region of Persia and the Himalayan ranges of India and has been cultivated in Iran, Afghanistan, Pakistan, North India, Armenia, Azerbaijan, Georgia, and the Mediterranean region for several millennia (Jurenka, 2008). Although grown in some regions of North America, its popularity as a consumer fruit has only recently reached the mainstream commercial markets of North America and the Western Hemisphere. In addition to its ancient historical uses, pomegranate is used in several systems of medicine for a variety of ailments. In the Indian *Ayurvedic* system of medicine, the pomegranate is prescribed as a general tonic and to treat diarrhea, ulcers, and parasites (Jurenka, 2008). Pomegranate is also an important part of the *Unani* system of medicine practiced in the Middle East and India where it is popularly used to treat diabetes (Jurenka, 2008). The recent spate in interest in the medicinal and nutritional properties of pomegranate stemmed from studies that suggested its anti-oxidant activity greater than that of green tea and red wine (Schubert et al., 1999; Gil et al., 2000; Noda et al., 2002). In humans, pomegranate juice consumption decreased low density lipoprotein (LDL) susceptibility to aggregation and retention (Aviram et al., 2000). In mice, oxidation of LDL by peritoneal macrophages was reduced by up to 90% after pomegranate juice consumption. This effect was associated with reduced cellular lipid peroxidation and superoxide release (Aviram et al., 2000). The up-take of oxidized LDL and native LDL by mouse peritoneal macrophages obtained after pomegranate juice administration was reduced by 20%. Pomegranate juice supplementation in mice reduced the number of foam cells and the size of atherosclerotic lesions. These observations suggest that pomegranate juice possesses potent anti-atherogenic effects in healthy humans and in atherosclerotic mice that could be attributable to its anti-oxidative properties. Following these observations, the general health benefits of pomegranate started to be vigorously explored and investigated (Jurenka, 2008; Adhami and Mukhtar, 2007; Afaq et al., 2005b; Adhami et al., 2009). Various products extracted from the pomegranate fruit have been found to be useful for treatment of: cardiovascular disease; diabetes; dental conditions; erectile dysfunction; ultraviolet (UV) radiation induced damages; and cancer and its prevention (Adhami et al., 2009; Jurenka, 2008).

2 Pomegranate Chemistry

Health benefits of pomegranates have largely been attributed to the presence of phytochemicals, the non-nutritive compounds that protect the plant from adverse effects of the environment. Its chemistry varies depending on the part (bark, fruit, leaves, and flowers) being analyzed. The soluble polyphenol content in the juice varies within the limits of 0.2–1.0%, depending on the variety, and includes mainly anthocyanins (such as cyanidin-3-glucoside, cyanidin-3,5-diglucoside, and delphindin-3-glucoside), catechins, ellagic tannins, and gallic and ellagic acids (Ben Nasr et al., 1996). The contents of total phenolics, flavonoids and proathocyanidins were found to be higher in peel than in the pulp (Ben Nasr et al., 1996). The large amount of phenolics contained in the peel has been suggested to impart strong antioxidant activity. The fruit being the edible part comprises 80% juice and 20% seed and is also the source of many active polyphenolic ingredients (Aviram et al., 2000).

Pomegranate juice is a rich source of anthocyanins and hydrolysable tannins (Reed et al., 2005). Positive reflectron mode Matrix-Assisted Laser Desorption/Ionization Time-of-Flight Mass Spectrometry (MALDI-TOF MS) results indicate the presence of six anthocyanins in pomegranate juice: pelargonidin 3-glucoside; cyanidin 3-glucoside; delphinidin 3-glucoside; pelargonidin 3,5-diglucoside; cyanidin 3,5-diglucoside; and delphinidin 3,5-diglucoside (Reed et al., 2005). MALDI-TOF MS also detected an oligomeric series of ellagitannins such as punicalin, pedunculagin, and punicalagin. The commercial processing for juice extraction involves the whole fruit including the peel, the arils, and the seeds and results in high ellagitannin content with approximately 2 g/L of punicalagins (Seeram et al., 2005). The commercially available pomegranate juice is rich in oligomers composed of 2–10 repeating units of gallic acid, ellagic acid, and glucose. There is a large variability in the amount of pomegranate metabolites among subjects which is attributed to differences in the microbial flora of the colon that are responsible for the metabolism of the ellagitannins (Cerda et al., 2004). Ellagitannins such as punicalagins undergo partial hydrolysis and spontaneous internal lactone formation to yield ellagic acid and are detected in only trace amounts in the blood (Larrosa et al., 2006a).

Many of the polyphenolic flavonoids are structurally similar to some mammalian estrogens and show weak estrogenic activity (Kuiper et al., 1998). These flavonoids, referred to as phytoestrogens, have been suggested to be linked to a lower incidence of hormonally dependent cancers of the breast and prostate. Elswijk et al. (2004) applied an on-line biochemical detection coupled to mass spectrometry (LC-BCD–MS) to profile the estrogenic activity in the pomegranate peel extract. The crude mixture was separated by HPLC, after which the presence of biologically active compounds, known or unknown, was detected by means of an on-line β-estrogen receptor (ER) bioassay. Quercetin, a compound possessing only weak estrogenic property (Elswijk et al., 2004), could be detected at a concentration level of 120 μM. Other widespread phytoestrogenic compounds like genistein, daidzein, kaempferol, and luteolin showed markedly lower concentrations (Elswijk et al., 2004).

3 Pomegranates and Cancer

Following the discovery of the anti-oxidant and health-promoting properties of pomegranates, there has been a surge in the studies examining cancer preventing potential of pomegranates (Table 11.1). The purpose of these studies is to

Table 11.1 Summary of laboratory and clinical studies with pomegranate in different in cancer types

Cancer type	Pomegranate fraction	Evidence (references)
Breast	Juice, seed-oil, fermented juice polyphenols, extract	Kim et al. (2002) Mehta and Lansky (2004), Toi et al. (2003), Jeune et al. (2005), Khan et al. (2009), Grossmann et al. (2010), Adams et al. (2010), Tran et al. (2010), Kuiper et al. (1998), Elswijk et al. (2004)
Prostate	Seed-oil, fermented juice polyphenols, extract, juice	Seeram et al. (2005), Lansky et al. (2005a,b), Albrecht et al. (2004), Seeram et al. (2007), Sartippour et al. (2008), Malik et al. (2005), Hafeez et al. (2008), Bin Hafeez et al. (2008), Hong et al. (2008), Rettig et al. (2008), Koyoma ey al. (2010), Kasimsetty et al. (2009), Pantuck et al. (2006)
Lung	Fruit extract	Khan et al. (2007a,b)
Colon	Seed-oil, juice	Kohono et al. (2004), Boateng et al. (2007), Adams et al. (2006), Larrosa et al. (2006), Saruwatari et al. (2008), Sharma (2010)
Skin	Seed-oil, fruit extract	Hora et al. (2003), Afaq et al. (2005a,b), Pacheco-Palencia et al. (2008), Afaq et al. (2009), Zaid et al. (2007), Syed et al. (2006)
Miscellaneous (leukemia)	Fresh and fermented juice	Mertens-Talcott and Percival (2005), Kawaii and Lansky (2004)

investigate potential benefits of pomegranates and identify active ingredients and their molecular targets that could be exploited for prevention and treatment of cancer. Ellagic acid found in many plants, and which has been demonstrated to exhibit strong anti-carcinogenic properties, is a major pomegranate ingredient. Following this discovery, many commercially available pomegranate extracts began to be "standardized to contain 40%" ellagic acid. However, focusing on ellagic acid standardization has been strongly argued (Lansky, 2006). It is generally viewed that pomegranate extract contains a blend of phytochemicals that work through a mechanism of synergy to promote cancer inhibition (Mertens-Talcott et al., 2005; Mertens-Talcott and Percival, 2005; Lansky et al., 2005a, b). The following sections will discuss the current literature on the studies of pomegranates against various cancers.

3.1 Pomegranates and Skin Cancer

The pomegranate fruit has been investigated for its anti-skin cancer activity (Hora et al., 2003; Afaq et al., 2005a, b; Pacheco-Palencia et al., 2008; Afaq et al., 2009; Zaid et al., 2007; Syed et al., 2006). Hora et al. (2003) investigated the effects of pomegranate seed oil on the development of skin tumors in a mouse model of chemical carcinogenesis. Skin tumors were initiated in 5-week-old, female CD-1 mice with an initial topical application of DMBA followed by bi-weekly promotion using 12-O-tetradecanoylphorbol 13-acetate (TPA). Tumor incidence was 100% in control mice compared to 93% in mice pretreated with 5% pomegranate seed oil prior to each TPA application (Hora et al., 2003). The average number of tumors per mouse was 20.8 in control compared to 16.3 per mouse in pomegranate seed oil-treated groups (Hora et al., 2003). The effect of pomegranate seed oil on TPA-stimulated ornithine decarboxylase (ODC) activity, an important event in skin cancer promotion, showed a 17% reduction in ODC activity. These initial observations suggested that pomegranate seed oil is a safe and effective chemopreventive agent against skin cancer (Hora et al., 2003). Anti-tumor-promoting effects of PFE were evaluated in a similar animal model of skin cancer development by Afaq et al. (2005a). Topical application of pomegranate fruit extract (PFE 2 mg/mouse) 30 min prior to TPA (3.2 nmole/mouse) application on mouse skin afforded significant inhibition, in a time-dependent manner, against TPA-mediated increase in skin edema and hyperplasia, epidermal ODC activity, and protein expression of ODC and cyclooxygenase-2 (Afaq et al., 2005a). PFE treatment also resulted in inhibition of TPA-induced phosphorylation of ERK1/2, p38 and JNK1/2, as well as activation of NF-κB (Afaq et al., 2005a). The effect of skin application of PFE on TPA-induced skin tumor promotion in DMBA-initiated CD-1 mouse was also investigated. In TPA-treated group, 100% of the mice developed tumors at 16 weeks on test, whereas at this time in PFE-treated group, only 30% of the mice exhibited tumors. Skin application of PFE prior to TPA application also resulted in a significant delay in latency period from 9 to 14 weeks and afforded protection when tumor data were considered in terms of tumor incidence and tumor multiplicity. These observations provide evidence that PFE possesses anti-skin-tumor-promoting effects in CD-1 mice by inhibiting conventional as well as novel biomarkers of TPA-induced tumor promotion.

Excessive exposure of solar ultraviolet (UV) radiation, particularly its UV-B component, to humans causes many adverse effects that include erythema, hyperplasia, hyperpigmentation, immunosuppression, photoaging and skin cancer. To investigate the effect of PFE for humans, Afaq et al. (2005b) determined its effect in normal human epidermal keratinocytes (NHEK) exposed UV-B. PFE (10–40 μg/mL) for 24 h before UV-B (40 mJ/cm^2) exposure dose dependently inhibited UV-B-mediated phosphorylation of ERKl/2, JNK1/2 and p38 protein (Afaq et al., 2005b). PFE treatment of NHEK also resulted in a dose- and time-dependent inhibition of UV-B-activation of NF-κB (Afaq et al., 2005b). These data demonstrated protective effects of PFE against UV-B radiation and provided a molecular basis for the observed effects. Pacheco-Palencia et al. (2008) investigated the protective effects of pomegranate fruit extract against UVA- and UVB-induced damage in SKU-1064 human skin fibroblast cells. Pomegranate extract (PE), in a range from 5 to 60 mg/L, was effective at protecting human skin fibroblasts from cell death following UV exposure which were attributed to a reduced activation of the pro-inflammatory transcription factor NF-κB, down-regulation of proapoptotic caspase-3, and an increased G0/G1 phase, associated with DNA repair (Pacheco-Palencia et al., 2008). However, higher polyphenolic concentrations

(500–10,000 mg/L) were needed to achieve a significant reduction in UV-induced reactive oxygen species levels and increased intracellular antioxidant capacity (from 1.9 to 8.6 μM Trolox equivalents/mL) (Pacheco-Palencia et al., 2008). Using reconstituted human skin (EpiDerm^{TM}), Afaq et al. (2009) determined the effect of pomegranate-derived products against UVB-mediated damages. Pretreatment of EpiDerm with pomegranate-derived products resulted in inhibition of UVB-induced: (i) cyclobutane pyrimidine dimmers; (ii) 8-dihydro-2′-deoxyguanosine (8-OHdG); (iii) protein oxidation; and (iv) proliferating cell nuclear antigen (PCNA) protein expression. Pretreatment of EpiDerm with pomegranate-derived products resulted in inhibition of UVB-induced: (i) collagenase (MMP-1); (ii) gelatinase (MMP-2, MMP-9); (iii) stromelysin (MMP-3); (iv) marilysin (MMP-7); (v) elastase (MMP-12); and (vi) tropoelastin. Gelatin zymography also revealed that pomegranate-derived products inhibited UVB-induced MMP-2 and MMP-9 activities (Afaq et al., 2009). Pomegranate-derived products also caused a decrease in UVB-induced protein expression of c-Fos and phosphorylation of c-Jun. These results highlight the various health promoting effects of pomegranate-derived products that may be useful against UVB-induced damage to the human skin. Zaid et al. (2007) evaluated the effect of polyphenol-rich pomegranate fruit extract (POMx) on UVB-induced oxidative stress and photoaging in human immortalized HaCaT keratinocytes. Pretreatment of HaCaT cells with POMx (10–40 μg/mL) inhibited UVB (15–30 mJ/cm^2)-mediated a decrease in cell viability, a decrease in intracellular glutathione content, and an increase in lipid peroxidation. Pretreatment of HaCaT cells with POMx also resulted in UVB-induced up-regulation of MMP-1, -2, -7 and -9, a decrease in TIMP-1, phosphorylation of MAPKs, and phosphorylation of c-jun. These results suggest that pomegrante protects HaCaT cells against UVB-induced oxidative stress and markers of photoaging.

PFE was tested for its possible preventive effects against UV-A which is the major portion of solar radiation reaching earth's surface and has been shown to lead to formation of benign and malignant tumors. UV-A exposure to NHEK led to an increase in phosphorylation of STAT3, AKT and ERK1/2 which were inhibited when cells were pretreated with PFE (60–100 μg/mL) for 24 h (Syed et al., 2006). PFE pretreatment also resulted in a dose-dependent inhibition in the phosphorylation of mTOR and p70S6K (Syed et al., 2006). These observations suggest that PFE is an effective agent for ameliorating UVA-mediated damages by modulating cellular pathways. Overall results suggest that pomegranate products are protective against UV induced damages to the skin and underscore their potential for use in topical applications.

3.2 Pomegranate and Prostate Cancer

The effects of pomegranate on prostate cancer have been investigated in the cell culture system, animal models, and in a phase-II clinical trial in humans. Various preparations of pomegranate, in the form of oils, fermented juice polyphenols, and pericarp polyphenols were tested on human prostate cancer cell growth both in vitro and in vivo (Seeram et al., 2005; Lansky et al., 2005a, b; Albrecht et al., 2004; Seeram et al., 2007; Sartippour et al., 2008; Malik and Mukhtar, 2006; Malik et al., 2005; Hafeez et al., 2008; Bin Hafeez et al., 2008). Each preparation inhibited growth of human prostate cancer LNCaP, PC-3, and DU 145 cells whereas normal prostate epithelial cells were significantly less affected (Albrecht et al., 2004). These effects were observed to be mediated by changes in cell cycle distribution and induction of apoptosis. Androgen-independent DU145 cells were treated with pomegranate cold pressed oil (35 μg/mL) and found to accumulate in the G2/M phase of the cell cycle that was associated with a significant up-regulation of the cyclin-dependent kinase inhibitor (cki) p21 and down-regulation of c-myc (Albrecht et al., 2004). In contrast, cell proliferation was inhibited predominantly by induction of apoptosis in PC-3 cells through a caspase 3-mediated pathway (Albrecht et al., 2004). All forms of pomegranate preparations were found to inhibit PC-3 cell invasion through Matrigel and to also inhibit the growth of PC-3 xenograft in athymic nude mice (Lansky et al., 2005a, b). These findings suggested an overall significant anti-proliferative and anti-tumor action of pomegranate-derived fractions against human prostate cancer. Components from pomegranate fruit each belonging to different representative chemical classes and showing known anti-cancer activities were tested as potential inhibitors of in vitro invasion of human prostate cancer cells in an assay employing Matrigel artificial membranes (Seeram et al., 2005, 2007; Sartippour et al., 2008). All compounds significantly inhibited invasion when employed individually at 4 μg/mL. Furthermore, when equally combined at the same dose, they showed a supra-additive inhibition of invasion (Lansky et al., 2005a).

Anti-proliferative and pro-apoptotic properties of PFE against human prostate cancer cells were demonstrated by the authors both in the cell culture system and in a xenograft mouse model (Malik and Mukhtar, 2006; Malik et al., 2005). Human prostate cancer PC-3 cells treated with PFE (10–100 μg/mL) for 48 h resulted in a dose-dependent inhibition of cell growth and induction of apoptosis (Malik et al., 2005). The induction of apoptosis and cell cycle arrest was associated with up-regulation of proapoptotic Bax and Bak, down-regulation of anti-apoptotic Bcl-XL and Bcl-2, induction of WAF1/p21 and KIP1/p27, a decrease in cyclins D1, D2, and E, and decrease in the protein expression of cyclin-dependent kinase-2, 4 and 6 (Malik et al., 2005). To demonstrate the efficacy of PFE in an in vivo setting, athymic nude mice were implanted with androgen-responsive CWR22Rν1 cells and given 0.1 and 0.2% (wt/vol) PFE in drinking water starting simultaneously after cell implantation (Malik et al., 2005). The selection of doses, 0.1 and 0.2%, was based on the assumption that a typical healthy individual (~70 kg) may be persuaded to drink 250 or 500 mL of pomegranate juice extracted from one or two fruits, respectively. Oral infusion of PFE to mice resulted in a significant inhibition in tumor growth as observed by prolongation of tumor appearance. Tumor volumes were consistently lower in mice that received PFE, with effects being dose-dependent and maximum inhibitory effect observed in the 0.2% PFE-fed group. Tumor growth inhibition was accompanied with a concomitant decrease in serum prostate-specific antigen and serum PSA levels were 70–85% lower in PFE fed mice as compared to water-fed mice (Malik et al., 2005). The reduction in prostate tumor growth with concomitant reduction in PSA levels observed in the xenograft model suggested that PFE may have clinical relevance.

Delphinidin, a major anthocyanidin in many pigmented fruits and vegetables and also present in pomegranates, was tested for its anti-cancer effects against human prostate cancer cells (Hafeez et al., 2008; Bin Hafeez et al., 2008). Delphinidin treatment to human prostate cancer cells led to a dose-dependent inhibition of cell growth while sparing normal human prostate epithelial cells (Bin Hafeez et al., 2008). Delphinidin treatment of cells resulted in a dose-dependent induction of apoptosis and arrest of cells in G2-M phase. This induction of apoptosis seemed to be mediated via activation of caspases because N-benzyloxycarbonyl-Val-Ala-Asp(OMe)-fluromethylketone, a general caspase inhibitor, significantly reduced apoptosis induced by delphinidin (Lansky, 2006). Delphinidin treatment of cells also resulted in a dose-dependent modulation in the NF-κB pathway. Delphinidin administration (2 mg, i.p. thrice weekly) to athymic nude mice implanted with human prostate cancer PC3 cells resulted in a significant inhibition of tumor growth that was associated with significant decrease in the expression of NF-κB/p65, Bcl2, and cell proliferation markers Ki67 and PCNA (Bin Hafeez et al., 2008). These data suggested a possibility that delphinidin could be developed as an agent for the management of human prostate cancer.

Prostate cancer initiates as an androgen dependent disease; however, advanced disease acquires an androgen-independent status that progress rapidly and is refractory to hormone conventional chemotherapeutic regimens. Hong et al. (2008) investigated the effects of pomegranate polyphenols, ellagitannin-rich extract and whole juice extract on the expression of genes for key androgen-synthesizing enzymes and the androgen-receptor. Genes HSD3B2 (3beta-hydroxysteroid dehydrogenase type 2), AKR1C3 (aldo-keto reductase family 1 member C3), and SRD5A1 (steroid 5alpha reductase type 1) were analyzed in LNCaP, LNCaP-AR, and DU-145 human prostate cancer cells. Pomegranate polyphenols inhibited gene expression and AR most consistently in the LNCaP-AR cell line where androgen receptor was over-expressed (Hong et al., 2008). These studies suggested that pomegranate polyphenols may be of particular importance in androgen-independent prostate cancer cells and the subset of human prostate cancers where the androgen receptor is up-regulated. In the LAPC4 xenograft model, pomegranate extract delayed the emergence of LAPC4 androgen-independent tumors in castrated mice through an inhibition of proliferation and induction of apoptosis (Rettig et al., 2008). Increase in NF-κB activity that occurred during the transition from androgen dependence to androgen independence was abrogated by pomegranate extract (Rettig et al., 2008). A recent study investigated the relationship between pomegranate-induced apoptosis in human prostate cancer and the insulin like growth factor/insulin like growth factor binding protein (IGF/IGFBP) axis (Koyoma et al., 2010). The IGF axis is critical for the regulation of apoptosis in many human cancer cell lines. Prostate cancer LAPC4 cells were treated with 10 μg/mL POMx, a highly potent pomegranate extract prepared from skin and arils (minus the seeds), and standardized to contain ellagitannin (37% punicalagins by HPLC). This treatment resulted in inhibition of cell proliferation and induction of apoptosis. Interestingly, co-treatment with POMx and IGFBP-3 revealed synergistic stimulation of apoptosis and additive inhibition of cell growth (Koyoma et al., 2010). This combination was also associated with increased JNK phosphorylation, and decreased Akt and mTOR activation, which is consistent with a growth inhibitory, pro-apoptotic function. Co-treatment with 100 ng/mL IGF-1 completely blocked apoptosis induction by POMx and IGF-I failed to inhibit POMx-induced apoptosis in cells lacking IGF-IR. POMx-treatment decreased IGF-1 mRNA expression in a dose-dependent manner indicating that its actions also involve tumor-specific suppression of IGF-1. These studies suggest that pomegranate components interact with the IGF axis and inhibit cancer development and progression.

The drug metabolizing enzyme cytochrome P450 CYP1B1 is involved in the activation of many carcinogens and in the metabolism of steroid hormones and has been suggested as a target for prostate cancer prevention. Kasimsetty et al. (2009) examined pomegranate ellagitannins and their microbial metabolites for their CYP1B1 inhibitory activity in a recombinant CYP1B1-mediated ethoxyresorufin-O-deethylase (EROD) assay. Urolithin A, a microbial metabolite, was the most potent uncompetitive inhibitor of CYP1B1-mediated EROD activity, exhibiting two-fold selectivity over CYP1A1, while urolithin B was a noncompetitive inhibitor with three-fold selectivity. The punicalins and punicalagins exhibited potent CYP1A1 inhibition with fivefold to tenfold selectivity over CYP1B1. Urolithins, punicalins, and punicalagins were tested for their 2,3,7,8-tetrachlorodibenzo-p-dioxin (TCDD)-induced CYP1 inhibitory activity in the 22Rv1 prostate cancer cell line. Urolithins A and B showed a decrease in their CYP1-mediated EROD inhibitory IC_{50} values upon increasing their treatment times from 30 min to 24 h Urolithin C, 8-O-methylurolithin A, and 8,9-di-O-methylurolithin C caused a potent CYP1-mediated EROD inhibition in 22Rv1 cells upon 24 h of incubation. Urolithins were observed to inhibit both the activity and expression of CYP1B1 which could have implications for prostate cancer prevention (Kasimsetty et al., 2009).

In a phase II clinical trial Pantuck et al. (2006) recruited patients with rising PSA and gave them 8 ounces of pomegranate juice daily until disease progression. PSA doubling time significantly increased with treatment from a mean of 15 months at baseline to 54 months post-treatment ($P<0.001$). A major drawback of this study was the absence of a proper placebo control; however, statistically significant prolongation of PSA doubling time suggested a potential of pomegranate for prevention of human prostate cancer (Pantuck et al., 2006). This initial clinical trial bears evidence in support of PFE because it suggests that pomegranate consumption may retard prostate cancer progression, which may prolong not only the survival but also improve the quality of life of patients.

3.3 Pomegranate and Breast Cancer

Studies in cell culture and mouse models suggest possible benefits of pomegranate juice against breast cancer risk (Sturgeon and Ronnenberg, 2010). These studies demonstrate that various constituents of pomegranates can inhibit aromatase and 17-β-hydroxysteroid dehydrogenase enzymes or have anti-estrogenic activity. Polyphenolic fractions from pomegranate fruit were assessed in vitro for their possible chemopreventive activity or as adjuvant in a therapeutic setting against human breast cancer cells (Kim et al., 2002). Polyphenols obtained from fermented juice at concentrations ranging from 100 to 1,000 μg/mL inhibited aromatase and 17-β-hydroxysteroid dehydrogenase type 1 activity by 60–80%. Human breast cancer cell lines MCF-7 and MB-MDA-231 cells were treated with fermented and fresh pomegranate juice. Polyphenols from fermented juice showed about twice the anti-proliferative effect as compared to polyphenols from fresh pomegranate juice. Pomegranate seed oil (100 μg/mL of medium) resulted in 90% inhibition of proliferation of MCF-7 cells. Invasion of MCF-7 cells across a Matrigel membrane was inhibited by 75% at 10 μg/mL of pomegranate seed oil (Kim et al., 2002). Pomegranate seed oil (50 μg/mL) also induced 54% apoptosis in MDA-MB-435 estrogen receptor negative metastatic human breast cancer cells. Fermented juice polyphenols resulted in 47% inhibition of cancerous lesion formation induced by the carcinogen 7,12-dimethylbenz[a]anthracene (DMBA) in a murine mammary gland organ culture (Kim et al., 2002). Mehta and Lansky (2004) further explored and compared the chemopreventive efficacy of a purified chromatographic peak of pomegranate fermented juice and also of whole pomegranate seed oil. Mouse mammary organ cultures were treated with pomegranate fermented juice polyphenols, a high-performance liquid chromatographic (HPLC) peak separated from fermented juice or pomegranate seed oil and on day 3, exposed to the carcinogen DMBA, and for 10 days treated with the putative pomegranate preparations. Fermented pomegranate juice resulted in a 42% reduction in the number of lesions compared with control, while the peak separated from the fermented juice and the pomegranate seed oil each resulted in an 87% reduction in number of tumorigenic lesions (Mehta and Lansky, 2004). The results suggested enhanced potential for the purified compound as well as pomegranate seed oil, both greater than pomegranate fermented juice polyphenols.

Toi et al. (2003) evaluated the anti-angiogenic potential of pomegranate polyphenols by measuring vascular endothelial growth factor (VEGF), interleukin-4 (IL-4), and migration inhibitory factor (MIF) in the conditioned media of MCF-7 or MDA-MB-231 human breast cancer cells, or immortalized normal human breast epithelial cells (MCF-10A). VEGF was strongly down-regulated in MCF-10A and MCF-7, and MIF up-regulated in MDA-MB-231, overall showing significant potential for down-regulation of angiogenesis by pomegranate fractions (Toi et al., 2003). These fractions further inhibited proliferation of human umbilical vein endothelial cells (HUVEC), myometrial, and amniotic fluid fibroblasts. A significant decrease in new blood vessel formation using the chicken chorioallantoic membrane (CAM) model was also observed. These findings demonstrate an anti-angiogenic potential of pomegranate fractions. The effect of pomegranate extracts in combination with genistein was investigated on the growth rate and apoptosis induction in human breast cancer cells MCF-7 (Jeune et al., 2005). Both pomegranate extracts and genistein had significant dose- and time-dependent cytotoxic effects on MCF-7 cells. The inhibition and apoptosis induction were significantly higher in the combination treatments than in the single treatments with either agent isolated (Jeune et al., 2005).

Because NF-κB is known to regulate several biological processes including tumorigenesis, Khan et al. (2009) hypothesized that PFEs may exert anticancer effects at least in part by modulating NF-κB activity. The aqueous PFE dose-dependently inhibited NF-κB-dependent reporter gene expression in aggressive breast cancer phenotypes while decreasing RhoC and RhoA protein expression. Inhibition of motility and invasion by PFEs, coincident with suppressed RhoC and RhoA protein expression, suggests a role for these defined extracts in lowering the metastatic potential of aggressive breast cancer species (Khan et al., 2009). Grossmann et al. (2010) investigated the potential ability of punicic acid to affect growth of both an estrogen insensitive breast cancer cell line (MDA-MB-231) and an estrogen sensitive cell line developed from the MDA-MB-231 cells (MDA-ERalpha7). Proliferation was inhibited 92 and 96% for MDA-MB-231 and MDA-ERalpha7 cells, respectively, compared to untreated cells by 40 μM punicic acid. Furthermore, punicic acid induced apoptosis in the MDA-MB-231 and MDA-ERalpha7 cells by 86 and 91%, respectively, compared to untreated control cells and disrupted cellular mitochondrial membrane potential. Punicic acid effects were partially blocked in the presence 20 μM of the antioxidant tocotrienol or the PKC inhibitor bisindolymaleimide I in both the MDA-MB-231 and MDA-ERalpha7 cells (Grossmann et al., 2010). Thus, punicic acid, a component of the pomegranate seed oil, has breast cancer inhibitor properties that are dependent on lipid peroxidation and the PKC pathway.

Adams et al. (2010) investigated the anti-aromatase activity and inhibition of testosterone-induced breast cancer cell proliferation by ellagitannin-derived compounds isolated from pomegranates. A panel of 10 ellagitannin-derived compounds including ellagic acid, gallagic acid, and urolithins A and B (and their acetylated, methylated, and sulfated analogues) was examined using a microsomal aromatase assay. Urolithin B was found to most effectively inhibit aromatase activity in a live cell assay. Proliferation assays also determined that urolithin B significantly inhibited testosterone-induced MCF-7 cell proliferation (Adams et al., 2010). Pomegranate seed linolenic acid isomers were evaluated as selective estrogen receptor modulators under in vitro conditions (Tran et al., 2010). Punicic acid inhibitory IC_{50} activity against estrogen receptor (ER)-α was 7.2 μM, for ER-β was 8.8 μM, and α-eleostearic acid inhibited ER-α/ER-β at 6.5/7.8 μM. Punicic acid and α-eleostearic acid induced ER-α and ER-β mRNA expression in MCF-7 but not in MDA-MB-231 (Tran et al., 2010). These data provide evidence that pomegranate components exhibit selective estrogen receptor modulatory activity and suggested a potential for pomegranate-derived compounds for the prevention of estrogen-responsive breast cancers.

3.4 Pomegranate and Colon Cancer

The effect of pomegranate seed oil (PGO) was studied in mice on the occurrence of colonic aberrant crypt foci (ACF) induced by azoxymethane (AOM) (Kohno et al., 2004; Boateng et al., 2007). Colonic tumors were induced in 6-week old male F344 rats by subcutaneous injections of AOM (20 mg/kg body weight) once a week for 2 weeks (Kohno et al., 2004). One week before the AOM treatment, mice were started on a diet containing 0.01, 0.1, or 1% PGO for 32 weeks. After 32 weeks, the incidence of colon tumors was 81% with a tumor multiplicity of 1.88/mice. Administration of PGO in the diet significantly inhibited the incidence and multiplicity of colonic adenocarcinomas; however, a dose-response relationship was not observed (Kohno et al., 2004). The inhibition of tumor incidence was associated with increased expression of peroxisome proliferator-activated receptor (PPAR) gamma protein in the non-tumor mucosa (Kohno et al., 2004). In another study (Boateng et al., 2007), rats received 20% pomegranate juice in drinking water and 3 weeks later received subcutaneous injections of AOM (16 mg/kg body weight at 7th and 8th weeks of age). Aberrant cryptic foci (ACF) measured on the 17th week were only 15.67 ± 1.86 in the pomegranate juice group compared to the control 171.67 ± 5.6 (Schubert et al., 1999). Total glutathione-S-transferase (GST) activity in the liver of the rats fed pomegranate juice was significantly ($p<0.05$) higher compared with the control, suggesting that pomegranate juice contributes to significant reductions in the formation of AOM-induced ACF (Boateng et al., 2007).

Adams et al. (2006) examined the effects of pomegranate juice on inflammatory cell signaling proteins in HT-29 human colon cancer cell line based on the fact that inflammation plays a key role in the development of colon cancer. At a concentration of 50 mg/L, pomegranate juice significantly suppressed TNFα-induced COX-2 protein expression by 79% and also reduced phosphorylation of the NF-kB/p65 subunit and its binding to the NF-κB response element. Pomegranate juice also abolished TNFα-induced AKT activation, needed for NF-κB activity (Adams et al., 2006). These data provided evidence that polyphenolic constituents in the pomegranate play an important role in the modulation of inflammatory signals in colon cancer cells.

Larrosa et al. (2006) observed that the anti-carcinogenic effect of dietary elagitannins could be mainly due to their hydrolysis product, elagic acid. Punicalagin was hydrolysed in the medium to yield elagic acid which entered into the cells, was metabolised to produce dimethyl-elagic acid, which then induced apoptosis via mitochondrial pathway in colon cancer Caco-2 cells but not in normal colon cells (Larrosa et al., 2006). Among several fruit juices tested (apple, peach, orange, pineapple, grapefruit, and pomegranate), pomegranate juice potently inhibited the sulfoconjugation of 1-naphthol in Caco-2 cells (Saruwatari et al., 2008). Punicalagin, the most abundant antioxidant polyphenol in pomegranate juice, was also found to strongly inhibit sulfoconjugation in Caco-2 cells with an IC_{50} of 45 μM. Phase II conjugation activity in the intestinal epithelium affects the bioavailability of drugs and other environmental xenobiotics. Pomegranate juice and punicalagin both inhibited phenol sulfotransferase activity in Caco-2 cells in vitro

(Saruwatari et al., 2008). These results suggest that constituents of pomegranate juice, most probably punicalagin, impair the enteric functions of sulfoconjugation and that this might have effects upon the bioavailability of drugs and other compounds present in food and in the environment and further, the effects might be related to the anti-carcinogenic properties of pomegranate juice.

Components of Wnt signaling pathways are known to play a pivotal role in human colon carcinogenesis, and inappropriate activation of the signaling cascade is observed in 90% of colorectal cancers. Sharma et al. (2010) investigated the effects of components of pomegranate extracts on Wnt signaling in a human 293T cell line using a luciferase reporter of canonical Wnt pathway-mediated transcriptional activation. The elagitannin extracts (IC_{50} = 28.0–30.0 μg/mL), ellagic acid (IC_{50} = 19.0 μg/mL; 63 μM), and urolithins (IC_{50} = 9.0 μg/mL; 39 μM) inhibited Wnt signaling, suggesting that ET-rich foods have potential against colon carcinogenesis (Sharma et al., 2010).

3.5 Pomegranate and Lung Cancer

The effects of PFE on lung tumorigenesis were examined by the authors both in vitro and in vivo (Khan et al., 2007a, b, 2008). Normal human bronchial epithelial cells (NHBE) and human lung carcinoma A549 cells were treated with PFE (50–150 μg/mL) for 72 h. While PFE resulted in a significant decrease in the viability of A549 cells, only minimal effects were observed on NHBE cells (Khan et al., 2007a). PFE treatment of A549 cells resulted in dose-dependent arrest of cells in G0/G1 phase of the cell cycle which was associated with induction of WAF1/p21 and KIP1/p27 and accompanied by decrease in the expression of downstream cell cycle regulatory proteins. PFE treatment also resulted in inhibition of several signaling pathways including MAPK PI3K/Akt and NF-κB. The effect of PFE was tested in mice implanted with A549 cells (Khan et al., 2007a). The appearance of tumors was observed in animals receiving water as early as 15 days post cell inoculation. This latency period was prolonged to 19 days in animals receiving PFE in drinking fluid. In mice that received water, the average tumor volume of 1,200 mm^3 was reached in 55 ± 2 days after tumor cell inoculation. At this time point, the average tumor volumes in the 0.1 and 0.2% PFE-fed groups were 621 and 540 mm^3, respectively (Khan et al., 2007a). The average tumor volume of 1,200 mm^3 was achieved in 67 ± 4 days after tumor cell inoculation in 0.1% PFE-fed group. The 0.2% PFE-fed group showed the most effective tumor growth inhibitory response where the targeted average tumor volume of 1,200 mm^3 was reached at 79 ± 3 days after tumor cell inoculation. These observations indicated that PFE could be a useful chemopreventive/chemotherapeutic agent against human lung cancer.

To further explore the benefits of PFE against lung tumorigenesis, the authors examined the effect of oral consumption of a human achievable dose of PFE in two mouse lung tumor protocols (Khan et al., 2007b). Benzo(a)pyrene [B(a)P] and

N-nitroso-tris-chloroethylurea (NTCU) were used to induce lung tumors, and PFE was given in drinking water to A/J mice. Lung tumor yield was examined on the 84th day and 140 days after B(a)P dosing and 240 days after NTCU treatment. Mice treated with PFE and exposed to B(a)P and NTCU had statistically significant lower lung tumor multiplicities than mice treated with carcinogens only (Khan et al., 2007b). Tumor reduction was 53.9 and 61.6% in the B(a)P + PFE group at 84 and 140 days, respectively, compared with the B(a)P group. The NTCU + PFE group had 65.9% tumor reduction compared with the NTCU group at 240 days (Khan et al., 2007b). Tumors from these animals were examined for effects on cell proliferation and various signaling pathways. Tumors had low proliferative indices as examined by ki-67 and PCNA staining. PFE treatment also resulted in inhibition of NF-κB, MAPK, and PI3K/Akt signaling. Since the mammalian target of rapamycin (mTOR) is downstream of both PI3K and Akt, it was determined that phosphorylation of mTOR was a result of PI3K/Akt activation (Khan et al., 2007b). Treatment with B(*a*)P and NTCU caused increased phosphorylation of mTOR at Ser^{2448}, whereas PFE administration resulted in inhibition of phosphorylation of mTOR. This observation was significant since the mTOR integrates mitogenic signals and intracellular nutrient levels to activate 4EBP1 and p70S6K that control protein translation and cell cycle progression. Phosphorylation of AMPKα, an upstream down-regulator of mTOR that was decreased in B(a)P and NTCU treated mice was restored in mice that received oral infusion of PFE (Khan et al., 2007b).

4 Future Perspective and Conclusions

Cancer continues to remain a leading cause of death in men in the United States and in many parts of Europe and the developing world. Although advances in diagnosis and treatment have substantially improved overall survival, there is general consensus that treatment options are limited and fraught with adverse side effects. Research into the use of non-toxic dietary ingredients is rapidly gaining ground and many natural agents are being investigated for possible use as cancer chemopreventive as well as cancer therapeutic agents. Various agents from dietary sources (both fruits and vegetables) have been identified with anti-cancer potential; however, to firmly establish their potential, in depth laboratory studies in appropriate pre-clinical models need to be conducted. This is essential for smooth transition into human clinical trials. Interest in pomegranate derived products, especially their anti-cancer properties, is largely attributed to initial experiments that reported antioxidant activity greater than that of red wine or even green tea. Pomegranate juice has shown an initial promise in a phase II clinical trial against prostate cancer and such studies need to be conducted in other cancers as well. While identifying individual active ingredients in the pomegranate juice would be ideal, it is interesting to note that many studies observed the extract or the juice to be more beneficial. This suggests the existence of a chemical synergy when using an extract. The use of

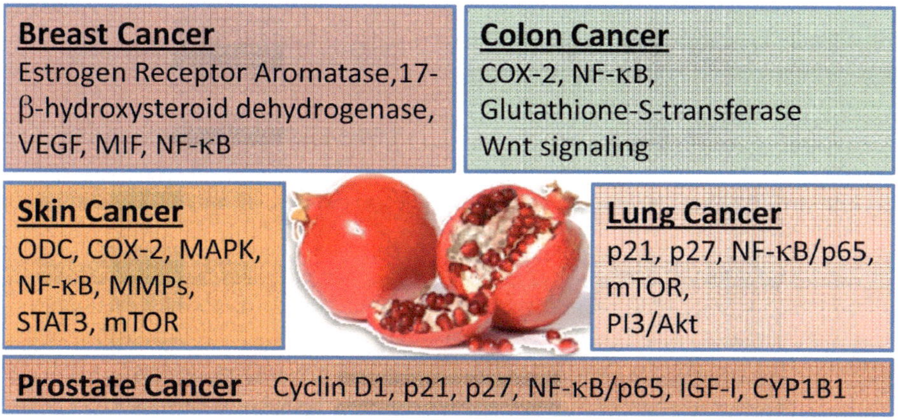

Fig. 11.1 Molecular targets identified for pomegranate against different cancer types

an extract rather than a purified compound could explain the inhibition of multiple targets (Fig. 11.1) observed in many studies and needs to be explored in clinical and epidemiological studies in the future.

Acknowledgements The original work from the author's (H.M.) laboratory outlined in this chapter was supported by United States Public Health Service Grants R01 CA 78809 and RO1 CA 120451.

References

Adams LS, Seeram NP, Aggarwal BB, Takada Y, Sand D, Heber D (2006) Pomegranate juice, total pomegranate ellagitannins, and punicalagin suppress inflammatory cell signaling in colon cancer cells. J Agric Food Chem 54:980–985

Adams LS, Zhang Y, Seeram NP, Heber D, Chen S (2010) Pomegranate ellagitannin-derived compounds exhibit antiproliferative and antiaromatase activity in breast cancer cells in vitro. Cancer Prev Res 3:108–113

Adhami VM, Khan N, Mukhtar H (2009) Cancer chemoprevention by pomegranate: laboratory and clinical evidence. Nutr Cancer 61:811–815

Adhami VM, Mukhtar H (2007) Anti-oxidants from green tea and pomegranate for chemoprevention of prostate cancer. Mol Biotechnol 37:52–57

Afaq F, Malik A, Syed D, Maes D, Matsui MS, Mukhtar H (2005b) Pomegranate fruit extract modulates UV-B-mediated phosphorylation of mitogen-activated protein kinases and activation of nuclear factor kappa B in normal human epidermal keratinocytes paragraph sign. Photochem Photobiol 81:38–45

Afaq F, Saleem M, Krueger CG, Reed JD, Mukhtar H (2005a) Anthocyanin- and hydrolyzable tannin-rich pomegranate fruit extract modulates MAPK and NF-kappaB pathways and inhibits skin tumorigenesis in CD-1 mice. Int J Cancer 113:423–433

Afaq F, Zaid MA, Khan N, Dreher M, Mukhtar H (2009) Protective effect of pomegranate-derived products on UVB-mediated damage in human reconstituted skin. Exp Dermatol 18:553–561

Albrecht M, Jiang W, Kumi-Diaka J, Lansky EP, Gommersall LM (2004) Pomegranate extracts potently suppress proliferation, xenograft growth, and invasion of human prostate cancer cells. J Med Food 7:274–283

Aviram M, Dornfeld L, Rosenblat M, Volkova N, Kaplan M, Coleman R, Hayek T, Presser D, Fuhrman B (2000) Pomegranate juice consumption reduces oxidative stress, atherogenic modifications to LDL, and platelet aggregation: studies in humans and in atherosclerotic apolipoprotein E-deficient mice. Am J Clin Nutr 71:1062–1076

1Ben Nasr C, Ayed N, Metche M (1996) Quantitative determination of the polyphenolic content of pomegranate peel. Z Lebensm Unters Forsch 203:374–378

Bin Hafeez B, Asim M, Siddiqui IA, Adhami VM, Murtaza I, Mukhtar H (2008) Delphinidin, a dietary anthocyanidin in pigmented fruits and vegetables: a new weapon to blunt prostate cancer growth. Cell Cycle 7:3320–3326

Boateng J, Verghese M, Shackelford L, Walker LT, Khatiwada J, Ogutu S, Williams DS, Jones J, Guyton M, Asiamah D, Henderson F, Grant L, DeBruce M, Johnson A, Washington S, Chawan CB (2007) Selected fruits reduce azoxymethane (AOM)-induced aberrant crypt foci (ACF) in Fisher 344 male rats. Food Chem Toxicol 45:725–732

Cerdá B, Espín JC, Parra S, Martínez P, Tomás-Barberán FA (2004) The potent in vitro antioxidant ellagitannins from pomegranate juice are metabolised into bioavailable but poor antioxidant hydroxy-6H-dibenzopyran-6-one derivatives by the colonic microflora of healthy humans. Eur J Nutr 43:205–220

Elswijk DA, Schobel UP, Lansky EP, Irth H, van der Greef J (2004) Rapid dereplication of estrogenic compounds in pomegranate (Punica granatum) using on-line biochemical detection coupled to mass spectrometry. Phytochemistry 65:233–241

Gil MI, Tomas-Barberan FA, Hess-Pierce B, Holcroft DM, Kader AA (2000) Antioxidant activity of pomegranate juice and its relationship with phenolic composition and processing. J Agric Food Chem 48:4581–4589

Grossmann ME, Mizuno NK, Schuster T, Cleary MP (2010) Punicic acid is an omega-5 fatty acid capable of inhibiting breast cancer proliferation. Int J Oncol 36:421–426

Hafeez BB, Siddiqui IA, Asim M, Malik A, Afaq F, Adhami VM, Saleem M, Din M, Mukhtar H (2008) A dietary anthocyanidin delphinidin induces apoptosis of human prostate cancer PC3 cells in vitro and in vivo: involvement of nuclear factor-kappaB signaling. Cancer Res 68: 8564–8572

Hong MY, Seeram NP, Heber D (2008) Pomegranate polyphenols down-regulate expression of androgen-synthesizing genes in human prostate cancer cells overexpressing the androgen receptor. J Nutriochem 19:848–855

Hora JJ, Maydew ER, Lansky EP, Dwivedi C (2003) Chemopreventive effects of pomegranate seed oil on skin tumor development in CD1 mice. J Med Food 6:157–161

Jeune MA, Kumi-Diaka J, Brown J (2005) Anticancer activities of pomegranate extracts and genistein in human breast cancer cells. J Med Food 8:469–475

Jurenka JS (2008) Therapeutic applications of pomegranate (Punica granatum L.): a review. Altern Med Rev 13:128–144

Kasimsetty SG, Bialonska D, Reddy MK, Thornton C, Willett KL, Ferreira D (2009) Effects of pomegranate chemical constituents/intestinal microbial metabolites on CYP1B1 in 22Rv1 prostate cancer cells. J Agric Food Chem 57:10636–10644

Kawaii S, Lansky EP (2004) Differentiation-promoting activity of pomegranate (Punica granatum) fruit extracts in HL-60 human promyelocytic leukemia cells. J Med Food 7:13–18

Khan GN, Gorin MA, Rosenthal D, Pan Q, Bao LW, Wu ZF, Newman RA, Pawlus AD, Yang P, Lansky EP, Merajver SD (2009) Pomegranate fruit extract impairs invasion and motility in human breast cancer. Integr Cancer Ther 8:242–253

Khan N, Afaq F, Kweon MH, Kim K, Mukhtar H (2007b) Oral consumption of pomegranate fruit extract inhibits growth and progression of primary lung tumors in mice. Cancer Res 67: 3475–3482

Khan N, Afaq F, Mukhtar H: (2008) Cancer chemoprevention through dietary antioxidants: progress and promise. Antioxid Redox Signal 10:475–510

Khan N, Hadi N, Afaq F, Syed DN, Kweon MH, Mukhtar H (2007a) Pomegranate fruit extract inhibits prosurvival pathways in human A549 lung carcinoma cells and tumor growth in athymic nude mice. Carcinogenesis 28:163–173

Kim ND, Mehta R, Yu W, Neeman I, Livney T, Amichay A, Poirier D, Nicholls P, Kirby A, Jiang W, Mansel R, Ramachandran C, Rabi T, Kaplan B, Lansky E (2002) Chemopreventive and adjuvant therapeutic potential of pomegranate (Punica granatum) for human breast cancer. Breast Cancer Res Treat 71:203–217

Kohno H, Suzuki R, Yasui Y, Hosokawa M, Miyashita K, Tanaka T (2004) Pomegranate seed oil rich in conjugated linolenic acid suppresses chemically induced colon carcinogenesis in rats. Cancer Sci 95:481–486

Koyama S, Cobb LJ, Mehta HH, Seeram NP, Heber D, Pantuck AJ, Cohen P (2010) Pomegranate extract induces apoptosis in human prostate cancer cells by modulation of the IGF-IGFBP axis. Growth Horm IGF Res 20:55–62

Kuiper JMGG, Lemmen JG, Carlsson B, Corton JC, Safe SH, van der Saag PT, van der Burg B, Gustafsson JÄ (1998) Interaction of estrogenic chemicals and phytoestrogens with estrogen receptor β. Endocrinology 139:4252–4263

Langley P (2000) Why a pomegranate? BMJ 321:1153–1154

Lansky EP, Harrison G, Froom P, Jiang WG (2005b) Pomegranate (Punica granatum) pure chemicals show possible synergistic inhibition of human PC-3 prostate cancer cell invasion across Matrigel. Invest New Drugs 23:121–122

Lansky EP, Jiang W, Mo H, Bravo L, Froom P, Yu W, Harris NM, Neeman I, Campbell MJ (2005a) Possible synergistic prostate cancer suppression by anatomically discrete pomegranate fractions. Invest New Drugs 23:11–20

Lansky EP (2006) Beware of pomegranates bearing 40% ellagic Acid. J Med Food 9:119–122

Larrosa M, Gonzalez-Sarrias A, Garcia-Conesa MT, Tomas-Barberan FA, Espin JC (2006a) Urolithins, ellagic acid-derived metabolites produced by human colonic microflora, exhibit estrogenic and antiestrogenic activities. J Agric Food Chem 54:1611–1620

Larrosa M, Tomás-Barberán FA, Espín JC (2006b) The dietary hydrolysable tannin punicalagin releases ellagic acid that induces apoptosis in human colon adenocarcinoma Caco-2 cells by using the mitochondrial pathway. J Nutriochem 17:611–625

Longtin R (2003) The pomegranate: nature's power fruit? J Natl Cancer Inst 95:346–348

Malik A, Afaq F, Sarfaraz S, Adhami VM, Syed DN, Mukhtar H (2005) Pomegranate fruit juice for chemoprevention and chemotherapy of prostate cancer. Proc Natl Acad Sci USA 102: 14813–14818

Malik A, Mukhtar H (2006) Prostate cancer prevention through pomegranate fruit. Cell Cycle 5:371–373

Mehta R, Lansky EP (2004) Breast cancer chemopreventive properties of pomegranate (Punica granatum) fruit extracts in a mouse mammary organ culture. Eur J Cancer Prev 13:345–348

Mertens-Talcott SU, Bomser JA, Romero C, Talcott ST, Percival SS (2005) Ellagic acid potentiates the effect of quercetin on p21waf1/cip1, p53, and MAP-kinases without affecting intracellular generation of reactive oxygen species in vitro. J Nutr 135:609–614

Mertens-Talcott SU, Percival SS (2005) Ellagic acid and quercetin interact synergistically with resveratrol in the induction of apoptosis and cause transient cell cycle arrest in human leukemia cells. Cancer Lett 218:141–151

Noda Y, Kaneyuki T, Mori A, Packer L (2002) Antioxidant activities of pomegranate fruit extract and its anthocyanidins: delphinidin, cyanidin, and pelargonidin. J Agric Food Chem 50: 166–171

Pacheco-Palencia LA, Noratto G, Hingorani L, Talcott ST, Mertens-Talcott SU (2008) Protective effects of standardized pomegranate (Punica granatum L.) polyphenolic extract in ultraviolet-irradiated human skin fibroblasts. J Agric Food Chem 56:8434–8441

Pantuck AJ, Leppert JT, Zomorodian N, Aronson W, Hong J, Barnard RJ, Seeram N, Liker H, Wang H, Elashoff R, Heber D, Aviram M, Ignarro L, Belldegrun A (2006) PhaseII study of pomegranate juice for men with rising prostate-specific antigen following surgery or radiation for prostate cancer. Clin Cancer Res 12:4018–4026

Reed JD, Krueger CG, Vestling MM (2005) MALDI-TOF mass spectrometry of oligomeric food polyphenols. Phytochemistry 66:2248–2263

Rettig MB, Heber D, An J, Seeram NP, Rao JY, Liu H, Klatte T, Belldegrun A, Moro A, Henning SM, Mo D, Aronson WJ, Pantuck A (2008) Pomegranate extract inhibits androgen-independent prostate cancer growth through a nuclear factor-kappaB-dependent mechanism. Mol Cancer Ther 7:2662–2671

Sartippour MR, Seeram NP, Rao JY, Moro A, Harris DM, Henning SM, Firouzi A, Rettig MB, Aronson WJ, Pantuck AJ, Heber D (2008) Ellagitannin-rich pomegranate extract inhibits angiogenesis in prostate cancer in vitro and in vivo. Int J Oncol 32:475–480

Saruwatari A, Okamura S, Nakajima Y, Narukawa Y, Takeda T, Tamura H (2008) Pomegranate juice inhibits sulfoconjugation in Caco-2 human colon carcinoma cells. J Med Food 11: 623–628

Schubert SY, Lansky EP, Neeman I (1999) Antioxidant and eicosanoid enzyme inhibition properties of pomegranate seed oil and fermented juice flavonoids. J Ethnopharmacol 66:11–17

Seeram NP, Adams LS, Henning SM, Niu Y, Zhang Y, Nair MG, Heber D (2005) In vitro antiproliferative, apoptotic and antioxidant activities of punicalagin, ellagic acid and a total pomegranate tannin extract are enhanced in combination with other polyphenols as found in pomegranate juice. J Nutriochem 16:360–367

Seeram NP, Aronson WJ, Zhang Y, Henning SM, Moro A, Lee RP, Sartippour M, Harris DM, Rettig M, Suchard MA, Pantuck AJ, Belldegrun A, Heber D (2007) Pomegranate ellagitannin-derived metabolites inhibit prostate cancer growth and localize to the mouse prostate gland. J Agric Food Chem 55:7732–7737

Sharma M, Li L, Celver J, Killian C, Kovoor A, Seeram NP (2010) Effects of fruit ellagitannin extracts, ellagic acid, and their colonic metabolite, urolithin A, on Wnt signaling. J Agric Food Chem 58:3965–3969

Sturgeon SR, Ronnenberg AG (2010) Pomegranate and breast cancer: possible mechanisms of prevention. Nutr Rev 68:122–128

Syed DN, Malik A, Hadi N, Sarfaraz S, Afaq F, Mukhtar H (2006) Photochemopreventive effect of pomegranate fruit extract on UVA-mediated activation of cellular pathways in normal human epidermal keratinocytes. Photochem Photobiol 82:398–405

Toi M, Bando H, Ramachandran C, Melnick SJ, Imai A (2003) Preliminary studies on the anti-angiogenic potential of pomegranate fractions in vitro and in vivo. Angiogenesis 6:121–128

Tran HN, Bae SY, Song BH, Lee BH, Bae YS, Kim YH, Lansky EP, Newman RA (2010) Pomegranate (Punica granatum) seed linolenic acid isomers: concentration-dependent modulation of estrogen receptor activity. Endocr Res 35:1–16

Zaid MA, Afaq F, Syed DN, Dreher M, Mukhtar H (2007) Inhibition of UVB-mediated oxidative stress and markers of photoaging in immortalized HaCaT keratinocytes by pomegranate polyphenol extract POMx. Photochem Photobiol 83:882–888

Chapter 12
Chemoprevention of Chronic Inflammatory Bowel Disease-Induced Carcinogenesis in Rodent Models by Berries

Allison Yang, Haonan Li, WanYing Zhang, Yeon Tae Chung, Jie Liao, and Guang-Yu Yang

Abstract Long-term chronic inflammation including inflammatory bowel disease is a well-recognized risk factor for cancer development. Fresh fruits, particularly berries, have been well documented as having protective effects against inflammation and cancer development. There are several key elements in the berries with functions against cancer, including vitamins (A, C, E, and folic acid), minerals (calcium and selenium), phenol compounds (particularly ellagic acid, ferulic acid, chlorogenic acid, coumaric acid, quercetin and anthocyanins), phytosterols (β-sitosterol, campesterol, and stigmasterol) and oligosaccharides. This chapter focuses on linking berries to chronic colitis-induced carcinogenesis from experimental evidence to potential usefulness on cancer prevention and treatment.

Keywords Anthocyanins · Animal model · Berry · Cancer · Carcinogenesis · Chemoprevention · Crohn's disease · Fiber · Fruit · Inflammation · Inflammatory bowel disease · Phytosterols · Oligosaccharides · Oxidative stress · Oxylipin · Ulcerative colitis

1 Introduction

Chronic inflammation is a well-recognized risk factor for human cancer development and at least one third of human cancer is in association with chronic inflammation. The inflammatory bowel diseases (IBD) are idiopathic and longstanding chronic inflammatory disease and are typical models of chronic inflammation-driven carcinogenesis. The IBD are comprised of two recognized entities: Crohn's disease and ulcerative colitis (UC). Both diseases are described as being mainly

G.-Y. Yang (✉)
Department of Pathology, Northwestern University Feinberg School of Medicine, Chicago, IL 60611, USA
e-mail: g-yang@northwestern.edu

G.D. Stoner, N.P. Seeram (eds.), *Berries and Cancer Prevention*,
DOI 10.1007/978-1-4419-7554-6_12,

gastrointestinal chronic inflammatory conditions, although they also both exhibit extraintestinal inflammatory manifestations. Crohn's disease is characterized by a discontinuous, transmural inflammatory process involved in both small and large bowel. Ulcerative colitis, on the other hand, is a continuous and diffuse pattern of inflammatory process extending proximally from the rectum and inflammation is limited to the mucosa only (Fuss et al., 2004). Although the incidence of IBD is low in the United States, the prevalence is dominant for this disease due to life-long disease process. The incidence of IBD ranges from 5 to 18 cases per 100,000 per year and is showing an upward trend. The peak incidence of IBD occurs in the third decade of life. Long-standing IBD patients have an increased risk of developing colorectal carcinoma. The cumulative risk of cancer development increases with the disease duration. Compared to the general population, UC patients have an overall 11-fold relative risk of cancer and a 38-fold increased risk if IBD is diagnosed before the age of 30 (Brostrom et al., 1987; Ekbom et al., 1990a; Kewenter et al., 1978; Prior et al., 1982).

In our daily English, "berry" is a term for any small edible fruit that is usually juicy, round or semi-oblong, brightly colored, sweet or sour, and does not have a stone or pit, although many seeds may be present. However, the botanical definition is that a berry is a simple fruit having seeds and pulp produced from a single ovary, which is further classified as a "true berry" and "modified berry". The typical "true berry" includes cranberries, elderberries, blueberries, and grapes. Interestingly, of the several types of common berries in daily life, many of them are not actual berries by the scientific definition. Blackberries are an aggregate fruit or a compound fruit composed of many drupelets, and strawberries are an aggregate accessory fruit. A compound fruit is one that develops from several ovaries in either a single flower or multiple flowers. An accessory fruit (sometimes called false fruit) is a fruit in which some of the flesh is derived not from the ovary but from some adjacent tissue, such as a strawberry. Some of the smaller pomes are sometimes referred to as berries, including hawberries.

The common berries, all colors of fruits, have significant, positive effects on multiple disease states including inflammation and cancer. Besides several essential and nutritional components found in berries such as vitamins, minerals and fiber, berries contain numerous bioactive components that provide health benefits that extend beyond basic nutrition. Berry colors are due to natural plant pigments that are composed of polyphenolic compounds (mainly including anthocyanins). Berry pigments are strong antioxidants. Recent research from laboratories has provided useful insights into the biological effects and underlying mechanisms of actions resulting from eating berries. Food-based cancer prevention studies, particularly of berries (black raspberries, blackberries or strawberries, etc.), exhibit anti-cancer properties in rodents and pilot clinical trials, as well from epidemiologic studies (Stoner, 2009). This chapter focuses on linking berries to chronic colitis-induced carcinogenesis from experimental evidence to potential usefulness on prevention and treatment of IBD and IBD related carcinomas in humans in the future.

2 Molecular Pathogenesis and Modeling of Inflammatory Bowel Disease-Induced Carcinogenesis

Colitis-induced colorectal cancer occurs in patients at a younger age than spontaneous colorectal cancer. It occurs more frequently as two or more synchronous primary cancers and may be more proximal in the colon. The risk of cancer is in association with duration of disease, increasing exponentially with longer duration (Lashner et al., 1989). In fact, after 10 years, the risk of cancer increases at a rate of 0.5–1% per year. The risk of cancer is also associated with extent of disease, increasing in patients with pancolitis compared to patients with left-sided disease only (Ekbom et al., 1990a; Sugita et al., 1991). The risk of cancer increases to 20- to 30-fold greater than in the general population for patients with pancolitis of greater than 10 year duration (Eaden, 2004). Even non-dysplastic areas of mucosal cells in ulcerative colitis have been shown to have genomic instability (Chen et al., 2003). The carcinomas are often infiltrative without obvious exophytic masses. Epithelial changes encompass a broad spectrum from inflammation-induced hyperplasia to dysplasia that is distinguished as low-grade or high-grade depending on cytologic features (Greenson, 2002). Flat dysplasia may ultimately lead to invasive carcinoma. Thus, morphologically, IBD-induced colorectal carcinogenesis follows a multi-step progression model. Manifestations of carcinogenesis are best understood within the context of the molecular pathogenesis and it also provides ample opportunity for prevention of colitis-driven carcinogenesis.

Several aspects of the chronic inflammatory process, including the overproduction of reactive oxygen species (ROS) and nitrogen species (RONS), overproduction/activation of key arachidonic acid (AA) metabolites and cytokines/growth factors and their associated signal transduction pathways, and immunity system dysfunction, may contribute to increased cancer risk. Targeting these key molecular events is crucial for the prevention and therapy of this disease and malignant transformation.

Comparisons of the molecular alteration profiles of sporadic and colitis-associated cancers have shown that the two types of cancer are similar in many of the gene alterations and overall processes. However, the timing and frequency of these alterations in colitis-associated cancers appear to be unique (Tomlinson et al., 1998; Thomas, 1993). Colitis-associated cancer is presumed to arise from an accumulation of genetic alterations in tumor suppressor genes (e.g., p53, p16, and APC), oncogenes (e.g., K-RAS), and DNA repair proteins (e.g., MSH2 and MLH1), as well as an overall loss of genomic stability (Seril et al., 2003). Comparisons of the molecular alteration profiles of sporadic and colitis-associated cancers have shown that the two types of cancer are similar in many of the gene alterations and overall processes. However, the timing and frequency of these alterations in UC-associated cancers appear to be unique (Tomlinson et al., 1998; Thomas, 1993). The best example is the tumor suppressor p53 gene. P53 is important in the cellular response to DNA damage due to exogenous and endogenous factors, including nitrosative and oxidative stress (Levine, 1997). *p53* mutations have been detected in nearly 70% of colitis-associated cancers and 20% of dysplastic lesions analyzed (Brentnall, 1994; Chaubert et al., 1994; Fogt et al., 1998; Harpaz et al., 1994; Holzmann et al., 1998; Hussain et al., 2000; Kern et al., 1994; Yin et al., 1993). Interestingly, the p53 mutation spectrum in colitis-induced cancer is dominated by mutations that may be caused by nitrosative and oxidative DNA modification (Chaubert et al., 1994; Kern et al., 1994; Holzmann et al., 1998; Harpaz et al., 1994; Yin et al., 1993; Greenblatt et al., 1994; Tornaletti and Pfeifer, 1995).

Multiple animal models of inflammatory bowel disease have been established. In general, these models can be mainly categorized into spontaneous, chemically induced, genetically engineered (transgenic or gene knock-out), and immunity adoptive transferring animal models. The genetically and chemically induced models of intestinal inflammation in rodents are commonly used models, despite their own limitations, because of their ready availability, rapid disease development, and potential for genetic manipulation (Warren and Watkins, 1994). The development of longstanding chronic IBD and IBD-induced dysplasia and carcinoma is observed in several strains of genetically engineered models and in chemically induced IBD models such as dextran sulfate sodium (DSS) induced chronic colitis model. These genetically and chemically induced models, studied in combination with specific genetic deficiencies, antioxidants, pharmacological enzyme inhibitors, and active anti-inflammatory food components have been proved useful in studying the mechanisms, treatment, and chemoprevention of IBD and IBD-induced carcinogenesis.

The two typical and the most commonly used rodent models of IBD-induced carcinogenesis are DSS-induced chronic ulcerative colitis in mice and spontaneous colitis in IL-10 knockout mice. The dextran sulfate sodium (DSS)-induced ulcerative colitis (UC) in rodents is the most commonly used colitis model. A unique colitis-carcinogenesis model in DSS-induced colitis is well established model in our lab. In this model, feeding of 2-fold iron diet to mice subjected to low dose, cyclic, long-term DSS treatment (to mimic flare-up and flare down inflammatory activity of UC in humans) increased colorectal carcinoma incidence from approximately 19% in mice with normal level of iron diet to approximately 88% in 2-fold iron diet (Seril et al., 2002). Feeding with the 2-fold iron diet mimics the consumption of an iron-rich diet by long-term UC patients who commonly have iron deficiency due to chronic mucosa inflammation and bleeding. Histopathological analysis reveals that similar to UC patients, most of the observed colonic adenocarcinomas were mucinous carcinomas as well polypoid adenocarcinoma and lymphoid follicle-associated adenocarcinoma (Fig. 12.1). Further studies indicate that iron increases cancer risk by enhancing epithelial cell proliferation, nitro-oxidative damage, and COX2 and 5-LOX up-regulation (Seril et al., 2005). Thus, DSS-induced and iron-enhanced UC-associated carcinogenesis in mice is a novel mouse model of inflammation-driven carcinogenesis without use of carcinogen (Seril et al., 2006).

IL-10 is an important regulatory anti-inflammatory cytokine and is involved in the colitis development. In IL-10 knockout mice, 100% of mice developed colitis after 3 months of age and histopathology reveals the transmural inflammation

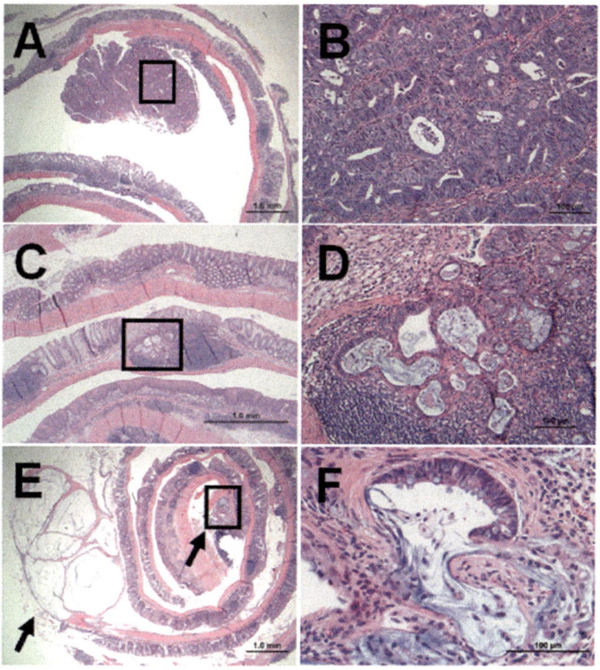

Fig. 12.1 Representative histopathology pictures of colitis-induced colonic adenocarcinoma: (**a** and **b**) polypoid well-differentiated adenocarcinoma, **b** is high magnification of *highlighted square* in **a**; (**c** and **d**) lymphoid follicle-associated adenocarcinoma, **d** is high magnification of *highlighted square* in **c**; and (**e** and **f**) invasive mucinous adenocarcinoma, **f** is high magnification of *highlighted square* in **e**

predominantly in the cecum that mimic Crohn's disease. Adenocarcinoma developed in 25% of IL-10 knockout mice after 3 months and 60% of after 6 months (Sturlan et al., 2001). Our data show that with administration of 2-fold iron diet, more than 80% of IL-10 knockout mice developed adenocarcinoma after 5 months, and morphologically the ulcerative moderately differentiated adenocarcinoma was commonly seen. Thus, IL-10 knockout mice mimic Crohn's disease and its induced carcinogenesis.

3 The Protective Effects of Berries Against Colitis and Colitis-Induced Cancer: Epidemiologic and Experimental Evidence

3.1 Epidemiologic Studies

There are numerous epidemiologic studies on the beneficial effects on consumption of fresh fruits/berries and colon cancer. However, there are a few studies on testing the relationship between berry consumption and inflammatory bowel disease which show that decreased consumption of fruit, fruit juice or vegetables has been reported among Crohn's disease patients (Kasper and Sommer, 1979; Thornton et al., 1979) and ulcerative colitis patients (Thornton et al., 1980). Several indirect epidemiologic studies indicate that the consumption of dietary fiber, especially the consumption of fiber from fruit, is negatively associated with the risk of IBD (Rawcliffe and Truelove, 1978; Reif et al., 1997). Epidemiologic studies imply that the fiber content of the fruit and vegetables is the protective factor; but whether other micronutrient components of these foods are effective is unclear. One study not only shows a negative association between fruit and vegetable consumption and IBD risk, but also there is a reduced risk associated with increased consumption of water, potassium (in Crohn's disease patients only), magnesium and vitamin C (Reif et al., 1997). On the other hand, fruit and vegetable intake being negatively associated with IBD patients may represent a response to the disease rather than an etiological factor. For example, low consumption of fruit and vegetables may be chosen by some patients or in some cases, even be advised to patients. Therefore, the beneficial effects and mechanism of fruits/berries and their active components against colitis and colitis-induced carcinogenesis need to be studied extensively in animal models as well in patients.

3.2 Experimental Studies

There are several studies on determining the effects of different berries or fruits on inflammatory bowel disease in mouse models, particularly using whole fruits or berries as dietary supplements. The protective effect of hawthorn fruit (Crataegifructus) has been observed on two murine colitis models: dextran sulfate sodium (DSS) and 2,4,6-trinitrobenzene sulfonic acid (TNBS) colitis (Fujisawa et al., 2005). Hawthorn fruit (2 g/kg body weight) in the diet protects animals from the reduction of body weight and colon length caused by colitis, increases hemoglobin count, and increases animal survival rates in these colitis animals. Further analysis indicates that Hawthorn fruit markedly decreases polymorphonuclear leukocytes infiltration and multiple erosive lesions in the colitis colon, as well improvement of leukotriene B4 (LTB4), a biochemical parameter of inflammation mass.

We have tested the effects of dietary supplementation of black raspberries on 2-fold dietary iron-enhanced spontaneous diffuse type colitis in IL-10 knockout mice (Liao et al., 2008). In IL-10 knockout mice, 100% of mice developed colitis after 3 months of age and histopathology revealed the transmural inflammation predominantly in the cecum. Five and ten percentage black raspberries are administered in the diet to mice starting at 4 weeks-old until termination of experiments at 23 weeks-old. Histopathologic analysis of chronic inflammatory activity in the colon showed dietary supplementation of berries significantly inhibited overall inflammatory index, including inflammation extent, ulcer formation, and epithelial hyperplasia (Fig. 12.2). Myeloperoxidase-labeled inflammatory cell infiltrates as a

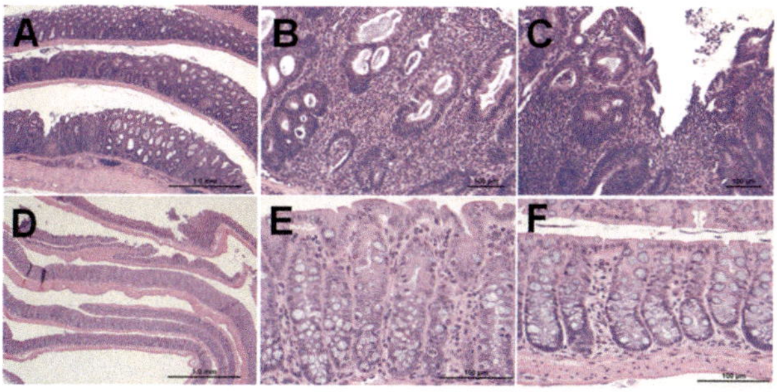

Fig. 12.2 Representative histopathology pictures of chronic colitis in IL-10 knockout mice: (**a**–**c**) representative photos of chronic active colitis without black raspberry treatment, photos from low magnification (**a**) to high maginification view (**b**–**c**), showing cryptitis and crypt abscess formation (**b**) as well focal erosion (**c**). (**d**–**f**) representative photos of chronic colitis with black raspberry treatment, photos from low magnification (**d**) to high maginification view (**e**–**f**), showing significant reduction of inflammatory activity (including cryptitis and crypt abscess and erosion)

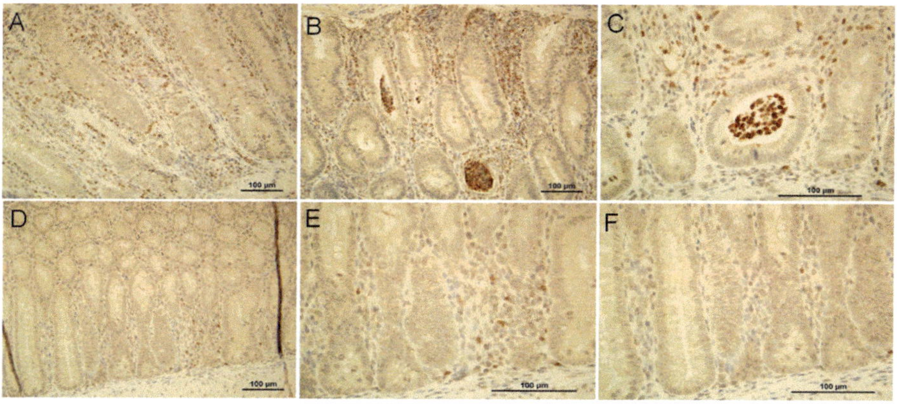

Fig. 12.3 Immunohistochemistry of myeloperoxidase-labeled inflammatory cell infiltrates in the colon. (**a**–**c**) chronic active colitis in IL-10 knockout mice: showing increased myeloperoxidase-labeled inflammatory cell infiltrates in the laminar propria (**a**), and cryptitis and crypt abscess (**b**–**c**). (**d**–**f**) chronic colitis in IL-10 knockout mice with black raspberry treatment: showing significant reduction of myeloperoxidase-labeled inflammatory cell infiltrates

unique inflammation biomarker, and is significantly reduced in the colitis colon in mice treated with 5 and 10% black raspberry (Fig. 12.3).

The most common edible berries in USA are blueberries and strawberries. Using DSS-induced acute colitis in rats, blueberry alone and in combination with probiotic strains significantly improved the disease activity index (DAI) of colitis (Osman et al., 2008). The severity of colitis is assessed based on the scoring of DAI including the parameters of body weight loss, stool consistency, and rectal bleeding (Murthy et al., 1993; Cooper et al., 1993). Reduction of DAI by blueberries is probably due to inhibited inflammatory process, particularly neutrophile infiltrates, and inflammation-caused oxidative stress.

Whether or not long term berry supplementation is effective on reducing the risk of cancer development in colitis is crucial. There are few experimental data available on this subject. Our data show that with administration of 2-fold iron diet, more than 80% of IL-10 knockout mice with colitis develop adenocarcinomas after 5 months iron diet treatment. The effects of dietary supplementation of black raspberries on spontaneous colitis-induced carcinogenesis in IL-10 knockout mice are further determined (Liao et al., 2008). Black raspberry supplementation in the diet to mice starting at 4 weeks old until termination of experiments at 23 weeks old showed significant reductions of colonic tumor incidence (38% [5/13 mice] and 30.8% [4/13 mice]) as observed in 5 and 10% berry supplemented groups, respectively, compared to IL-10 KO control mice (colorectal tumor incidence is 71.4% [10/14 mice]). This study indicates that black raspberries as a food-based prevention agent may have a potential for prevention of inflammation-driven carcinogenesis.

4 Key Active Components of Berries in Prevention of Colitis and Colitis-Induced Cancer in Rodent Models

Berries contain a broad range of beneficial and high nutritional contents, including dietary fiber, vitamins, and essential minerals, as well phytonutrients (particularly the flavonoid compounds including anthocyanins, ellagitannins and quercetin). There is a marked difference in the nutrient contents among different berries, or even in the same type of berry grown in different geographic locations. Obviously, berry phytonutrients and fibers are crucial active components in protecting humans from chronic disease including chronic inflammatory disease and cancer. In this chapter, we mainly focus on experimental evidence on the protective role of phytonutrients and fibers against colitis and colitis-induced carcinogenesis.

4.1 Berry-Derived Fiber, Especially Fructooligosaccharides, as a Crucial Probiotic Against Colitis

Short-chain fatty acids, including butyrate, propionate and lactate, are produced in the colon as a consequence of bacterial fermentation of dietary fiber by certain bacteria species including luminal Bifidobacterium, Eubacterium and Lactobacillus species (Stewart et al., 2008). Short-chain fatty acids are easily absorbed by the colonic mucosa and are an important source of nutrients for metabolism by colonic epithelial cells; additionally, they are a unique energy source for colonic epithelial cells (D'Argenio and Mazzacca, 1999; Chapman, 2001). Functionally they are trophic to the intestinal mucosa, stimulate water and sodium absorption in the colon, and induce enzymes that promote mucosal restitution. In addition, a direct anti-inflammatory role of short-chain fatty acid, such as butyrate, may be attributable to targeting nuclear factor-KF-*k*B that prevents the transcription of pro-inflammatory mediators (Segain et al., 2000). The short-chain fatty acids also inhibit lymphocyte activation and proliferation and myeloperoxidase activity in neutrophils, which directly causes tissue destruction (Chapman, 2001; Liu et al., 2001).

Fructooligosaccharides, as important components of fruit fiber, exhibit more rapid fermentation than long-chain inulin and production of more short-chain fatty acid (Stewart et al., 2008). Blueberries and raspberries contain large amount of fructooligosaccharides (Muir et al., 2009). Animal experiments demonstrate that probiotics and blueberries reduce the severity of dextran sulfate sodium (DSS)-induced colitis (Osman et al., 2008), and a pectic polysaccharide from cranberries exhibits a protective effect against acetic acid-induced colitis in mice (Popov et al., 2006). An open-label, parallel-grouping, randomized study of another dietary fiber, Platago ovata seeds, shows an equal efficacy to mesalazine in maintaining remission in patients with ulcerative colitis (Fernandez-Banares et al., 1999). A small clinical trial of fructooligosaccharides on Crohn's disease shows that supplementation with fructooligosaccharides increases faecal bifidobacteria concentrations, modifies mucosal dendritic cell function, and also decreases Crohn's disease activity (Lindsay et al., 2006). Thus, more studies in this exciting area, particularly the large, randomized, and placebo controlled clinical trials are needed.

4.2 Berry-Derived Anthocyanins as an Active Phytonutrient Against Inflammation and Carcinogenesis

Edible berries all of colors are rich sources of anthocyanins which are responsible for the red, violet, purple, and blue color of the berries. Anthocyanins exhibit a wide range of biologic effects and health benefits, largely due to its antioxidant function. It also presents with the therapeutic benefits on the integrity of genomic DNA, inhibition of inflammatory process, and chemoprevention of carcinogenesis (Wang and Stoner, 2008).

Berry-derived anthocyanins are water-soluble glycosides of polyhydroxyl and polymethoxyl derivatives of 2-phenylbenzopyrylium. pH is a responsible factor for the color and chelating ability of anthocyanins. Anthocyanins naturally exist at low pH as intense colors such as red or orange and are highly electron deficient, which leads to their potent activity toward chelating free radicals and oxygen reactive species. Various anthocyanin-containing extracts or anthocyanin-rich fractions from fruits and berries have been investigated for their chemopreventive and therapeutic potential for various chronic diseases including inflammation and cancer. Experimental evidence shows that anthocyanins, as a strong antioxidant, inhibit several inflammatory diseases including endotoxin-induced uveitis in mice (Yao et al.), airway inflammation and hyperresponsiveness in a murine asthma model (Park et al., 2007), and lung inflammation induced by carrageenan in rats (Rossi et al., 2003). Our study showed that ethanol extract of black raspberry (anthocyanin-rich fractions) markedly inhibited spontaneous colitis in IL-10 knockout mice. Mechanistic studies showed that anthocyanin-rich fraction significantly restored colitis- induced inflammatory gene profiles.

5 Molecular Target or Mechanism of Berry and Its Extract on Inhibiting Inflammation and Carcinogenesis

The key aspects of molecular targets of berry and its extracts include: (1) modulation of anti-oxidative capacities; (2) inhibition of aberrant arachidonic acid metabolism; and (3) modulation of carcinogene and inflammation-activated signaling and gene expression profile, particularly in cell proliferation, apoptosis and angiogenesis.

5.1 Anti-Inflammation-Induced Nitro-Oxidative Stress

The role of inflammation-induced oxidative stress and cellular damage in inflammatory process as well its induced carcinogenesis has been discussed extensively (Ames et al., 1995; Feig et al., 1994; Poulsen et al., 1998; Wink et al., 1998). Various biological reactions are known to generate reactive oxygen and nitro-oxide species (RONS), including superoxide anion, hydrogen peroxide and hydroxyl radicals, nitric oxide (NO), and peroxynitrite (Beckman et al., 1990; Jacob and Burri, 1996; Peskin, 1997). Superoxide and nitric oxide play a critical role by directly causing cellular injury or by taking part in the formation of highly reactive hydroxyl radicals and peroxynitrite radicals. The increased activities and accumulation of leukocytes (neutrophils and macrophages) during the inflammatory process result in a greatly enhanced generation of RONS (Babbs, 1992; Grisham, 1994). In inflammatory bowel disease patients, abundant neutrophil and macrophage infiltration into the local inflamed mucosa contributes to an increase in the production of RONS, and inflammatory cells may also carry iron to the inflamed area, which further enhances oxidative damage (Babbs, 1992; Holmes et al., 1998; Herulf et al., 1998; Reynolds et al., 1995). RONS have been shown to cause DNA strand breaks (which facilitate chromosomal translocation), oxidative modification of DNA bases (e.g. 8-OHdG), deamination of 5-methylcytosine, lipid peroxidation, protein oxidation, and altered gene expression (Ames et al., 1995; Feig et al., 1994; Poulsen et al., 1998; Wink et al., 1998).

Berries rank highly among fruit for their oxygen radical absorbance capacity value (ORAC). Both anthocyanins and flavonoid glycosides are responsible for the red, violet, purple, and blue color of the fruits/berries as the natural pigmentation and exhibit a wide range of antioxidant protection and therapeutic benefits. Several experimental evidence and pilot clinical trials have shown the protective effect of berries against oxidative stress. Dietary consumption of blueberry polyphenolics is significant protection against free radicals and oxidative stress within red blood cells in vivo (Youdim et al., 2000), and black raspberry shows a significant antioxidant protection in the gut epithelium of weanling pigs due to its high anthocyanin content (Wu et al., 2006). A pilot study in eight elderly women shows that with comparative assessment on total antioxidant status in serum following consumption of strawberries, spinach, red wine, or vitamin, the consumption of the foods enriched in antioxidant phenolic compounds markedly increases the serum antioxidant capacity in these elderly women (Cao et al., 1998).

Using DSS or TNBS induced colitis mouse model, a strong activity of anthocyanins or flavonoid phenolic compounds from fruits/berries against inflammation-induced oxidative stress have been demonstrated in several studies. The common and novel biomarkers used for detecting the oxidative stress are malondialdehyde (MDA) for lipid peroxidation, nitrotyrosin formation for nitro-oxidative protein damage, and 8-oxo-2-deoxyguanosine for oxidative stress-caused DNA damage. DSS treatment enhances RONS productions, and free radicals induce oxidative DNA damage in colonic mucosa (Seril et al., 2003, 2006). Supplementation with phenolic compounds from fruits/berries inhibits colitis-caused lipid peroxidation, measured as MDA, and reduces free radical-caused oxidized-DNA, measured by ratio of 8-oxodG/dG (Osman et al., 2008). The studies from our lab showed 5% black raspberry or ethanol berry extract (enriched anthocyanins) markedly reduced nitrotyrosin formation in the macrophages as well colonic epithelial cells in colitis. These results further support the antioxidative function of berries and their extracts. However, whether or not inhibition of oxidative DNA damage is correlated with reduction of specific gene mutation and genetic instability remains to be investigated further.

5.2 Inhibition of Aberrant Oxylipin Metabolic Profile

One of the pivotal molecules in inflammation is arachidonic acid, which when released in response to tissue injury simplistically has three potential metabolic fates. It can be metabolized by the Cyclooxygenase (COX), Lipoxygenase (LOX), and cytochrome P450 epoxygenases pathways resulting in the production of prostaglandins, leukotrienes and epoxyeicosanoids, respectively, and plays a crucial role in the inflammatory process (Fig. 12.4). These eicosanoids play vital roles in the maintenance of gastrointestinal integrity, wound healing, and inflammation. Inflammatory bowel disease (IBD) is associated with increased prostaglandin synthesis and prostaglandin synthase activity (Sharon et al., 1978; Rampton et al., 1980), and mucosal expression of COX-2 correlates with IBD disease activity (Hendel and Nielsen, 1997; Raab et al., 1995; Singer et al., 1998). However, the clinical use of nonsteroidal anti-inflammatory drugs (NSAINs) exacerbates IBD (Kaufmann and Taubin, 1987). NSAIDs and COX-2- inhibitors (e.g., celecoxib) have, for the most part, been shown to be harmful in animal models of IBD as well (Berg et al., 2002; Reuter et al., 1996). These findings may be explained by the ideas that COX-2 and PGE2 inhibition leads to inhibit cell proliferation and delay the ulcer healing and leads to shunt AA substrates to other pathways, particularly to the inflammatory 5-LOX-LTB_4 pathway to enhance inflammatory cell infiltrates in the inflamed ulcer (Flamand et al., 2002; Ham et al., 1983; Harizi et al., 2002; Planaguma et al., 2002).

Cross talk among the pathways in the arachidonate and other lipid cascades is likely to be a general phenomenon. A shift in eicosanoids from a pattern generally initiating and propagating inflammation to a pattern of resolution of inflammation would be an important strategy for anti-inflammatory process (Inceoglu et al., 2007).

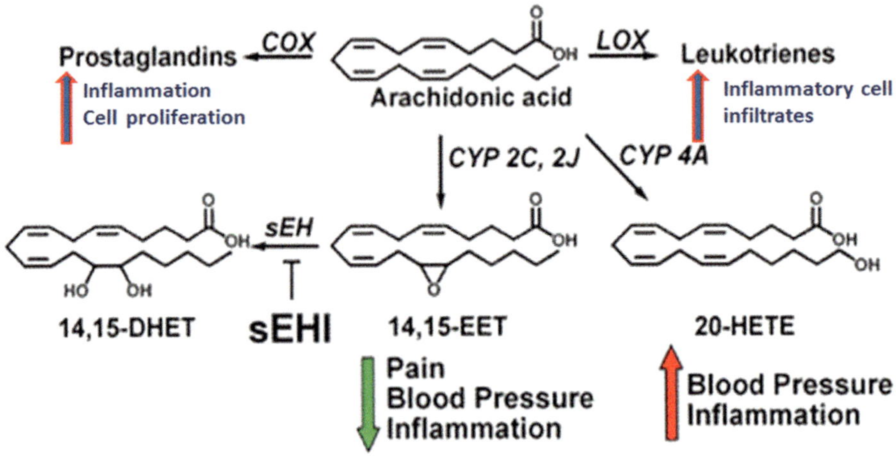

Fig. 12.4 Metabolites and their functions of arachidonic acid metabolic pathways

An epidemiologic study indicates consumption of fruit and vegetables in adolescents significantly reduces inflammation and oxidative stress, including reduction of 15-keto-dihydro-PGF(2alpha) metabolite (urinary 8-iso prostaglandin F(2alpha), an F(2)-isoprostane) (Holt et al., 2009). Several studies exhibit inhibitory effects of phenolic compounds from fruits and berries on suppressing COX2, LOX, and iNOS gene expression and their products including PGE2, LTB4, and NO (Stoner, 2009; Wang and Stoner, 2008). Our study on global transcript gene profile indicates that supplementation with black raspberry inhibits colitis-upregulated phospholipase A2 and soluble expoxide hydrolase. Therefore, modulation of the arachidonate and other lipid cascades or metabolic pathways would be more important in inhibiting inflammation and overcome the side effect of COX inhibitors.

5.3 Modulation of Inflammation or Carcinogen-Activated Gene Expression Profile, Particularly Focusing on Inflammation and Cancer Signaling Including Apoptosis, Proliferation and Angiogenesis

Abnormal up-regulation of the inflammatory protein, NF-κB, is a common occurrence in many cancers, and inhibitors of this signaling pathway usually exhibit significant chemopreventive potential (Stoner, 2009; Wang and Stoner, 2008; Stoner et al., 2008). Interestingly, through their ability to inhibit the mRNA and/or protein expression levels of NF-κB and various interleukins, the anthocyanins have exhibited anti-inflammatory effects in multiple cell types in vitro (Stoner, 2009; Wang and Stoner, 2008).

Using molecular biology approach, particularly the global transcriptional gene array technology, numerous molecular targets of berry have been identified. Studies from Stoner's lab show that 462 of the 2,261 carcinogen-N-nitrosomethylbenzylamine (NMBA)-dysregulated genes in rat esophagus are restored to near-normal levels of expression by treatment of black raspberry. The crucial genes among berry-regulated 462 genes are related to multiple aspects of biologic function and pathways, mainly involved in phase I and II metabolism, oxidative damage, and oncogenes and tumor suppressor genes that regulate apoptosis, cell cycling, and angiogenesis (Stoner et al., 2008). Topical application of a bioadhesive black raspberry gel modulates gene expression in human premalignant oral lesions (Mallery et al., 2008), and shows twenty-seven genes, including RNA processing, signal transduction, and inflammatory pathways are uniformly down-regulated by black raspberries. The up-regulation of proapoptotic and terminal differentiation pathways are also observed in a subset of patients responding to the application of the berry gel.

Using transcriptional gene array analysis with 24,611 gene probes, we have demonstrated that 797 genes show the significant expression level changes in IL-10 knockout mice compared to wild-type mice; among these altered genes, 168 genes are being further modulated by berry supplementation (Liao, 2009). Further pathway analysis among these regulated gene profiles shows that dietary berries mainly regulates gene expression profiles involved in inflammatory processes and T cell activation, arachidonic acids metabolism, as well as interleukins and chemokine signaling.

6 Summary and Conclusion

The consumption of fresh berries beneficially affected inflammation and its associated carcinogenesis are beginning to be understood. Yet, given the nutritional beneficial functions on human health, it would be important to determine specifically biologic effect or molecular targets of berry and each of its active components, particularly the interactions among the bioactive components (including phenolic compounds, soluble and insoluble fibers, essential minerals, and vitamins) on biologic function.

Several molecular events involved in chronic inflammatory process may contribute to multistage progression of human cancer development, including the overproduction of reactive oxygen and nitrogen species, overproduction/activation of key arachidonic acid metabolites and cytokines/growth factors, and immunity system dysfunction (Wong and Harrison, 2001). Multiple animal models of inflammatory bowel disease have been established, and in general, these models provide a unique function to further elucidate molecular targets of bioactive components of berry on chronic inflammatory process as well on inflammation-induced carcinogenesis. In addition, the identified molecular targets by berries would be crucial biomarkers useful for clinical trial in humans in the future.

Chronic inflammation is one of the most important factors contributing to human cancer (Coussens and Werb, 2002). Inflammatory bowel disease (IBD), including ulcerative colitis (UC) and Crohn's disease (CD), is a typical chronic inflammatory disease with significantly increased risk for the development of cancer (Collins et al., 1987; Debinski and Kamm, 1997; Ekbom et al., 1990b). The development of dysplasia and adenocarcinoma in inflammatory bowel disease patients is likely due to long-standing inflammation (Debinski and Kamm, 1997; Collins et al., 1987; Riddell et al., 1983). The histopathogenesis of chronic colitis-induced carcinogenesis follows a multiple step progression model from inflamed and hyperplastic epithelia to dysplasia and adenocarcinoma (Riddell et al., 1983). The average duration of long-standing inflammatory bowel disease is approximately 30 years (Russel and Stockbrugger, 1996), providing ample opportunity for having the significant clinical trials on the prevention and treatment of this inflammatory disease and its induced carcinogenesis. The animal experimental studies have provided rational that berry, as a food-based preventive agent, has high potential for the prevention of inflammation-related carcinogenesis in the colon.

Acknowledgement The related studies are partially supported by NIH R01 grant (CA104741).

References

Ames BN, Gold LS, Willett WC (1995) The causes and prevention of cancer. Proc Natl Acad Sci USA 92(12):5258–5265

Babbs CF (1992) Oxygen radicals in ulcerative colitis. Free Radic Biol Med 13:169–181

Beckman JS et al (1990) Apparent hydroxyl radical production by peroxynitrite: implications for endothelial injury from nitric oxide and superoxide. Proc Natl Acad Sci USA 87(4):1620–1624

Berg DJ et al (2002) Rapid development of colitis in NSAID-treated IL-10-deficient mice. Gastroenterology 123(5):1527–1542

Brentnall TA et al (1994) Mutations in the p53 gene: an early marker of neoplastic progression in ulcerative colitis. Gastroenterology 107:369–378

Brostrom O et al (1987) The risk of colorectal cancer in ulcerative colitis. An epidemiologic study. Scand J Gastroenterol 22(10):1193–1199

Cao G et al (1998) Serum antioxidant capacity is increased by consumption of strawberries, spinach, red wine or vitamin C in elderly women. J Nutr 128(12):2383–2390

Chapman MA (2001) The role of the colonic flora in maintaining a healthy large bowel mucosa. Ann R Coll Surg Engl 83(2):75–80

Chaubert P et al (1994) K-ras mutations and p53 alterations in neoplastic and nonneoplastic lesions associated with longstanding ulcerative colitis. Am J Pathol 144:767–775

Chen R et al (2003) DNA fingerprinting abnormalities can distinguish ulcerative colitis patients with dysplasia and cancer from those who are dysplasia/cancer-free. Am J Pathol 162(2): 665–672

Collins RH Jr, Feldman M, Fordtran JS (1987) Colon cancer, dysplasia, and surveillance in patients with ulcerative colitis. A critical review. N Engl J Med 316(26):1654–1658

Cooper HS et al (1993) Clinicopathologic study of dextran sulfate sodium experimental murine colitis. Lab Invest 69(2):238–249

Coussens LM, Werb Z (2002) Inflammation and cancer. Nature 420(6917):860–867

Debinski H, Kamm MA (1997) Natural History of Ulcerative Colitis. In: Allan RN et al (ed) Inflammatory Bowel Diseases, Churchill Livingstone, New York, NY, pp 463–474

D'Argenio G, Mazzacca G (1999) Short-chain fatty acid in the human colon. Relation to inflammatory bowel diseases and colon cancer. Adv Exp Med Biol 472:149–158

Eaden J (2004) Review article: colorectal carcinoma and inflammatory bowel disease. Aliment Pharmacol Ther 20(Suppl 4):24–30

Ekbom A et al (1990a) Ulcerative colitis and colorectal cancer. A population-based study. N Engl J Med 323(18):1228–1233

Ekbom A et al (1990b) Ulcerative colitis and colorectal cancer. A population-based study. N Engl J Med 323:1229–1233

Feig DI, Reid TM, Loeb LA (1994) Reactive oxygen species in tumorigenesis. Cancer Res 54(Suppl 7):1890s–1894s

Fernandez-Banares F et al (1999) Randomized clinical trial of Plantago ovata seeds (dietary fiber) as compared with mesalamine in maintaining remission in ulcerative colitis. Spanish Group for the Study of Crohn's Disease and Ulcerative Colitis (GETECCU). Am J Gastroenterol 94(2):427–433

Flamand N et al (2002) Cyclic AMP-mediated inhibition of 5-lipoxygenase translocation and leukotriene biosynthesis in human neutrophils. Mol Pharmacol 62(2):250–256

Fogt F et al (1998) Comparison of p53 immunoexpression with allelic loss of p53 in ulcerative colitis-associated dysplasia and carcinoma. Oncol Rep 5:477–480

Fujisawa M et al (2005) Protective effect of hawthorn fruit on murine experimental colitis. Am J Chin Med 33(2):167–180

Fuss IJ et al (2004) Nonclassical CD1d-restricted NK T cells that produce IL-13 characterize an atypical Th2 response in ulcerative colitis. J Clin Invest 113(10):1490–1497

Greenblatt MS et al (1994) Mutations in the p53 tumor suppressor gene: clues to cancer etiology and molecular pathogenesis. Cancer Res 54:4855–4878

Greenson JK (2002) Dysplasia in inflammatory bowel disease. Semin Diagn Pathol 19(1):31–37

Grisham MB (1994) Oxidants and free radicals in inflammatory bowel disease. Lancet 344: 859–861

Ham EA et al (1983) Inhibition by prostaglandins of leukotriene B4 release from activated neutrophils. Proc Natl Acad Sci USA 80(14):4349–4353

Harizi H et al (2002) Cyclooxygenase-2-issued prostaglandin e(2) enhances the production of endogenous IL-10, which down-regulates dendritic cell functions. J Immunol 168(5): 2255–2263

Harpaz N et al (1994) p53 protein expression in ulcerative colitis-associated colorectal dysplasia and carcinoma. Hum Pathol 25:1069–1074

Hendel J, Nielsen OH (1997) Expression of cyclooxygenase-2 mRNA in active inflammatory bowel disease. Am J Gastroenterol 92(7):1170–1173

Herulf M et al (1998) Increased luminal nitric oxide in inflammatory bowel disease as shown with a novel minimally invasive method. Scand J Gastroenterol 33:164–169

Holmes EW et al (1998) Glutathione content of colonic mucosa: Evidence for oxidative damage in active ulcerative colitis. Dig Dis Sci 43:1088–1095

Holt EM et al (2009) Fruit and vegetable consumption and its relation to markers of inflammation and oxidative stress in adolescents. J Am Diet Assoc 109(3):414–421

Holzmann K et al (1998) Comparative analysis of histology, DNA content, p53 and Ki-ras mutations in colectomy specimens with long-standing ulcerative colitis. Int J Cancer 76:1–6

Hussain SP et al (2000) Increased p53 mutation load in noncancerous colon tissue from ulcerative colitis: a cancer-prone chronic inflammatory disease. Cancer Res 60(13):3333–3337

Inceoglu B et al (2007) Soluble epoxide hydrolase inhibition reveals novel biological functions of epoxyeicosatrienoic acids (EETs). Prostaglandins Other Lipid Mediat 82(1-4):42–49

Jacob RA, Burri BJ (1996) Oxidative damage and defense. Am J Clin Nutr 63(6):985S–990S

Kasper H, Sommer H (1979) Dietary fiber and nutrient intake in Crohn's disease. Am J Clin Nutr 32(9):1898–1901

Kaufmann HJ, Taubin HL (1987) Nonsteroidal anti-inflammatory drugs activate quiescent inflammatory bowel disease. Ann Intern Med 107(4):513–516

Kern SE et al (1994) Molecular genetic profiles of colitis-associated neoplasms. Gastroenterology 107:420–428

Kewenter J, Ahlman H, Hulten L (1978) Cancer risk in extensive ulcerative colitis. Ann Surg 188(6):824–828
Lashner BA, Silverstein MD, Hanauer SB (1989) Hazard rates for dysplasia and cancer in ulcerative colitis. Results from a surveillance program. Dig Dis Sci 34(10):1536–1541
Levine AJ (1997) p53, the cellular gatekeeper for growth and division. Cell 88:323–331
Liao J, Li-Shu Wang YTC, Yang A, Stoner G, Yang G-Y (2008) Inhibition of chronic colitis-induced carcinogenesis in IL-10 knockout mice by dietary supplementation of black raspberries. Cancer Prev Res 1(Suppl 7):PR–13
Liao J, Chung YT, Yang A, Stoner G, Yang G-Y (2009) Modulation of inflammatory gene expression profile and inhibition of chronic colitis-induced carcinogenesis by dietary supplementation of black raspberries in IL-10 knockout mice. Proc of AACR 100th Annual Meeting, Colorado, April, 100:56
Lindsay JO et al (2006) Clinical, microbiological, and immunological effects of fructo-oligosaccharide in patients with Crohn's disease. Gut 55(3):348–355
Liu Q et al (2001) Effect of sodium butyrate on reactive oxygen species generation by human neutrophils. Scand J Gastroenterol 36(7):744–750
Mallery SR et al (2008) Topical application of a bioadhesive black raspberry gel modulates gene expression and reduces cyclooxygenase 2 protein in human premalignant oral lesions. Cancer Res 68(12):4945–4957
Muir JG et al (2009) Measurement of short-chain carbohydrates in common Australian vegetables and fruits by high-performance liquid chromatography (HPLC). J Agric Food Chem 57(2): 554–565
Murthy SN et al (1993) Treatment of dextran sulfate sodium-induced murine colitis by intracolonic cyclosporin. Dig Dis Sci 38(9):1722–1734
Osman N et al (2008) Probiotics and blueberry attenuate the severity of dextran sulfate sodium (DSS)-induced colitis. Dig Dis Sci 53(9):2464–2473
Park SJ et al (2007) Anthocyanins inhibit airway inflammation and hyperresponsiveness in a murine asthma model. Food Chem Toxicol 45(8):1459–1467
Peskin AV (1997) Interaction of reactive oxygen species with DNA. A review. Biochemistry (Mosc) 62(12):1341–1347
Planaguma A et al (2002) Aspirin (ASA) regulates 5-lipoxygenase activity and peroxisome proliferator-activated receptor alpha-mediated CINC-1 release in rat liver cells: novel actions of lipoxin A4 (LXA4) and ASA-triggered 15-epi-LXA4. Faseb J 16(14):1937–1939
Popov SV et al (2006) Preventive effect of a pectic polysaccharide of the common cranberry Vaccinium oxycoccos L. on acetic acid-induced colitis in mice. World J Gastroenterol 12(41):6646–6651
Poulsen HE, Prieme H, Loft S (1998) Role of oxidative DNA damage in cancer initiation and promotion. Eur J Cancer Prev 7(1):9–16
Prior P et al (1982) Cancer morbidity in ulcerative colitis. Gut 23(6):490–497
Raab Y et al (1995) Mucosal synthesis and release of prostaglandin E2 from activated eosinophils and macrophages in ulcerative colitis. Am J Gastroenterol 90(4):614–620
Rampton DS et al (1980) Rectal mucosal prostaglandin E release and electrolyte transport in ulcerative colitis. Adv Prostaglandin Thromboxane Res 8:1621–1625
Rawcliffe PM, Truelove SC (1978) Breakfast and Crohn's disease–I. Br Med J 2(6136):539–540
Reif S et al (1997) Pre-illness dietary factors in inflammatory bowel disease. Gut 40(6):754–760
Reuter BK et al (1996) Exacerbation of inflammation-associated colonic injury in rat through inhibition of cyclooxygenase-2. J Clin Invest 98(9):2076–2085
Reynolds PD et al (1995) Nitric oxide in ulcerative colitis. Lancet 345(8947):448 discussion 449
Riddell RH et al (1983) Dysplasia in inflammatory bowel disease: standardized classification with provisional clinical applications. Hum Pathol 14:931–966
Rossi A et al (2003) Protective effects of anthocyanins from blackberry in a rat model of acute lung inflammation. Free Radic Res 37(8):891–900
Russel MGVM, Stockbrugger RW (1996) Epidemiology of inflammatory bowel disease: an update. Scand J Gastroenterol 31:417–427

Segain JP et al (2000) Butyrate inhibits inflammatory responses through NFkappaB inhibition: implications for Crohn's disease. Gut 47(3):397–403

Seril DN et al (2002) Dietary iron supplementation enhances DSS-induced colitis and associated colorectal carcinoma development in mice. Dig Dis Sci 47(6):1266–1278

Seril DN, Liao J, Yang G-Y, Yang CS (2003) Oxidative stress and ulcerative colitis-associated carcinogenesis: studies in AQ3 humans and animal models. Carcinogenesis 24(3):353–362

Seril DN et al (2005) Systemic iron supplementation replenishes iron stores without enhancing colon carcinogenesis in murine models of ulcerative colitis: comparison with iron-enriched diet. Dig Dis Sci 50(4):696–707

Seril DN, Liao J, West AB, Yang GY (2006) High-iron diet: foe or feat in ulcerative colitis and ulcerative colitis-associated carcinogenesis. J Clin Gastroenterol 40(5):391–397

Sharon P et al (1978) Role of prostaglandins in ulcerative colitis. Enhanced production during active disease and inhibition by sulfasalazine. Gastroenterology 75(4):638–640

Singer II et al (1998) Cyclooxygenase 2 is induced in colonic epithelial cells in inflammatory bowel disease. Gastroenterology 115(2):297–306

Stewart ML, Timm DA, Slavin JL (2008) Fructooligosaccharides exhibit more rapid fermentation than long-chain inulin in an in vitro fermentation system. Nutr Res 28(5):329–334

Stoner GD et al (2008) Carcinogen-altered genes in rat esophagus positively modulated to normal levels of expression by both black raspberries and phenylethyl isothiocyanate. Cancer Res 68(15):6460–6467

Stoner GD (2009) Foodstuffs for preventing cancer: the preclinical and clinical development of berries. Cancer Prev Res 2(3):187–194

Sturlan S et al (2001) Interleukin-10-deficient mice and inflammatory bowel disease associated cancer development. Carcinogenesis 22(4):665–671

Sugita A et al (1991) Colorectal cancer in ulcerative colitis. Influence of anatomical extent and age at onset on colitis-cancer interval. Gut 32(2):167–169

Thomas HJ (1993) The timing of p53 inactivation in chronic ulcerative colitis. Gastroenterology 104(6):1889–1891

Thornton JR, Emmett PM, Heaton KW (1979) Diet and Crohn's disease: characteristics of the pre-illness diet. Br Med J 2(6193):762–764

Thornton JR, Emmett PM, Heaton KW (1980) Diet and ulcerative colitis. Br Med J 280(6210):293–294

Tomlinson I et al (1998) A comparison of the genetic pathways involved in the pathogenesis of three types of colorectal cancer. J Pathol 184(2):148–152

Tornaletti S, Pfeifer GP (1995) Complete and tissue-independent methylation of CpG sites in the p53 gene: implications for mutations in human cancers. Oncogene 10:1493–1499

Wang LS, Stoner GD (2008) Anthocyanins and their role in cancer prevention. Cancer Lett 269(2):281–290

Warren BF, Watkins PE (1994) Animal models of inflammatory bowel disease. J Pathol 172(4):313–316

Wink DA et al (1998) The multifaceted roles of nitric oxide in cancer. Carcinogenesis 19(5): 711–721

Wong NA, Harrison DJ (2001) Colorectal neoplasia in ulcerative colitis-recent advances. Histopathology 39(3):221–234

Wu X, Pittman HE 3rd, Prior RL (2006) Fate of anthocyanins and antioxidant capacity in contents of the gastrointestinal tract of weanling pigs following black raspberry consumption. J Agric Food Chem 54(2):583–589

Yao N, Lan F, He RR, Kurihara H (2010) Protective effects of bilberry (*Vaccinium myrtillus L.*) extract against endotoxin-induced uveitis in mice. J Agric Food Chem. 58(8):4731–4736

Yin J et al (1993) p53 point mutaions in dysplastic and cancerous ulcerative colitis lesions. Gastroenterology 104:1633–1639

Youdim KA et al (2000) Polyphenolics enhance red blood cell resistance to oxidative stress: in vitro and in vivo. Biochim Biophys Acta 1523(1):117–122

Part IV
Berry Chemoprevention in High-Risk Populations

Chapter 13
Cancer Prevention in Humans at High-Risk for Development of Cancer: Prevention of Oral Dysplasia in Humans by Berry Formulations

Susan R. Mallery and Meng Tong

Abstract Oral epithelial dysplasia, which is the precursor lesion for oral squamous cell carcinoma (oral SCC), presents an ideal opportunity for chemoprevention. First, oral dysplastic lesions are visible and can therefore be readily monitored during both the trial and recall phases of treatment. Secondly, in the event that local delivery chemoprevention will be used, the direct visibility enables agent placement. The current standard of care for lesions of moderate dysplasia or higher is complete blade excision or laser ablation. Unfortunately, many of these lesions are recalcitrant to treatment and recur despite the surgeon obtaining microscopically clear margins. Such patients would greatly benefit from effective chemopreventive therapy. The vast majority of oral epithelial dysplasia clinical trials to date, which relied on systemic administration of the chemopreventive, have been largely ineffective due to an inability to obtain therapeutically effective levels of compound at the treatment site without eliciting systemic toxicities. In contrast, a local delivery strategy of an effective chemopreventive compound will provide a therapeutic advantage by providing effective local concentrations without deleterious systemic side effects.

Keywords Oral epithelial dysplasia · Local delivery formulations · Oral dysplasia chemopreventive trials · Indicators of therapeutic efficacy

a. Oral epithelial dysplasia: clinical features and current strategies for management. Oral squamous cell carcinoma (OSCC), which arises from the surface oral epithelium, comprises 90% of the cancers that occur in the oral cavity (Bagan et al., 2010). Analogous to other carcinomas, OSCCs do not develop de novo, but subsequent to cumulative metabolic and molecular alterations that occur during the characterized progression from mild-moderate-severe epithelial dysplasia to carcinoma-in-situ to invasive oral OSCC (Fig. 13.1). While tobacco and alcohol use

S.R. Mallery (✉)
Division of Oral Maxillofacial Surgery, Pathology and Anesthesiology, College of Dentistry, The Ohio State University, Columbus, OH 43210, USA
e-mail: mallery.1@osu.edu

G.D. Stoner, N.P. Seeram (eds.), *Berries and Cancer Prevention*,
DOI 10.1007/978-1-4419-7554-6_13,

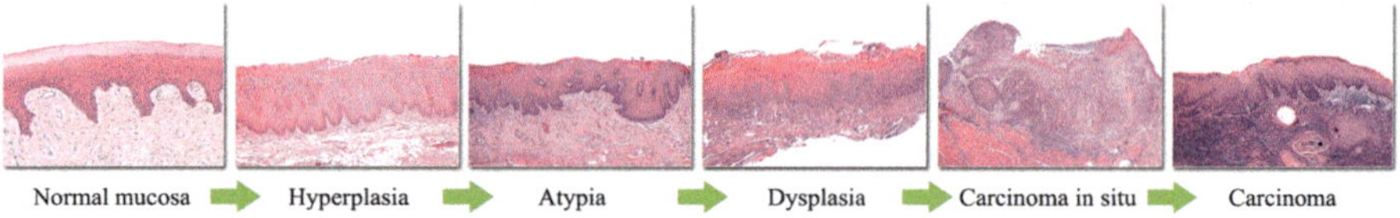

Fig. 13.1 As with any epithelial malignancy, oral squamous cell carcinoma does not occur de novo, but as the result of a series of developmental perturbations that arise during the transition from normal tissue to invasive squamous cell carcinoma. Hyperplasia, which has no preneoplastic potential, is characterized by an overall thickening of the spinous layer (acanthosis) and increased keratin production (hyperkeratosis). Atypia represents an indeterminate stage with some irregular maturation; however, these changes maybe either reactive or preneoplastic. Dysplasia, which represents a recognized preneoplastic process that may progress to squamous cell carcinoma, shows disturbances that progress from basilar third (*mild*) to approximately 50% of epithelial thickness (*moderate*) to full thickness changes (*severe*). Carcinoma in situ is a squamous cell carcinoma that has not yet invaded the basement membrane. Overt squamous cell carcinoma is characterized by the presence of invasive nests and cords of tumor tissue in the underlying connective tissue

are the best established oral cancer risk factors, other recognized OSCC risk factors include infection with oncogenic strains of human papillomaviruses (HPVs 16, 18, 31, 33, and 35), sunlight exposure and subsequent UVB damage (cancers of the lip vermilion zone), immunodeficiencies (most frequently AIDS patients), betel nut chewing, and nutritional deficiencies, notably iron deficiency anemia (Scully and Bagan, 2009; Rodriguez et al., 2004; Vigneswaran et al., 1995; Gillison et al., 2008; Goon et al., 2009; Chen et al., 2008; Richie et al., 2008). Although epithelial dysplasia can occur throughout the mouth, the three "pooling areas" are the anterior floor of mouth and ventral tongue, posterior-lateral tongue, and retromolar pad-anterior tonsillar pillar comprising the high-risk, high-incidence sites (Neville and Day, 2002; Waldron and Shafer, 1975; Islam et al., 2010). Involvement of other oral locations such as gingiva (older female patients), buccal mucosa (betel nut chewers) and tonsillar-pharyngeal (oncogenic HPV strains) are more prevalent in certain patient populations (Neville and Day, 2002; Waldron and Shafer, 1975; Islam et al., 2010).

Oral epithelial dysplasia displays variable clinical presentations. While the adherent white plaque with crisply defined clinical borders (often referred to as "leukoplakia") is probably the best-recognized, other appearances are more heterogeneous and include mixed red-white (speckled), ulcerative, and verrucous variants (Kramer et al., 1978; Greer, 2006). Erythroplakic lesions, which clinically appear velvety-red, represent the most ominous presentation as 90% of erythroplakic lesions display severe epithelial dysplasia, or worse, following biopsy (Reichart and Philipsen, 2005). Microscopic evaluative criteria including cellular and nuclear pleomorphism, basal cell crowding and hyperplasia, prominent nucleoli, premature keratinization, decreased cellular adherence, mitotic activity superior to the basal cell layer, increased mitotic indices and/or abnormal mitotic figures, and drop-shaped, bulbous epithelial rete ridges have been established to assist in the diagnosis of oral epithelial dysplasia (Neville et al., 2009). These histologic features, in conjunction with the microscopic extent of disease, (perturbations limited to basal third [mild dysplasia], approximately 50% epithelial thickness [moderate dysplasia], full thickness changes [severe dysplasia], cancer that has not yet invaded the basement membrane [carcinoma-in-situ]) are used to determine the final microscopic diagnosis.

Complete removal of lesional tissue, either by blade excision or laser ablation, is the current standard of care for oral premalignant lesions with a histopathologic diagnosis of moderate epithelial dysplasia or higher. While this treatment caveat sounds very straightforward, there are currently two major problems encountered in the management of oral epithelial dysplasia. First, approximately 30% of oral dysplastic epithelial lesions recur despite the fact that the surgeon obtained clinically and microscopically-clear surgical margins (Arduino et al., 2009; Mehanna et al., 2009). Secondly, while histologic indicators such as higher grade and molecular markers such as loss of heterozygosity at tumor suppressor gene loci are associated with a more aggressive clinical course, we are currently unable to predict which premalignant oral lesions will progress to overt OSCC. Consequently, patients are faced with the need for frequent recall examinations, repeated surgeries, and the associated morbidities including pain and anxiety. Provided these current treatment limitations and the fact that oral dysplastic lesions arise in a visibly accessible location (which enables direct clinical monitoring), there has been and continues to be a high level of interest in oral cancer chemoprevention.

b. Early vitamin A metabolite (isotretinoin) oral cancer chemoprevention trials. The hallmark oral cancer chemopreventive trial, lead by Hong et al. (1986), evaluated the effects of a vitamin A metabolite 13-cis-retinoic acid (isotretinoin) (1-2 mg/kg daily), on oral leukoplakia. Trial results were promising as 67% of the participants' lesions demonstrated significant decreases in size and 54% of the treated lesions showed a reversal of dysplasia (relative to a 10% response rate in both categories in the placebo group). Based on Hong et al.'s positive results, a subsequent trial by Lippman et al. (1993) evaluated a lower isotretinoin "maintenance" dose, with the goal to preserve responsiveness while concurrently reducing deleterious effects. Treatment entailed an initial inductive, high dose isotretinoin phase, followed by a reduced dose maintenance therapy using either isotretinoin or β-carotene. The results showed decreased levels of disease progression and a longer duration to disease progression in the isotretinoin maintenance therapy cohort. Despite the reduced isotretinoin dosage, treatment-associated morbidities were still observed in this second trial (Lippman et al., 1993). Furthermore, interpretation of these two isotretinoin studies' data is complicated by the fact that an appreciable number of participants' leukoplakic lesions were classified as "hyperplasia not otherwise specified" (Hong et al., 1986; Lippman et al., 1993). While dysplastic lesions have an established malignant transformation potential, reactive hyperplastic lesions do not (Silverman et al., 1984; Scuibba, 1995). Consequently, inclusion of reactive hyperplastic lesions would skew the results towards a more positive outcome (Silverman et al., 1984; Scuibba, 1995). Many participants in these isotretinoin trials developed deleterious effects that ranged from mild (cheilitis, skin dryness, and facial erythema) to moderate (conjunctivitis and hypertriglyceridemia) to advanced (Grade III and IV toxicities) (Hong et al., 1986; Lippman et al., 1993).

These adverse effects, in conjunction with the recognition that oral cancer chemoprevention will likely entail treatment for a sustained period of time, prompted the evaluation of other prospective chemopreventive compounds and dosing strategies.

c. Subsequent vitamin A derivative studies. From an epithelial growth perturbation standpoint, natural and synthetic vitamin A derivatives elicit many positive effects including induction of terminal differentiation and apoptosis (Freemantle et al., 2003; Smith and Saba, 2005; Hail et al., 2006). The ultimate outcome of treatment (induction of terminal differentiation and/or apoptosis) reflects dose obtained at the treatment site, duration of treatment, and specific vitamin A compound under evaluation (Shah et al., 1983; Garewal et al., 1990; Epstein and Gorsky, 1999; Garewal et al., 1999). Due to its reduced toxicity profile and ability to induce effects via both retinoid receptor and receptor-independent routes, the synthetic retinoid N-(4-hydroxyphenyl) retinamide (4-HPR) has been employed in several oral cancer chemoprevention trials (Chiesa et al., 2005; Lippman et al., 2006; William et al., 2009). In 2005, Chiesa et al. published results from a long-term study that evaluated the effects of low-dose treatment (200 mg 4-HPR daily versus no treatment for 1 year) for individuals following surgery for white oral lesions which included both hyperkeratoses (classified as "benign") and dysplasias. The primary end-point was to assess whether or not the 4-HPR protected against the subsequent development of oral cancer. The data implied that 4-HPR administration protected against new lesion development and suppressed local lesional recurrence for approximately 7 months. The high number of participants' lesions classified as benign hyperkeratosis prior to treatment raises concerns regarding the ability to determine the actual extent of chemopreventive effectiveness (Chiesa et al., 2005).

M.D. Anderson's researchers directed two additional 4-HPR oral cancer chemoprevention trials (Lippman et al., 2006; William et al., 2009). The first study, which was based on the premise that 4-HPR can induce apoptosis via a RAR-independent route, assessed the effects of 4-HPR on retinoid-resistant oral dysplastic lesions (Lippman et al., 2006). Results from this study showed that 34% of the participants had a partial reduction in clinical lesion size following administration of 200 mg 4-HPR for 3 months, and 9 of the 12 clinically responsive oral lesions progressed within 9 months of discontinuation of 4-HPR. While it was initially speculated that 4-HPR would elicit its effects regardless of the presence or absence of RAR receptors, the data indicated that 4-HPR elicited apoptosis was receptor mediated. Consequently, the investigators speculated that the levels of 4-HPR achieved at the treatment site were insufficient to induce apoptosis by a receptor independent route (Lippman et al., 2006). More recently, (William et al., 2009) evaluated the effects of high-dose 4-HPR (900 mg/m^2 b.i.d. in 3 week cycles, with 1 week on drug, 2 weeks off) on oral leukoplakic lesions. The trial was discontinued at week 12 following conduction of the clinical responses and plasma analyses as only 20% of the evaluated patients had achieved a partial response. The histologic effects noted were: 2 patients' lesions decreased grade, 7 had no change, and 6 lesions increased grade. It was concluded that 4-HPR, provided in the dosage used for this trial, was ineffective in the management of premalignant oral lesions (William et al., 2009). Notably, as none of these 4-HPR trials evaluated the levels of 4-HPR achieved in oral mucosa, it is impossible to determine whether the modest therapeutic responses reflect agent ineffectiveness or an inability to obtain therapeutically relevant compound levels at the treatment site.

d. Results from additional recent chemopreventive trials. Based on the findings that cyclooxygenase 2 is frequently elevated in premalignant and malignant epithelial lesions, NCI sponsored several target-tissue site Celecoxib trials. Accordingly, Papdimitrakopoulou et al. (2008) assessed the effects of either placebo (n=18), or two doses (100 mg, n=17) or 200 mg (n=15) Celecoxib twice daily for 3 months on oral dysplastic lesions. Six additional patients received 400 mg Celecoxib b.i.d. in an unblinded study extension. While pre and post treatment biopsies were obtained on all patients, levels of Celecoxib at the oral tissue treatment site were not obtained. No differences at either the clinical or microscopic levels were observed among the forty nine (46 randomized and 3 open label) evaluable participants. The results showed that there was a 33% clinical improvement in the placebo arm relative to a 31% in the Celecoxib cohort. It was therefore concluded that Celecoxib was ineffective in the management of premalignant oral epithelial lesions (Papadimitrakopoulou et al., 2008).

A recent natural product based clinical trial evaluated the chemopreventive effects of three doses of green tea extract capsular formulations (500, 750, 1,000 mg/m^2, delivered t.i.d.) relative to placebo capsules (Tsao et al., 2009). Only a portion of the participants had lesions that were microscopically premalignant in nature while others' lesions were diagnosed as hyperkeratosis and hyperplasia. The results showed trends towards increased clinical responsiveness in the green tea extract cohorts, with responsiveness improving with higher doses. Pharmacokinetic analyses were limited to plasma and caffeine was used as a surrogate marker as the levels of ECGC were too erratic for monitoring. No differences among the groups were observed with regard to progression to OSCC (Tsao et al., 2009).

e. Oral cancer chemoprevention trials that used local delivery of chemopreventive compounds. It is well established that local delivery methods can provide a "pharmacologic advantage" by their ability to deliver therapeutically relevant compound levels at the treatment site without eliciting adverse systemic effects (Sood et al., 2005). Furthermore, local mucosal delivery avoids first-pass metabolism, which eliminates compound modification by liver enzymes and the need for compound perfusion from the systemic circulation to the overlying epithelium (Sood et al., 2005). Previous local delivery oral cavity chemoprevention trials have evaluated gel and rinse formulations as well as injection of recombinant adenoviruses (Epstein and Gorsky, 1999; Rudin et al., 2003; Li et al., 2009; Mulshine et al., 2004). In 1999, Epstein and Gorsky conducted a trial to evaluate the effects of topical application of a 0.05% vitamin A (tretinoin) acid gel on oral leukoplakic lesions. Positive aspects of this study included topical application as well as confirmation that at least 10 of the 26 participants had dysplastic lesions prior to treatment. Trial results showed that 3 participants' lesions decreased in grade, 3 remained stable, and 4 progressed.

Negative components of the Epstein and Gorsky study included the fact that only 10 persons had pretreatment biopsies, frequency of gel application did not appear closely controlled, and participants were permitted to continue smoking over the duration of the trial.

Studies by Rudin et al. (2003) employed mouthwash-mediated delivery of an attenuated adenovirus ONYX-015, which had been shown to be cytotoxic to cells with mutated p53. Although results of this study were encouraging (histologic regression of the dysplastic lesions in 37% of the 19 patients), the trial was discontinued after 2 of the 7 patients evaluated demonstrated circulating adenoviral antibody titers. The strategy used by Rudin et al. was to employ the adenovirus to selectively eradicate cells carrying a mutant p53 gene. Conversely, Li et al.'s (2009) study, which also used an adenoviral vector, desired to insert wild type p53 into dysplastic oral epithelial cells. The treatment entailed sequential injections over 15 days (injections on days 1, 4, 7, 10 and 13 days). While intraepithelial injection of fluid would likely induce acantholysis between the lesional epithelial cells which could result in necrosis and cell death, this study did not include injection of a vaccine vehicle control group. Trial results showed that 82% (18 of 22) of patients developed tissue necrosis following injections, which confirms this supposition. Although approximately one third of the participants developed adverse systemic effects including fever, increased white blood counts, and flu-like symptoms, no participants were monitored for circulating antibodies against the adenoviral vector. Notably, beneficial clinical effects, as determined by absence of lesional recurrence, were observed up to 24 months following adenoviral injection treatment; thereby implying wild-type p53 had been integrated into the transient amplifying epithelial cell pool (Li et al., 2009).

Mulshine et al. (2004) evaluated the chemopreventive efficacy of a rinse that contained the cyclooxygenase (COX) inhibitor, Ketorolac. The premise for this study was that Kerotolac had been shown to inhibit prostaglandin production in gingival crevicular fluid for over 12 h. It was therefore speculated that a Ketorolac rinse could suppress oral mucosal cyclooxygenase activities without eliciting gastrointestinal side effects. While no toxicities were observed, comparable decreases in lesional sizes were observed in the Ketorolac relative to placebo rinses (30 and 32% for Ketorolac and placebo, respectively). The authors speculated that a variety of factors, including capacity of the COX inhibitor to penetrate cornified surface epithelial layer to reach the proliferating basal cells, could have affected the clinical outcome (Mulshine et al., 2004).

f. Preclinical black raspberry studies that support BRB are promising agents for oral cancer chemoprevention. Although additional sections in this text will present the preclinical BRB studies in more detail, it is important to discuss the highlights, particularly in the context as to why these data are promising for oral cancer chemoprevention. Currently, oral dysplastic lesional histologic grade and specific molecular perturbations, such as LOH and promoter methylation at key sites, are the best predictive indicators regarding the potential for progression to malignancy (Gao et al., 2004; Papadimitrakopoulou and Hone, 2000). Clinical correlative studies have also shown the contributions of angiogenesis, and elevated levels of the high-output proinflammatory enzymes inducible nitric oxide synthase (iNOS) and cyclooxygenase-2 (COX-2) in progression of oral dysplastic lesions (Papadimitrakopoulou and Hone, 2000; Brennan et al., 2007; Chan et al., 1999; Gallo et al., 2002; Conelly et al., 2005). The contribution of tobacco-associated carcinogens in the development of HNSCC is well-accepted (Johnson, 2001). Consequently, suppression of production of complete angiogenic cytokines such as VEGF, reduction in iNOS and COX-2 functions, and suppression of tobacco-associated carcinogen bioactivation could have a beneficial impact in oral cancer chemoprevention.

A series of data obtained from a variety of cell models, including human head and neck squamous cell carcinoma cells, have shown that BRB and anthocyanin-enriched BRB extracts demonstrate a variety of chemopreventive effects including inhibition of tobacco-associated carcinogen cell transformation and transcription factor activation, suppression of autologous VEGF production, promotion of apoptosis and differentiation, and inhibition of iNOS function (Xue et al., 2001; Huang et al., 2002; Rodgrigo et al., 2006). Additional mechanistic studies determined that the BRB cyanidin glycoside enriched fraction provided the greatest chemopreventive impact (Hecht et al., 2006) and this extract suppressed VEGF production by targeting the Akt pathway (Huang et al., 2006).

The studies conducted by Kresty et al. (2001) which demonstrated that BRB inhibited in a dose-dependent fashion DNA adduct formation and tumor formation in a rat model of esophageal carcinogenesis, established the framework for subsequent in vivo analyses. Additional evaluations using this rat esophageal model showed BRB reduced nitrosomethylbenzylamine-induced angiogenesis and down-regulated iNOS, COX-2 and c-Jun (Chen et al., 2006a, b). Other investigations, which substantiated the earlier in vitro findings of Hecht et al. (2006), confirmed that BRB anthocyanins suppress rat esophageal tumorigenesis (Wang et al., 2009).

g. Formulation and characterization of a mucoadhesive gel for oral cancer chemoprevention. There are several reasons that oral epithelial dysplasia is a disease that is readily amenable to local chemopreventive therapy. First, the target site for oral cancer chemoprevention is localized. Secondly, the pharmacologic advantage obtained by local delivery provides the ability to achieve therapeutically-relevant oral cavity levels without inducing systemic toxicities. Lastly, the fact that the mouth is visually accessible enables clinical monitoring and permits the patient to directly apply the chemopreventive agent to lesional tissue.

Many current oral cavity formulations, such as Temovate®, are aqueous-based gels. Aqueous gels are compatible with the moist oral environment and provide clinically effective up-take at the treated site. Furthermore, dosing strategies for oral mucosa (i.e., multiple doses throughout the day), are optimal for maintenance of therapeutic local levels. Although gel-based formulations have been shown to be well-tolerated and effective in the mouth, prior to clinical applications it is necessary to confirm stability of the therapeutic compounds in the gel delivery vehicle (Mallery et al., 2007). Anthocyanins, which represent the predominant BRB phenolic compounds, have been demonstrated to provide a significant portion of BRB's chemopreventive impact (Tian et al., 2006; Hecht et al., 2006). Consequently, the four BRB anthocyanins (cyanidin 3-rutinoside, cyanidin 3-xylosylrutinoside, cyanidin 3-glucoside, and cyanidin 3-sambubioside) were the compounds that were monitored during the prototype gel formulation studies and the subsequent clinical trial. Results revealed that both pH and temperature affect anthocyanin stabilities (Mallery et al., 2007). Not surprisingly, anthocyanins are more stable at an acidic pH (3.5) which promoted formation of their naturally occurring, more stable, flavylium cation conformation (Mallery et al., 2007). Similarly, lower temperatures (4°C), which increased flavylium cation stability, also preserved anthocyanin integrity (Mallery et al., 2007). Evaluation of a prototype gel (5% BRB w/w, pH 6.5., 0.5 gm applied to the floor of the mouth) confirmed that gel-delivered BRB anthocyanins were readily absorbed into oral mucosa as 6 of 9 human subjects contained detectable BRB anthocyanin plasma levels 5 min following gel application (Mallery et al., 2007).

h. Results of pilot clinical trial to assess efficacy of the BRB mucoadhesive gel on oral premalignant lesions. Our labs recently completed a pilot Phase I/II oral cancer chemoprevention trial to assess chemopreventive efficacy of a bioadhesive gel that contained 10% BRB (w/w) on microscopically confirmed premalignant oral lesions (Shumway et al., 2008; Mallery et al., 2008). Thirty total individuals participated in this trial (20 with premalignant epithelial lesions and 10 normal controls) which entailed topical application of 0.5 gm of BRB (10% BRB w/w, pH 3.5) gel to the lesional site (or designated control area) q.i.d. for 6 weeks. Results from this trial demonstrated that topical BRB gel application significantly decreased loss of heterozygosity indices at loci associated with tumor suppressor genes, uniformly suppressed genes associated with RNA processing, growth factor recycling, inhibition of apoptosis, and significant reduced COX-2 levels in lesional epithelium (Shumway et al., 2008; Mallery et al., 2008). In a patient subset, gel application decreased lesional histologic grade, reduced lesional clinical size (Fig. 13.2), decreased vascular densities in the superficial connective tissues, and induced genes associated with epithelial differentiation (Mallery et al., 2008).

i. Results from pharmacokinetic and metabolism studies of BRB, with a focus on black raspberry anthocyanins. The extent of chemopreventive efficacy derived from topical BRB gel application showed appreciable interpatient differences (Ugalde et al., 2009). Possible factors that could affect gel-based therapeutic effects include absorption, penetration into target tissue, and local tissue metabolism of key BRB constituents. Pharmacokinetic analyses were therefore conducted on healthy volunteers to determine the biodistribution of the four black raspberry anthocyanins in saliva, oral mucosal tissue, and plasma following oral mucosal gel application. The pharmacologic advantage achieved by local delivery was demonstrated in these studies as significantly higher levels of BRB anthocyanins were detected in the donors' saliva and oral tissues relative to their matched plasma samples (Ugalde et al., 2009). These PK data also showed appreciable donor-related variations in anthocyanin up-take and retention in the mouth; findings which could reflect

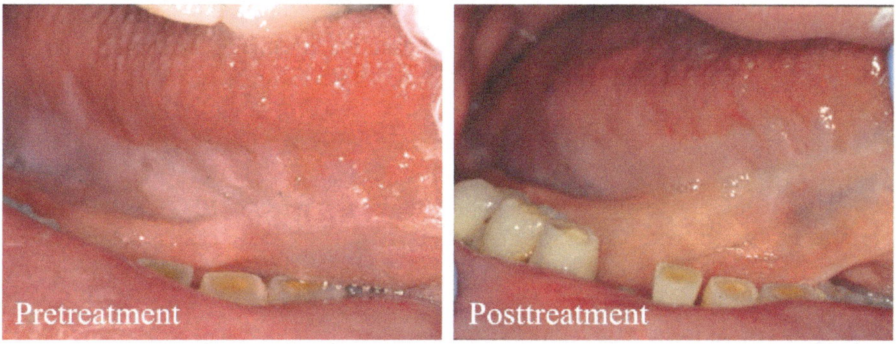

Fig. 13.2 A subset of the participants in the BRB mucoadhesive gel clinical trial showed marked clinical and histologic improvements following a 6-week application of the 10% berry gel. The pretreatment clinical appearance of this ventral tongue lesion shows marked hyperkeratosis with crisp demarcation of lesional tissue i.e. "leukoplakia" that was confirmed to be premalignant from the pretreatment biopsy. Clinical regression, as evidenced by overall loss in lesional tissue delineation and reduction in hyperkeratosis, is evident in the post-treatment photograph (These two clinical photographs are reproduced from the Fig. 2 which was published in Clinical Cancer Research 2008,14:2425). This patient also demonstrated a decrease of two histologic grades in his post-treatment biopsy

pH, production, and clearance of saliva as well as local anthocyanin metabolism. Provided the confirmed presence of glycosidase activity in human saliva (and its presence in oral microflora), local anthocyanin bioactivation (i.e., removal of associated sugars to obtain the aglycone and cyaniding), occurs in the mouth (Walle et al., 2005). Due to its replacement of bulky sugar moieties with hydroxyl groups, it is probable that cyanidin possesses superior antioxidant activities relative to its parent anthocyanin (Walle et al., 2005; Prior and Wu, 2006). Removal of the sugar moieties, however, also decreases compound stability (Fleschhut et al., 2006). Consequently, cyanidin is rapidly converted to its corresponding phenolic acid which is protocatechuic acid, which may also retain antioxidant properties (Walle et al., 2005). Provided the extensive heterogeneity in humans' metabolic enzymes, and the recognized antioxidant scavenging benefit of conversion to cyanidin, interpatient variations in glycosidase activities likely impacted therapeutic efficacies (Prior and Wu, 2006; Walle et al., 2005). Studies are ongoing to characterize enzymatic profiles of other anthocyanin-related metabolic enzymes in human oral tissues. Finally, to our knowledge, previous oral cavity chemoprevention trials have not assessed chemopreventive constituent levels at the target treatment site. Our data, which confirm that topical application provides significantly higher local relative to systemic anthocyanin levels, supports the pharmacologic advantage-local delivery premise.

j. Chemopreventive aspects to be addressed by an ongoing NCI-supported BRB gel chemoprevention trial. Ohio State University is serving as the institutional lead for a multi-center, placebo-controlled BRB gel oral cancer chemoprevention trial. This study will partner with investigators at the Universities of Louisville and North

Carolina, Chapel Hill and will be conducted under a FDA-approved Investigational New Drug for the 10% BRB gel. Many of the same parameters, such as histological grade, LOH indices, angiogenesis, COX-2 and iNOS levels, assessed in the pilot trial will also be evaluated in this current study. Several key modifications, which include: increase in trial duration from 6 to 12 weeks; determination of pretreatment oral mucosal anthocyanin bioactivation profiles; inclusion of an investigator; and participant blinded, placebo gel cohort, have been introduced. This study should commence patient accrual late spring 2010, with projected completion within 18 months of study initiation.

References

Arduino PG, Surace A, Carbone M et al (2009) Outcome of oral dysplasia: a retrospective hospital-based study of 207 patients with a long follow-up. J Oral Pathol Med 38:540–544

Bagan J, Sarrion G, Jimenez Y (2010) Oral cancer: clinical features. Oral Oncol. doi:10.1016/j.oraloncology.2010.03.009

Brennan M, Migliorati CA, Lockhart PB et al (2007) Management of oral epithelial dysplasia: a review. Oral Surg Oral Med Oral Pathol Oral Radiol Endod 103(S19):e1–e12

Chan G, Boyle JO, Yang EK et al (1999) Cyclooxgenase-2 expression is up-regulated in squamous cell carcinoma of the head and neck. Cancer Res 59:991–994

Chen YJ, Chang JT, Liao CT et al (2008) Head and neck cancer in the betel quid chewing area: recent advances in molecular carcinogenesis. Cancer Sci 99:1507–1514

Chen T, Hwang H, Rose ME et al (2006a) Chemopreventive properties of black raspberries in N-Nitrosomethylbenzylamine-Induced rat esophageal tumorigenesis: down-regulation of Cyclooxygenase-2, inducible nitric oxide synthase, and c-Jun. Cancer Res 66:2853–2859

Chen T, Rose ME, Hwang H et al (2006b) Black raspberries inhibit N-nitrosomethylbenzylamine (NMBA)-induced angiogenesis in rat esophagus parallel to the suppression of COX-2 and iNOS. Carcinogenesis. 27:2301–2307

Chiesa F, Tradati N, Gregolato R et al (2005) Randomized trial of fenretinide (4-HPR) to prevent recurrences, new lacalizations, and carcinomas in patients operated on for oral leukoplakia: Long term results. Int J Cancer 115:625–629

Connelly ST, Macabeo-Ong M, Dekker N et al (2005) Increased nitric oxide levels and iNOS over-expression in oral squamous cell carcinoma. Oral Oncol 41:261–267

Epstein JB, Gorsky M (1999) Topical application of vitamin A to oral leukoplakia. Cancer 86: 921–927

Fleschhut J, Kratzer F, Rechkemmer G et al (2006) Stability and biotranformation of various anthocyanins in vitro. Eur J Nutr 45:7–18

Freemantle SJ, Spinella MJ, Dmitrovsky E (2003) Retinoids in cancer therapy and chemoprevention: promise meets resistance. Oncogene 22:7305–7315

Gallo O, Masini E, Bianchi B et al (2002) Prognostic significance of cyclooxygenase-2 pathway and angiogenesis in head and neck squamous cell carcinoma. Hum Pathol 33:708–714

Gao S, Worm J, Guldberg P et al (2004) Loss of heterozygosity at 9q33 and hypermethylation of the DBCCR1 gene in oral squamous cell carcinoma. Br J Cancer 91:760–764

Garewal HS, Katz RV, Meyshens F et al (1999) B-carotene produces sustained remissions in patients with oral leukoplakia results of a multicenter prospective trial. Arch Otolaryngol Head Neck Surg 125:1305–1310

Garewal HS, Meyskens FLJ, Killen D et al (1990) Response of oral leukoplakia to beta-carotene. J Clin Oncol 8:1715–1720

Gillison ML, Souza GD, Westra W et al (2008) Distinct risk factor profiles for human papillomavirus type 16-positive and human papillomavirus type 16-negative head and neck cancers. J Natl Cancer Inst 100:407–420

Goon PK, Stanley MA, Ebmeyer J et al (2009) HPV & head and neck cancer: a descriptive update. Head Neck Oncol 1:36

Greer RO (2006) Pathology of malignant and premalignant oral epithelial lesions. Otolaryngol Clin North Am 39:249–275

Hail N Jr, Kim HJ, Lotan R (2006) Mechanisms of fenretinide-induced apoptosis. Apoptosis 11:1677–1694

Hecht SS, Huang C, Stoner GD et al (2006) Identification of cyanidin glycosides as constituents of freeze-dried black raspberries which inhibit anti-benzo[a]pyrene-7,8-diol-epoxide induced NFκB and AP-1 activity. Carcinogenesis 27:1617–1626

Hong WK, Endicott J, Itri LM et al (1986) 13-cis-retinoic acid in the treatment of oral leukoplakia. N Engl J Med 315:1501–1505

Huang C, Huang Y, Hu W et al (2002) Inhibition of benzo(a)pyrene diol-epoxide-induced transactivation of activated protein 1 and nuclear factor κB by black raspberry extracts. Cancer Res 62:6857–6863

Huang C, Li J, Song L, Zhang D et al (2006) Black raspberry extracts inhibit Benzo(a)Pyrene Diol-Epoxide-induced activator Protein 1 activation and VEGF transcription by targeting the phosphotidylinositol 3-Kinase/Akt pathway. Cancer Res 66:581–587

Islam MN, Kornberg L, Veenker E, et al (2010) Anatomic site based ploidy analysis of oral premalignant lesions. Head Neck Pathol 4:10–14

Johnson N (2001) Tobacco use and oral cancer: a global perspective. J Dent Educ 65:328–339

Kramer IR, Lucas RB, Pindborg JJ et al (1978) Definition of leukoplakia and related lesions: an aid to studies on oral precancer. Oral Surg Oral Med Oral Pathol 46:518–539

Kresty LA, Morse MA, Morgan C et al (2001) Chemoprevention of esophageal tumorigenesis by dietary administration of lyophilized black raspberries. Cancer Res 61:6112–6119

Li Y, Li L-J, Zhang S-T, Wang L-J et al (2009) In vitro and clinical studies of gene therapy with recombinant human Adenovirus-p53 inject for oral leukoplakia. Clin Cancer Res 15:6724–6731

Lippman SM, Batsakis JG, Toth BB et al (1993) Comparison of low-dose isotretinoin with beta carotene to prevent oral carcinogenesis. N Engl J Med 328:15–20

Lippman SM, Lee JJ, Martin JW et al (2006) Fenretinide activity in retinoid-resistant oral leukoplakia. Clin Cancer Res 12:3109–3114

Mallery SR, Stoner GD, Larsen PE et al (2007) Formulation and in-vitro and in-vivo evaluation of a mucoadhesive gel containing freeze dried black raspberries: implications for oral cancer chemoprevention. Pharm Res 24:728–737

Mallery SR, Zwick JC, Pei P et al (2008) Topical application of a bioadhesive black raspberry gel modulates gene expression and reduces cyclooxygenase 2 protein in human premalignant oral lesions. Cancer Res 68:4945–4957

Mehanna HM, Rattay T, Smith J et al (2009) Treatment and follow-up of oral dysplasia - a systematic review and meta-analysis. Head Neck 31:1600–1609

Mulshine JL, Atkinson JC, Greer RO et al (2004) Randomized, double-blind, placebo-controlled phase IIB trial of the cyclooxygenase inhibitor ketorolac as an oral rinse in oropharyngeal leukoplakia. Clin Cancer Res 10:1565–1573

Neville BW, Damm DD, Allen CM et al (2009) Epithelial pathology. In: Oral and maxillofacial pathology, 3rd edn. Sauders Elsevier, St. Louis

Neville BW, Day TA (2002) Oral cancer and precancerous lesions. CA Cancer J Clin 52:195–215

Papadimitrakopoulou VA, Hong WK (2000) Biomolecular markers as intermediate end points in chemoprevention trials of upper aerodigestive tract cancer. Int J Cancer. 88:852–855

Papadimitrakopoulou VA, William WN, Dannnberg AJ et al (2008) Randomized phase II study of celecoxib in oral premalignant lesions. Clin Cancer Res 14:2095–2101

Prior RL, Wu X (2006) Anthocyanins: Structural characteristics that result in unique metabolic patterns and biological activities. Free Rad Res 40:1014–1028

Reichart PA, Philipsen HP (2005) Oral erythroplakia-a review. Oral Oncol. 41:551–561

Richie JP Jr, Kleinman W, Marina P et al (2008) Blood iron, glutathione, and micronutrient levels and the risk of oral cancer. Nutr Cancer 60:474–482

Rodgrigo KA, Rawal Y, Renner RJ et al (2006) Suppression of the tumorigenic phenotype in human oral squamous cell carcinoma cells by an ethanol extract derived from freeze-dried black raspberries. Nutrition And Cancer 54:58–68

Rodriguez T, Altieri A, Chatenoud L et al (2004) Risk factors for oral and pharyngeal cancer in young adults. Oral Oncol 40:207–213

Rudin CM, Cohen EE, Papadimitrakopoulou VA et al (2003) An attenuated adenovirus, ONYX-015, as mouthwash therapy for premalignant oral dysplasia. J Clin Oncol 21:4546–4552

Scuibba JJ (1995) Oral leukoplakia. Crit Rev Oral Biol Med 6:147–160

Scully C, Bagan J (2009) Oral squamous cell carcinoma: overview of current understanding of aetiopathogenesis and clinical implications. Oral Dis 15:388–399

Shah JP, Strong EW, DeCosse JJ et al (1983) Effect of retinoids on oral leukoplakia. Am J Surg 146:466–470

Shumway BS, Kresty LA, Larsen PE et al (2008) Effects of a topically applied bioadhesive berry gel on loss of heterozygosity indices in premalignant oral lesions. Clin Cancer Res 14: 2421–2430

Silverman S Jr, Gorsky M, Lozada F (1984) Oral leukoplakia and malignant transformation. A follow-up study of 257 patients. Cancer 53:563–568

Smith W, Saba N (2005) Retinoids as chemoprevention for head and neck cancer: where do we go from here? Crit Rev Oncol Hematol 55:143–152

Sood S, Shiff SJ, Yang CS et al (2005) Selection of topically applied non-steroidal anti-inflammatory drugs for oral cancer chemoprevention. Oral Oncol 41:562–567

Tian Q, Gusti MM, Stoner GD et al (2006) Urinary excretion of black raspberry (Rubus occidentalis) anthocyanins and their metabolism. J Agric Food Chem 54:1467–1472

Tsao AS, Liu D, Martin J et al (2009) Phase II randomized, placebo-controlled trial of green tea extract in patients with high-risk oral premalignant lesions. Cancer Prev Res 2:931–941

Ugalde CM, Liu Z, Ren C et al (2009) Distribution of anthocyanins delivered from a bioadhesive black raspberry gel following topical application in normal healthy volunteers. Pharm Res 26:977–986

Vigneswaran N, Tilashalski K, Rodu B et al (1995) Tobacco use and cancer. A reappraisal. Oral Surg Oral Med Oral Pathol Oral Radiol Endod 80:178–182

Waldron CA, Shafer WG (1975) Leukoplakia revisited. A clinicopathologic study 3256 oral leukoplakias. Cancer 36:1386–1392

Walle T, Browning AM, Steed LL et al (2005) Flavonoid glucosides are hydrolyzed and thus activated in the oral cavity. J Nutr 135:48–52

Wang L-S, Hecht SS, Carmella SG et al (2009) Anthocyanins in black raspberries prevent esophageal tumors in rats. Cancer Prev Res 2:84–93

William WN Jr, Lee J, Lippman SM et al (2009) High-dose fenretinide in oral leukoplakia. Cancer Prev Res 2:22–26

Xue H, Aziz RM, Sun N et al (2001) Inhibition of cellular transformation by berry extracts. Carcinogenesis 22:351–356

Chapter 14
Cancer Prevention in Populations High At-Risk for the Development of Oral Cancer: Clinical Trials with Black Raspberries

Thomas J. Knobloch, Bruce C. Casto, Amit Agrawal, Steven K. Clinton, and Christopher M. Weghorst

Abstract It is estimated that oral cancers will present with more than 400,000 new cases worldwide, establishing this malignancy as the sixth most common cancer globally. In association with the "field" effects of these epithelial neoplasias, oral cancers are marked by high frequencies of local invasion and recurrence, and 5-year survival times of less than 60% depending upon the stage of the initial lesion. Epidemiological studies support the hypothesis that a decreased oral cancer incidence is associated with lifestyle changes, including diminished exposure to alcohol and tobacco and increased dietary incorporation of fruits and vegetables. Food-based approaches to cancer prevention, including dietary exposure to black raspberries, emphasize the potential for complex mixtures of bioactive food components to inhibit several processes and mechanistic states within a multistep oral carcinogenesis archetype. Both pre-clinical and clinical models of black raspberry administration have demonstrated a striking capacity of black raspberries and their derivatives to specifically modulate gene transcriptional profiles in a manner that favors oral cancer prevention strategies.

Keywords Oral cancer · Clinical trial · Black raspberries · Chemoprevention · Dietary intervention · Biomarkers · Nutraceutical · Whole-food intervention · Cancer risk reduction · Phytochemical · Bioactive food components

---

T.J. Knobloch (✉)
Division of Environmental Health Sciences, College of Public Health, The Ohio State University, Columbus, OH 43210, USA
e-mail: knobloch.1@osu.edu

C.M. Weghorst (✉)
Division of Environmental Health Sciences, College of Public Health, The Ohio State University, Columbus, OH 43210, USA
e-mail: weghorst.2@osu.edu

G.D. Stoner, N.P. Seeram (eds.), *Berries and Cancer Prevention*,
DOI 10.1007/978-1-4419-7554-6_14,

Abbreviations

CCND1	Cyclin D1
CDKN2A	Cyclin-dependent kinase inhibitor 2A, p16INK4A and p14ARF; *FHIT*, fragile histidine triad gene
g	*Grams*
HNSCC	*Head and neck squamous cell carcinoma*
LOH	Loss of heterozygosity
LBR	Lyophilized black raspberries
OSCC	Oral squamous cell carcinoma
qRT-PCR	Quantitative real time reverse transcription polymerase chain reaction
RASSF1A	RAS-association domain family 1, isoform A
RB1	Retinoblastoma
TP53	Tumor protein p53

1 Oral Cancer

1.1 Oral Cancer Background

Oral squamous cell carcinomas (OSCCs) are the most common manifestation of head and neck squamous cell carcinomas (HNSCCs) and are projected to account for more than 400,000 new cases worldwide (Parkin et al., 2005; Lippman et al., 2005; Jemal et al., 2004). In the United States, it is estimated that in 2009 there were 35,720 new OSCC cases and 7,600 deaths as a result of oral cancers, with incidence rates more than two to threefold greater in men than women (Parkin et al., 2002; American Cancer Society, 2009). Although OSCCs have demonstrated a consistent decrease of 2% per year in men since 1980, and in women since 1990 (American Cancer Society, 2009) in the United States, deleterious global trends are likely to persist as the incidence of smoking increases worldwide.

Oral cancer patients with early stage disease often present with minimal clinical symptoms. Consequently, oral cancers are characterized by high rates of local invasion and frequent lymph node metastases (Sasaki et al., 2005; Garzino-Demo et al., 2006) that are likely associated with the late clinical presentation and delayed diagnosis of these lesions. The concept of oral and other intraepithelial neoplasias (IEN) arising not from "isolated cellular phenomenon," but instead due to "an anaplastic tendency involving many cells at once" was proposed by Slaughter (1944, 1946) to describe the multicentric tumor capacity of the at-risk oral landscape. In a seminal paper, Slaughter et al. (1953) formally designated "field cancerization" as the hypothesis that exposure to carcinogens resulted in alterations that are present throughout the epithelia of OSCC patients, and that these "fields" could result in the genesis of multiple independent lesions and multifocal tumors. These authors originally proposed that multiple oral cancer lesions could develop from distinct, independent cell clones. These "field" effects have been further defined to include oral cancer lesions that are distant from the cancer fields but derived from expansion of an original "field" clone. Braakhuis et al. (2003) described each "field" as consisting of a carcinogen-exposed stem cell that acquired genetic defects and generated a patch. A patch now represented a clonal population of the original stem cell and its altered daughter cells. The patch accumulated additional genetic defects, acquired a growth advantage over the normal epithelium, and transitioned into an expanding preneoplastic field. Eventually, further molecular alterations and clonal divergence resulted in the development of tumors within this new field. Indeed, 20% of OSCC patients will present with a local recurrent malignant lesion within 18 months following surgical resection for cure, while 22–42% will present with a second primary tumor within 5–8 years (Cooper et al., 1989; Schwartz et al., 1994; Leon et al., 1999).

Unfortunately, despite ongoing advances in surgical and therapeutic strategies, the overall survival rate for OSCCs has not appreciably changed for several decades and remains less than 60% at 5-years following diagnosis. In OSCC cases involving locoregional invasion, the survival rate deceases to 35% at 5 years. Furthermore, rigorous multimodal treatment strategies (surgical resection, adjuvant radiation and/or chemotherapy) often result in significant physical disfiguration, diminished mastication and swallowing, and impaired speech. The sum of these physical and functional consequences can be the formation of substantial psychosocial disabilities with respect to appearance and self-esteem.

Case-control studies and epidemiological data have demonstrated a causal relationship between oral cancers and exposure to tobacco carcinogens (Decker and Goldstein, 1982; Reibel, 2003; Mao et al., 2004). While alcohol use is an independent risk factor for developing OSCCs, the combined use of tobacco and alcohol markedly amplifies the risk for oral cancer development (IARC Working Group on the Evaluation of Carcinogenic Risks to Humans, 2004) and may account for nearly 75% of all oral cancers (Wynder and Stellman, 1977; Mashberg et al., 1993). Other risk factors for oral cancers include dietary deficiencies and positivity for human papillomas virus (HPV). HPV, primarily HPV16 ($\sim$90%), can be detected in 20–25% of all HNSCC and 50–85% of oropharynx cancers. (Gillison and Shah, 2001; Kreimer et al., 2005; IARC Working Group on the Evaluation of Carcinogenic Risks to Humans, 2007; Adelstein et al., 2009). In addition, conflicting data exists as to the potential risk modifying effects of marijuana for HNSCCs (Zhang et al. 1999; Gillison et al., 2000; Liang et al., 2009). What is becoming increasingly clear from the current knowledge base is the significant influence of lifestyle on cancer risk. The American Institute for Cancer Research (Glade, 1999; Wiseman, 2008) estimates that up to 50% of oral cancers can be prevented by appropriate modifications to diet and lifestyle factors. Lifestyle changes include tobacco cessation, moderation in alcohol consumption, proper exercise, weight control measures, and avoidance of high-risk sexual behaviors. Diet and health guidelines for cancer prevention include a recommendation for plant-based foods, including low-starch fruits and vegetables that are enriched in polyphenolics, flavonoids, and antioxidants, that have demonstrated an association with a decreased risk of oral cancer development (Glade, 1999; IARC Working Group on the Evaluation of Carcinogenic Risks to Humans, 2004; Wiseman, 2008).

1.2 Molecular Biology of Oral Cancer

Oral cancer progresses through a multistep process of carcinogenesis whereby an accumulation of genetic deficiencies, risk modifying behaviors, and gene-environmental interactions culminate in a malignant phenotype. A series of stepwise genetic alterations, including mutations, deletions, loss of heterozygosity, genome instability, and aneuploidy are well documented in established tumor suppressors and proto-oncogenes in OSCCs (Forastiere et al., 2001; Lippman et al., 2005). Furthermore, epigenetic modifications, most notably methylation status changes in CpG islands, have been established as important markers of neoplastic progression in OSCCs. Additionally, OSCCs are more than just isolated tumorigenic epithelial cells. The complex interactions between, at-risk "field effect" epithelial cells, premalignant epithelial cells, malignant epithelial cells, infiltrating immune cells, stromal cells, and the extracellular matrix within the tumor microenvironment generate metabolic changes that drive the tumorigenic process. Deregulated communication between components of the tumor microenvironment promote the progression of the oral malignancy and facilitate the transition from at-risk normal cells to benign, dysplastic, premalignant, malignant, and metastatic cell types. The complete tumor microenvironment provides angiogenesis factors to maintain tumor oxygen levels and promote growth, and invasion factors that ultimately lead to metastasis.

Following exposure to the initial environmental insult, a chromosomal LOH occurs at 9p21 (*CDKN2A*; p16INK4A and p14ARF) and 3p14 (*FHIT*) and *RASSF1A*, followed by LOH at 4q, 8p, 11q13 (*CCND1*), 13q14 (*RB1*), 14q, 17p13 (*TP53*), and finally LOH at 8q, 13p, and 18q (Califano et al., 1996; Lippman et al., 2005; Choi and Myers, 2008) (Fig. 14.1). Additionally, epigenetic changes at the *CDKN2A* locus result in promoter hypermethylation and inactivation of p16. The importance of the *CDKN2A* locus to oral carcinogenesis is further emphasized by the common occurrence of p16 inactivating mutations in HNSCCs and premalignant lesions (Yeudall et al., 1994; Reed et al., 1996; Papadimitrakopoulou et al., 1997; Lang et al., 1998). Therefore, the p16 tumor suppressor is notably targeted for inactivation by three distinct mechanisms: LOH, mutation/microdeletion, and DNA hypermethylation. Similarly, the *TP53* locus is targeted by LOH and mutations that result in an absent or dysfunctional p53 tumor suppressor, while both *FHIT* and *RASSF1A* are subject to LOH and hypermethylation at the remaining allele. Loss of function in mutant p53 further promotes oral carcinogenesis by diminishing a cell's ability to repair genomic damage and regulate appropriate passage through the cell cycle. In contrast, while the *CCND1* locus is subject to LOH, it is also a region of genomic amplification (11q13) resulting in over-expression of the cyclin D1 oncogene and forced progression through the cell cycle. Further over-expression of *PTGS2* (COX2; prostaglandin-endoperoxide synthase 2 [prostaglandin G/H synthase and cyclooxygenase]) and activated *EGFR* (epidermal growth factor receptor) advance the malignant potential of the increasingly dysfunctional oral cells (Fig. 14.1).

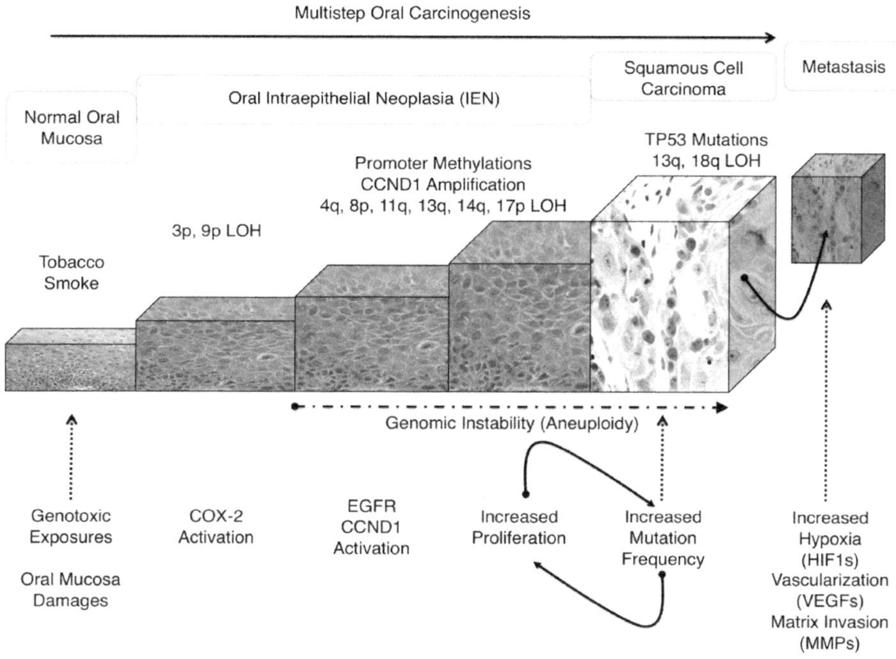

Fig. 14.1 Multistep oral carcinogenesis model. Following initial environmental exposures, oral epithelial cells concurrently and sequentially acquire characteristic genomic and epigenomic alterations. Mutations, loss of heterozygosity, gene amplification, and deregulated gene promoter methylation results in the inappropriate expression and activation of cellular factors that circumvent normal growth control mechanisms. Aberrant orchestration of inflammation, proliferation, and vascularization promotes conditions that ultimately favor invasion and metastatic spread

1.3 Prevention of Oral Cancer by Whole Foods

Diet as a risk reduction strategy for the development of diseases, including cancer, has long been associated with traditional medicinal practices and folk remedies. Yan Yonghe, a physician living in China during the Song Dynasty (960–1279), wrote the Jisheng Fang ("Life Helping Formulae") to provide instructions for promoting health and well-being. These formulae and remedies leveraged the powers of whole foods and their derivatives against the insults of disease, including what we now recognize as Fang's description of esophageal cancer. In 1908, Roger Williams suggested in his book, *The Natural History of Cancer with Special Reference to its Causation and Prevention*, that excess consumption of red meats and "other cofactors ... deficient exercise, and probably also a lack of sufficient fresh vegetable food" was associated with the development of cancer. Williams recognized that these observations were of "paramount importance in the aetiology of cancer." Early epidemiological studies examining the association between diet and cancer by Orr (1933) and Stocks (1933) identified nutritional factors such as low consumption of fruits and vegetables as risk factor components for cancer. For many years, food-based cancer risk reduction strategies were relegated to the "complementary and alternative medicine" categories of intervention, with strong anecdotal evidence, but a perceived lack of rigorous, hypothesis-testing investigation. Since Michael Sporn defined his concept of chemoprevention in 1976 (Sporn, 1976; Sporn et al., 1976) there has been increasing interest, scientific effort, and national funding directed towards defining the capacity of various whole foods and their bioactive components to modify oral cancer risk.

It has become increasingly evident that the incidence and development of OSCCs is the consequence of the complex interaction between environmental exposures, genetic factors, and epigenetic signals. Environmental carcinogens, such as those found in tobacco products, have been shown repeatedly to alter the genetic state of exposed cells. The consequence of these uncorrected genotoxic damages is inappropriately regulated cell growth and the manifestation of a malignant phenotype. One obvious approach to oral cancer prevention is through risk reduction strategies that emphasize modifiable lifestyle changes, such as cessation of tobacco product use and restricted alcohol consumption. It has been estimated that smoking-related diseases alone cost the US more than 196 billion dollars each year (American Cancer Society, 2009). Smoking represents the single largest preventable cause of disease and premature death worldwide and has been notably associated with enhanced risks of heart disease, stroke, chronic lung disease, cancers of the lung, larynx, esophagus, stomach, bladder, cervix, pancreas, kidneys leukemia, and oral cavity (American Cancer Society, 2009). Unfortunately, many individuals are unable or unwilling to commit to the lifestyle changes necessary to effectively decrease cancer risk.

Cancer chemoprevention can be defined as the use of natural compounds, synthetic agents, or dietary constituents, in combination or alone, to inhibit, delay, or reverse the multistep carcinogenic process (Stoner et al., 1997; Kelloff et al., 1999; Sporn et al., 1976; Sporn, 1976). Because OSCC progression can exhibit a prolonged period of dysplastic and premalignant lesion development, an extended window of chemopreventive opportunity is available to introduce cancer risk reduction strategies. Since OSCCs develop in a multistep process over a 10–20 year period of time that involves the accumulation of decisive genetic events and epigenetic modifications, there are many points at which to initiate a cancer risk reduction intervention (Fig. 14.1). It becomes possible for chemopreventive agents to target distinct mechanistic states within OSCC progression, including initiation, promotion, and progression. Chemoprevention can be described as addressing distinct at-risk environs. Primary prevention focuses on protective measures in healthy patients who are at elevated risk for oral cancer, such as tobacco users. Secondary prevention involves high at-risk patients who have manifested a premalignant condition, such as oral leukoplakia. Tertiary prevention encompasses OSCC patients who have presented an initial malignant lesion, been treated for cure, and want to prevent the occurrence of a second primary tumor (Hong et al., 2000). Oral cancer is well suited for examining the potential of chemopreventive intervention strategies for several reasons. First, the oral cavity provides an anatomical location that facilitates non-intrusive access to the tissues at risk. Cancer prevention agents can be directly administered to localized restricted areas, oral tissues can be readily obtained for analyses, and measurements of exposure and outcome can be effectively acquired. Second, high at-risk populations represented by users of tobacco and alcoholic products are easily identified and readily available.

1.4 Food-Based Phytochemicals and Cancer Prevention

Food-based approaches to cancer prevention emphasize the potential for complex mixtures of bioactive food components to inhibit several processes and mechanistic states within the multistep carcinogenesis model. Just as oral cancers represent a complex malignant microenvironment and not simple deregulated epithelia, so do whole food-based bioactive mixtures reveal the elaborate orchestration of individual preventive compounds. While a number of preventive agents have been identified in foods, many other constituents remain to be isolated and evaluated for chemopreventive efficacy. Additionally, the specific mechanisms by which food components inhibit, delay, or revert malignant phenotypes have yet to be described in detail. In contrast to whole food focused strategies, single-agent approaches to cancer chemoprevention parallel pharmaceutical models and emphasizes an understanding of specific mechanisms of action at discrete carcinogenic stages. These studies can be systematically designed and rigorously controlled for content and outcome measurements. However, in "field effect" cancers such as OSCCs with different at-risk cell types in overlapping stages of carcinogenic progression and multiple deregulated pathways, there may be distinct advantages to the combinatorial exposure of bioactive components to reducing tumor development. Therefore, whole food-based interventions benefit from the concurrent exposure of at-risk oral tissues to several bioactive agents that affect multiple metabolic and signaling pathways. The use of whole foods in cancer prevention studies allows the examination of multiple food component interactions and models dietary and nutritional contributions to cancer risk.

1.5 Black Raspberries as a Cancer Prevention Agent

The rationale for the use of black raspberries as a cancer risk reduction agent for OSCCs originates from widespread epidemiological studies in which fruit and vegetable consumption is inversely related to oral cancer incidence (Pavia et al., 2006). Programs such as the Center for Disease Control and Prevention's (CDC) national "Healthy People 2010" initiative strives to increase the proportion of Americans consuming daily ≥ 2 servings of fruits and ≥ 3 servings of vegetables, respectively (US Department of Health and Human Services, 2000). Among fruits, black raspberries (*Rubus occidentalis*) are of particular interest due to their complement of compounds with demonstrated chemopreventive activity, including fiber, vitamin A, vitamin C, vitamin E, folate, calcium, selenium β-sitosterol, ellagic acid, ferulic acid, bioflavonoids (quercetin), ellagitannins and anthocyanins (cyanidin 3-glucoside, cyanidin 3-sambubioside, cyanidin 3-rutinoside and cyanidin 3-xylosylrutinoside) (Stoner, 2009). The anthocyanin content of black raspberries (Tian et al., 2006; He et al., 2009; Stoner, 2009) contributes a marked antioxidant activity to these fruits (Wang and Lin, 2000; Kresty et al., 2001; Moyer et al., 2002), a feature common to many food-based chemopreventive agents.

As of 2010, only two published clinical trials had been conducted to evaluate pharmacokinetics and biomarker modulation following administration of dietary LBR in human subjects. First, in a Phase I study, Stoner et al. (2005) examined the tolerability and pharmacokinetics of 11 healthy subjects who consumed 45 g of LBR powder daily for 1 week. Maximum concentrations of polyphenolic antioxidants were measured 1–2 h following LBR administration in plasma and 0–4 h in urine. Less than 1% of these bioactivity markers were absorbed and detected in urine. Second, in a Phase IIA study, Kresty et al. (2006) evaluated biomarkers in Barrett's esophagus patients who consumed 32 g (females) or 45 g (males) of LBR powder daily for 6 months. An interim analysis of 10 patients demonstrated a reduction in oxidative stress, as measured by the thromboxane/endoperoxide receptor antagonist 8-epi-prostaglandin F2alpha and the free radical-induced oxidative DNA damage biomarker 8-hydroxy-2′-deoxyguanosine. No significant toxicities or serious adverse events were reported in either study. Three additional Phase I studies (OSU0497, OSU06132, OSU07085) by Weghorst et al. (2004, 2006, 2008) are in progress to profile transcriptional changes in oral tissues following the short-term administration of dietary LBR in pre-surgical OSCC patients. The daily dosing regimens of 4.3 g (OSU0497, OSU06132) and 8 g (OSU07085) of LBR are markedly decreased with respect to the preceding studies, and are designed to leverage an extended localized exposure to the oral cavity.

1.6 Pre-clinical Studies with Black Raspberries in Human Oral Cancer Cells

As a transitional step from pre-clinical animal cancer prevention studies (see Casto et al. in Chapter 10: Inhibition of Oral Cancer in Animal Models by Berries), an alcohol extract of LBR (LBR-OH) (Xue et al., 2001) was assessed for its ability to suppress cell growth and induce gene expression changes, and consequently reveal its chemopreventive potential, using human oral cavity cells in vitro.

1.6.1 Black Raspberry Extract and Human Oral Cancer Cell Proliferation

A passage-limited, non-immortalized human oral cell line (TE1177) was established by D'Ambrosio et al. (2000) from epithelium surgically removed during a tonsillectomy and recapitulated a normal oral phenotype. The immortalized but non-tumorigenic 83-01-82SCC (designated "SCC83") cell line was derived from a human OSCC of the tongue and presents as a surrogate premalignant in vitro model Lee et al., 1997; D'Ambrosio et al., 2000, 2001). Both TE1177 and SCC83 have been well studied for their response to phytochemical and chemopreventive agents. In order to assess growth inhibitory potential of the LBR-OH, cells were seeded into 96-well tissue culture plates containing complete growth medium. After 24 h, the culture medium was replaced with fresh medium containing medium alone (proliferation/growth control), 10% DMSO alone (delivery control), or dilutions of the LBR-OH (up to 300 μg/mL) dissolved in 10% DMSO. The final concentration of DMSO in the culture medium was 0.2%. On every alternate day, the culture medium was replaced with fresh medium containing the LBR extract or delivery vehicle. On day 7 when the proliferation control (unexposed) cells reached confluence, cell proliferation was measured by proxy using a second generation tetrazolium salt cleavage assay (WST-1). The tetrazolium salt 4-[3-(4-iodophenyl)-2-(4-nitrophenyl)-2H-5-tetrazolio]-1,3-benzene disulfonate is cleaved to formazan by cellular enzymes (Berridge et al., 1996). The metabolic activity of viable cells is reflected by the overall activity of cellular mitochondrial dehydrogenases, and subsequently, by the amount of formazan cleavage product formed in the assay. The colorimetric changes are quantified using a scanning multiwell spectrophotometer and directly correlates to the number of metabolically active cells in the sample.

While no significant changes in cell proliferation were observed with any concentration of LBR extract in the normal oral epithelium TE1177 cells, LBR extract decreased cellular proliferation of the premalignant SCC83 cells in a dose-dependent manner to a maximum inhibition of 45% (Knobloch et al., 2003, unpublished; Han et al., 2005) (Fig. 14.2). These in vitro assays demonstrated the differential growth inhibitory effects of bioactive LBR components on human oral premalignant cells compared to cells derived from normal oral epithelium. These in vitro findings demonstrated an ability of the bioactive phytochemical components of LBR to selectively target non-normal oral epithelial cells and supported a hypothesis that the cells in human oral lesions would be responsive to growth inhibitory (cancer preventive) signaling mediated by LBR in a clinical setting.

1.6.2 Modulation of In Vitro Gene Expression Profiles Associated with Oral Carcinogenesis

Concurrent cell cultures for growth inhibition evaluation and total RNA isolation were performed using SCC83 cells exposed to 200 μg/mL of LBR-OH. Affymetrix GeneChip Human Genome Arrays (HG-U133 Plus 2.0 Arrays) containing 1,300,000 unique oligonucleotide features representing >47,000 transcripts and approximately 39,000 genes were used to transcriptionally profile changes in gene expression between the vehicle control (0.2% DMSO) and LBR-OH samples. The resulting Affymetrix CEL files, which store an intensity value ± standard deviations and the number of pixels used to calculate the intensity value for each feature on the probe array, were processed by DNA-Chip Analyzer (dChip) software (Li and Wong, 2001; Parmigiani et al., 2003), gcRMA adjustments for background

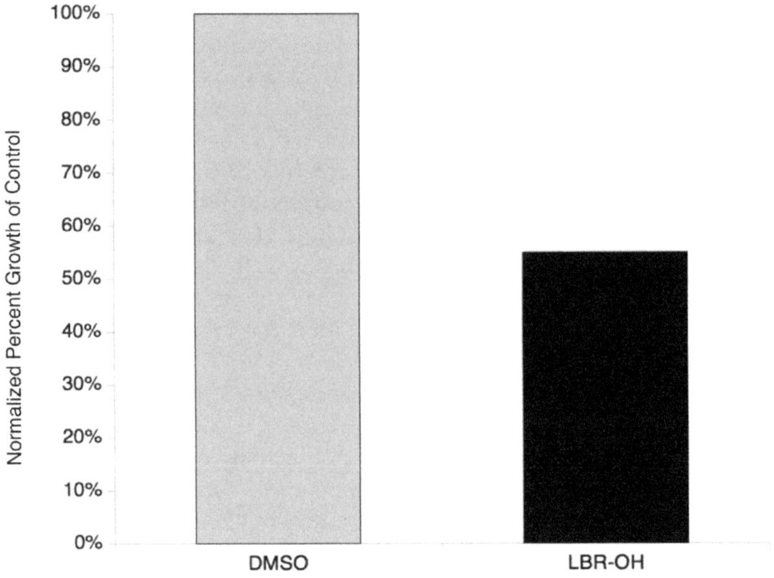

Fig. 14.2 LBR-dependent growth inhibition in SCC83 Cells. SCC83 oral premalignant epithelial cells demonstrate a growth inhibition of 45% following a 4-day exposure to 200 μ/mL LBR-OH compared to 0.2% DMSO exposed control cells. Cellular proliferation and viability was assessed using a WST-1 colorimetric assay (Roche Applied Science, Indianapolis, IN) (Knobloch et al., 2003 unpublished, Han et al., 2005)

intensities including optical noise and non-specific binding, and custom statistical routines. The NIH Database for Annotation, Visualization and Integrated Discovery (DAVID)(Knobloch et al., 2008; Dennis et al., 2003; Huang et al., 2009) was used for initial characterization of the unbiased, global GeneChip probe ID data set.

A sample of 1,429 unique Affymetrix probe sets demonstrated a significant and >1.5-fold change in gene expression between DMSO-treated and LBR-OH exposed premalignant oral cells. Conversion of the Affymetrix probe IDs by DAVID generated a list of 1,281 annotated DAVID IDs (GENE_SYMBOL) for use in subsequent modeling. Initially, Functional Annotation Clustering, a term-centric modular enrichment analysis, was performed for the DAVID IDs of interest. Over-representation of duplicated genes was minimized by calculating one tail Fisher Exact Probability Value (EASE score) statistics only on non-redundant DAVID IDs. The in vitro data set was parsed into clusters of functionally related annotations and groups of related gene–term relationships, including cell cycle, cell proliferation, cell adhesion, transcription negative, transcription positive, histone transferase activity, phosphoprotein, cell differentiation, and apoptosis (Knobloch et al., 2008, unpublished) (Table 14.1). DAVID Gene-Enrichment algorithms were used to characterize the input genes for strong statistical associations (EASE Score) with certain categorical terms. Within the DAVID modeling system, a *P*-Value ≤ 0.05 is considered strongly enriched for a specific annotation category.

Table 14.1 LBR-OH-dependent DAVID Functional Annotation Groups

DAVID functional annotation term[a]	Category	Gene count	Gene (%)	p-value	Enrichment[b]
Phosphoprotein	SP_PIR_KEYWORDS[c,d]	501	39.1	<0.000001	1.70
Gene expression	GOTERM_BP_ALL[e]	306	24.2	<0.000001	1.27
Cell differentiation	GOTERM_BP_ALL	148	11.6	<0.005	1.20
Post-translational protein modification	GOTERM_BP_ALL	140	10.9	<0.00001	1.40
Negative regulation of biological process	GOTERM_BP_ALL	124	9.8	<0.000001	1.61
Positive regulation of biological process	GOTERM_BP_ALL	110	8.7	<0.000001	1.53
Cell cycle	GOTERM_BP_ALL	110	8.7	<0.0001	1.89
Cell death	GOTERM_BP_ALL	82	6.5	<0.0005	1.50
Cell adhesion	GOTERM_BP_ALL	82	6.5	<0.0001	1.63
Cell proliferation	GOTERM_BP_ALL	72	5.7	<0.005	1.22
Response to DNA damage stimulus	GOTERM_BP_ALL	36	2.8	<0.005	1.70

[a]Database for Annotation, Visualization and Integrated Discovery (DAVID).
[b]Gene Ontology database, biological process analysis.
[c]SwissProt (SP) and Protein Information Resource (PIR) databases, keyword analysis.
[d]Derived from Functional Annotation chart parsed for terms with more than 50 members.
[e]Gene Ontology database, biological process analysis.

1.7 Clinical Studies with Black Raspberries in Oral Cancer Patients

1.7.1 Phase I Clinical Trial: Pre-surgical Model

A number of hypotheses and specific aims were proposed for the investigational Phase 1 OSCC/LBR clinical trial (OSU0497) initiated by Weghorst et al. (2004). First, it was essential to evaluate the willingness of newly diagnosed OSCC patients to participate in a food-based cancer prevention study. Second, it was important to assess the feasibility of administering LBR in an oral troche (dissolvable lozenge) delivery format to pre-surgical OSCC patients. Third, the study would obtain data to document self-reported adherence to a 4.3 g/day LBR regimen during a pre-operative period. Fourth, once again using self-reporting metrics, the study would measure adherence to a prescribed low phenolic diet during the LBR intervention period. Fifth, as is the intent of a Phase I design, the study sought to monitor the safety, toxicity, and adverse advents associated with LBR intervention using standard US Department of Health and Human Services criteria (US Department of Health and Human Services, 2009). Sixth, a cohort of participant samples would be used to generate a preliminary transcriptional profile of LBR-dependent gene expression changes following short-term, low-dose administration of the LBR troches.

Patients suspected of exhibiting stage I–IV OSCCs (Sobin et al., 2009) following clinical examination were approached as prospective OSU0497 participants. Patients were presented with a summary of the current Phase I study, provided informed consent, and were enrolled as participants pending histopathologic analysis of biopsied tissues. Following pathological confirmation of an appropriate oral lesion, participants were provided a detailed explanation of the study and afforded an opportunity to ask questions. Biopsied tissues included the OSCC tumor (T1), adjacent non-tumor tissue (A1), and distant (contralateral and/or >3 cm from surgical margin) high at-risk normal tissue (N1). OSU0497 participants were supplied with LBR troches, study guidelines and instructions, and a food/tobacco use diary. OSCC patients participating in the OSU0497 protocol administered three LBR troches 4× per day for a period of time, as determined by their physician's accepted standard of care practices, prior to surgical resection for cure. On the evening prior to surgery, participants ceased administration of LBR troches. During surgical resection for cure, LBR-exposed biospecimens corresponding to tumor (T2), adjacent non-tumor (A2), and distant high at-risk normal (N2) tissues were collected and stored pending subsequent analysis.

Pre-surgical Model Subject Population

Patients over the age of 18 years with newly diagnosed, biopsy-confirmed OSCC (stages I–IV) were potentially eligible for the OSU0497 Phase I trial. Enrollment criteria included that the patient must already be planned for surgical resection of their tumor, be able to take nutrition or medications orally, and present no prior history of intolerance (including hypersensitivity or allergy) to berry or berry-containing products. Although there are no known or expected adverse effects of LBR upon the unborn fetus, women of child-bearing potential must have a negative serum or urine pregnancy test prior to enrollment. Exclusion criteria included a history of intolerance to berry or berry-containing products, pregnancy, and inability to grant informed consent. Participants were excluded from the use of COX-1 or COX-2 inhibitors, high dose multivitamins, herbal supplements, and/or medications/supplements intimate to their clinical condition that could be discontinued, or strict vegetarian (vegan) dietary practices, since these compounds and behaviors could similarly target the mechanisms postulated for LBR exposure. Finally, OSU0497 participants must not have received chemotherapy or radiation adjuvant therapy prior to their surgery or be planned for such adjuvant therapies. Participants in the OSU0497 study were also categorized according to geographical catchment area as either representing an Appalachian or non-Appalachian demographic population segment. The Appalachian community represents an underserved health care population and is characterized by an elevated incidence of lung and bronchial cancers whose risk factors overlap with those for oral cancer. The incidence and mortality of OSCC among males and females in rural Appalachian regions are higher than those found in non-Appalachian regions of the same states (Casto et al., 2009). These trends are postulated to be associated with Appalachian lifestyle factors, including alcohol consumption, tobacco use, dietary and nutritional deficiencies, and a reflection of Appalachian region as a medically underserved region. Access and availability to proper oral health care may be an important factor contributing to a delayed recognition of untreated premalignant oral lesions in the Appalachian population (Casto et al., 2009).

Pre-surgical Model Selection of Dose and Delivery Method

Selection of an appropriate LBR dose was based on an equivocal quantity extrapolated (based upon accessible oral cavity surface area) from pre-clinical animal studies that demonstrated a significant reduction (44%) in the number of oral cavity tumors (Casto et al., 2002). The equivalent dose of orally administered LBR for humans was estimated at 4.3 g per day. In order to prolong the duration of oral mucosa contact and potential bioactive component delivery, troches were compounded for delayed dissolution using industry standard methods. Each square troche was 25 × 25 mm and contained 358 mg LBR plus inert ingredients and binders, including starch, hydroxypropyl methylcellulose, microcrystalline cellulose, magnesium stearate, polyethylene glycol, and carnauba wax. Three LBR troches were self-administered *q.i.d.* for an accumulated daily dose of 4.3 g. The daily LBR dosage exposures in OSU0497 are far less than the amounts of LBR previously administered to either healthy participants (45 g/day) (Stoner et al., 2005) or Barrett's esophagus patients (32–45 g/day) without toxicity (Kresty et al., 2006). In the short-term exposure, low dose LBR trial (OSU0497), each troche contributed approximately 1.5 whole black raspberries weight for weight (w/w) equivalents, or a cumulative daily dosing equivalent of 15 whole black raspberries. In the case of oral cavity exposure, the effective LBR dose was based on comparative surface area rather than total body weight and focused on a targeted locoregional delivery instead of systemic dissemination.

Pre-surgical Model Source and Storage of Black Raspberries

In order to effectively study LBR-dependent gene expression profiles in human oral cavity tissues, it is crucial to ensure that the food-based parental agent used is as standardized as possible. A single source of whole black raspberries (Jewel variety) were mechanically harvested as a single lot, washed, and immediately frozen at −20°C on a single day. The micronutrient and phytochemical content of the parental crop harvested in different years is markedly reproducible (Stoner, 2009). The frozen whole black raspberries are lyophilized in a commercial grade VirTis

Sublimator Freeze Dryer (SP Industries, Inc; Warminster, PA). The freeze-dried black raspberries are subsequently ground into a powder and stored at −20°C. Since black raspberries contain approximately 90% water, the lyophilized product is about 1:10 w/w equivalent of wet black raspberries (i.e., 4.3 g of LBR ≅ 43 g of whole black raspberries).

Pre-surgical Model Clinical Protocols

All oral cavity tissue specimens were acquired following appropriate patient informed consent using accepted standard of care practices and an institutional review board (IRB) approved protocol (Federal regulations 45 CFR 46.103, 46.107, 46.109, 46.113). Biospecimens representative of post-exposure LBR tumor (T2), non-tumor adjacent tissue (A2), and high at-risk distant normal tissue (N2) were obtained, and correspond to patient-matched tissues (T1, A1, N1) obtained at the time of participant enrollment. Following biopsy, tissues were immediately prepared for histopathology and immunohistochemistry (10% neutral buffered formalin fixation), nucleic acid enrichment (Ambion RNAlater and liquid nitrogen stabilization), protein isolation (liquid nitrogen), and anthocyanin/ellagic acid content (5% formic acidification and liquid nitrogen storage).

Pre-surgical Model Evaluation of Black Raspberry Components in Oral Cavity Tissues

Representative malignant oral tissues were evaluated for the presence of known LBR components [cyanidin 3-*O*-glucoside, cyanidin 3-*O*-sambubioside, cyanidin 3-*O*-(2^G-xylosylrutinoside) and cyanidin 3-*O*-rutinoside] by high performance liquid chromatography electrospray ionization mass spectrometry and tandem mass spectroscopy (HPLC ESI/MS/MS). Both cyanidin 3-*O*-(2^G-xylosylrutinoside) and cyanidin 3-*O*-rutinoside were readily detected in the oral tissue at the time of surgical resection, more than 8 h after the last LBR troche exposure. Whether these cyanidin glycosides represent accumulated LBR component deposition or reflect only the most acute LBR exposure remains under active investigation.

Pre-surgical Model Assessment of Oral Carcinogenesis-Associated Biomarkers

Preliminary evaluation of an interim cohort of OSU0497 participants supports the hypothesis that transcriptional biomarkers of cellular growth, cell-cell communication, inflammation, and apoptosis are significant LBR-exposure-dependent indicators of favorable chemopreventive outcomes (Whitmore et al., 2008, unpublished). Affymetrix HG-U133 Plus 2.0 GeneChip Arrays were used to assess an interim cohort (n=10 participants) of OSU0497 patient-matched tissues (n=40) and dChip Software was used to convert Affymetrix CEL files for subsequent analyses. Custom computer routines were developed to normalize the data, estimate differential expression, and provide statistical testing measures. The log-ratio

Y of perfect match (PM) to mismatch (MM) was used for initial probe expression as follows: Y=ln(PM/MM). Since PM/MM may vary systematically in the absence of true expression, Y was centered (averaged) for each array to zero, and designated Y_C. The median M of the centered Y_C pair-wise readings for each probe set on an array was used as a summary measure of expression. The median, not mean, was used to guard against undue outlier influences. This normalization step proposes that probe-pair effects within each probe set is random, and therefore, well represented by a central statistic such as the median (Whitmore et al., 2008, unpublished). Significantly modulated LBR-responsive genes were analyzed using DAVID and interrogated against current knowledge databases to generate a subset of putative LBR-dependent expression biomarkers (n=90) which was consistent with a favorable oral carcinogenesis inhibiting activity. These 90 transcriptional biomarkers and an additional six normalizing, or "housekeeping", genes were arrayed onto custom microfluidic cards (4×96, 384-well format) and analyzed by qRT-PCR such that patient-matched tissues (N1, N2, T1, T2) were concurrently processed. Further analysis of the microfluidic card derived qPCR data generated a novel concise set ($n \cong 15$) of LBR-responsive gene expression biomarkers with which to analyze the complete OSU0497 patient tissue sets. This novel gene expression profile set is characterized by inclusion in KEGG categories (Kanehisa et al., 2010) encompassing the p53 signaling pathway, apoptosis, cell cycle, cell growth and death, replication and repair, MAPK signaling pathway, and arachidonic acid metabolism (Knobloch et al., 2010, unpublished). The utility of these LBR-dependent transcriptional changes as diagnostic or prognostic biomarkers remains to be systematically described using the complete OSU0497 clinical study dataset.

1.7.2 Phase I/II Clinical Trial: Post-surgical Model

Interim analysis of OSU0497 demonstrated that short-term clinical LBR exposure to pre-surgical OSCC patients resulted in the modulation of transcriptional profiles in both cancer cells and high at-risk "normal" oral tissues (Knobloch et al., 2010, unpublished). Furthermore, the LBR-dependent changes were in a direction that would favor inhibition or reversal of neoplastic progression. The hypothesis of the ongoing Phase I OSU06132 and OSU07085 clinical trials is that long-term daily exposure of LBR to post-surgical OSCC patients will modulate the expression of genes critical to oral oncogenesis in high at-risk tissues. These transcriptional profiles may provide diagnostic or prognostic biomarker panels for estimating the role of LBR-dependent oral cancer prevention.

An LBR Long-Term Exposure Post-surgical Clinical Model Assessing OSCC Recurrence in an Underserved Population

The Appalachian region includes 420 counties, 13 states and nearly 25 million people along more than 1,000 miles from southern New York to northeastern

Mississippi (Appalachian Regional Commission, 2010). May people living within the Appalachian region are characterized as representing an underserved population with marked health disparities. As mentioned previously, the incidence and mortality of OSCC among rural Appalachians are higher than present in non-Appalachian states and elevated relative to those found in non-Appalachian regions of the same states (Casto et al., 2009). Furthermore, overall poor nutrition and deficient oral health care are often associated with the primary risk factors of alcohol and tobacco use. It has been estimated that 50–60% of patients who present with primary oral tumors will subsequently develop local-regional recurrences, 20% of which will occur within the first 18 months following surgical resection for cure. The OSU06132 protocol was developed to address the hypothesis that long-term exposure to LBR in Appalachian OSCC patients would result in a decreased incidence of recurrent and/or second primary oral tumors.

An LBR Long-term Exposure Post-surgical Randomized Clinical Model Assessing Persistent Expression of Oral Carcinogenesis Biomarkers

The randomized Phase IB/IIA post-surgical OSU07085 model enrolls participants following surgical resection for cure of stage I or II HNSCCs. Daily cumulative LBR doses (0, 4, 8 g) in two delivery systems (troche and saliva substitute) are given for 6 months after post-surgical recovery. Oral epithelial brush biopsies (OralCDx), whole blood, urine, and saliva are collected at selected time points and evaluated for outcomes of adherence/exposure, safety/toxicity, and capacity to modulate specific gene expressions profiles associated with carcinogenic progression. The active OSU07085 clinical trial will address several specific aims. First, the study determines the ability of post-surgical HNSCC patients to adhere to the chemoprevention trial design and defines the tolerability and potential adverse events of long-term LBR administration. Second, the investigation defines the association between LBR exposure, dose and delivery vehicle, and the up-take of LBR components into oral tissues. Third, the ability of LBR to regulate gene expression in high at-risk oral tissues in post-surgical HNSCC patients is examined. Fourth, the trial analyzes the persistence of gene expression changes following cessation of long-term LBR exposure.

Post-surgical Model Subject Population

Study participants in the OSU07085 Phase IB/IIA post-surgical clinical trial were previously diagnosed with stage I or stage II HNSCC and experienced surgical resection for cure without further adjuvant therapy. Enrollees were randomized into six treatment groups by daily LBR dose (0, 4, or 8 g) and delivery system (troche or methylcellulose-based saliva substitute) and monitored for a period of 6 months. Oral cavity brush biopsies, saliva, blood, and urine were collected at selected time points and evaluated for outcomes relative to compliance/exposure, safety/toxicity, and biomarker assessment. Furthermore, a cohort of former OSCC survivors will be followed for 2 years post-LBR intervention to evaluate the persistence of gene modulation and potential cancer risk reduction efficacy.

Post-surgical Model Selection of Dose and Delivery Methods

Two LBR delivery modalities (troche or saliva substitute) and three daily cumulative doses (0, 4, or 8 g) were implemented in the OSU07085 randomized, placebo-controlled study. The placebo control dose (0 g, 4× per day), low dose (1 g, 4× per day), and high dose (2 g, 4× per day) delivery systems will be assessed with respect to participant adherence to the study design, as well as relative to tissue concentrations of LBR components, histopathology, and biomarker/molecular outcomes.

Post-surgical Model Clinical Protocols

All oral cavity tissue specimens were acquired following appropriate patient informed consent in accordance with National Cancer Institute guidelines (http://www.cancer.gov/clinicaltrials) and the recommendations of the Internal Review Board at The Ohio State University. The OSU07085 study aims to determine the adherence of post-surgical HNSCC patients to the clinical trial design expectations, define long-term LBR tolerability, and report possible LBR-associated adverse effects in this patient cohort. OSU07085 will document participant compliance with long-term, self-administration of LBR troches or saliva substitute, as well as patient ability to successfully attend a series of pre-scheduled standard of care medical appointments. Adherence to the long-term LBR administration schedule will be assessed by maintenance of a daily Food Consumption Diary, participant interviews, and LBR component analysis in biospecimens. Concurrently, the frequency and severity of adverse events according to the US Department of Health and Human Services "Common Toxicity Criteria for Adverse Events" (2009) will be described as necessary, as will any additional specific issues related to dental and oral health. Oral tissue biospecimens representative of high at-risk normal tissue will be obtained at the time of participant enrollment (baseline) and subsequently, at every standard of care scheduled follow-up appointment interval of 6–8 weeks. Additionally, saliva, blood, and urine samples will be collected at these time points. Following long-term (6 months) exposure to the OSU06132 agents, serialized oral brush biopsies will be obtained at the time of last trial agent administration and weekly thereafter for 4 weeks in order to assess the short-term persistence of transcriptional regulation following cessation of the OSU07085 agent. Additionally, oral brush biopsies will be obtained at 6, 12, 18, and 24 months following cessation of LBR administration to evaluate long-term persistence, or lack thereof, of LBR-associated gene expression changes.

Post-surgical Model Evaluation of Black Raspberry Components in Oral Cavity Tissues

Biochemical indicators of LBR exposure, including cyanidin glycosides, will be assessed in oral brush biopsy specimens using HPLC ESI/MS (see "Pre-surgical Model Evaluation of Black Raspberry Components in Oral Cavity Tissues" for details).

Post-surgical Model Assessment of Oral Cancer-Associated Biomarkers

The OSU07085 study will assess the ability of LBR to modulate transcriptional profiles that would favor the inhibition, delay, or reversal of oral carcinogenesis in the high at-risk normal oral tissues of post-surgical HNSCC patients. These studies will evaluate LBR-dependent transcriptional biomarkers first characterized in high at-risk normal tissues derived from OSCC patients following short-term LBR exposure (see Pre-surgical Model, Knobloch et al., 2010). Oral brush biopsy tissues will be evaluated by qRT-PCR for differential gene expression changes as a function of LBR dose and delivery modality, and further interrogated for possible associations with clinical covariates. Furthermore, the persistence of LBR-dependent transcriptional changes following cessation of long-term LBR exposure will be evaluated, as will preliminary rates of OSCC recurrence and/or second primary oral cancer in a participant cohort over a 2 year interval. Moreover, oral brush biopsies will be collected from any suspect recurrent/second primary lesions and evaluated for both transcriptional biomarkers of LBR-exposure and the gene expression pattern of established OSCC-associated genes.

1.8 Black Raspberries, Cancer Prevention, and Future Directions

In 1773, the aphorisms of American inventor and statesman, Benjamin Franklin, were collected into Poor Richard's Almanack. Perhaps no greater quote attributed to Franklin is that "an ounce of prevention is worth a pound of cure," and this philosophy remains at the core of cancer risk reduction and prevention strategies today. The transition from preclinical animal and in vitro models forms the foundation of translational clinical science and practice. Characterization of bioactive food components and their possible pharmacologic derivatives must continually proceed through in vitro systems, in vivo models, and in situ applications. The basic science and translational studies described in this Chapter provide an essential foundation for the design parameters of a future Phase III randomized clinical trial. However, since the quintessential food-based cancer prevention strategies require life-style changes, there remain significant roadblocks as investigators move forward in the field. It is through multidisciplinary cooperation, sustained basic science funding, interactive partnerships with clinical trial participants, and strategic policy changes that food-based cancer prevention will become a realistic outcome.

References

Adelstein DJ, Ridge JA, Gillison ML, Chaturvedi AK, D'Souza G, Gravitt PE, Westra W, Psyrri A, Kast WM, Koutsky LA, Giuliano A, Krosnick S, Trotti A, Schuller DE, Forastiere A, Ullmann CD (2009). Head and neck squamous cell cancer and the human papillomavirus: summary of a National Cancer Institute State of the Science Meeting, November 9–10, 2008, Washington, DC. Head Neck 31:1391–1422

American Cancer Society. Cancer Facts & Figures 2009. Atlanta: American Cancer Society; 2009

Appalachian Regional Commission (2010) http://www.arc.gov/

Berridge MV, Tan AS, McCoy KD, Wang R (1996) The Biochemical and cellular basis of cell proliferation assays that use tetrazolium salts. Biochemica 4:14–19

Braakhuis BJM, Tabor MP, Kummer JA, Leemans CR, Brakenhoff RH (2003) A genetic explanation of Slaughter's concept of field cancerization: evidence and clinical implication. Cancer Res 63:1727–1730

Califano J, van der Riet P, Westra W, Nawroz H, Clayman G, Piantadosi S, Corio R, Lee D, Greenberg B, Koch W, Sidransky D (1996) Genetic progression model for head and neck cancer: implications for field cancerization. Cancer Res 56:2488–2492

Casto BC, Kresty LA, Kraly CL, Pearl DK, Knobloch TJ, Schut HA, Stoner GD, Mallery SR, Weghorst CM (2002) Chemoprevention of oral cancer by black raspberries. Anticancer Res 22:4005–4015

Casto BC, Sharma S, Fisher JL, Knobloch TJ, Agrawal A, Weghorst CM (2009) Oral cancer in Appalachia. J Health Care Poor Underserved 20:274–285

Choi S, Myers JN (2008) Molecular pathogenesis of oral squamous cell carcinoma: implications for therapy. J Dent Res 87:14–32 Review

Cooper JS, Pajak TF, Rubin P, Tupchong L, Brady L, Leibel SA, Laramore GE, Marcial VA, Cox JD (1989) Second malignancies in patients who have head and neck cancer: incidence, effect on survival and implications based on the ROTG experience. Int J Radiat Oncol Biol Phys 17:449–456

Decker J, Goldstein JC (1982) Risk factors in head and neck cancer. N Engl J Med 306:1151–1155

Dennis G Jr, Sherman BT, Hosack DA, Yang J, Gao W, Lane HC, Lempicki RA (2003) DAVID: Database for Annotation, Visualization, and Integrated Discovery. Genome Biol 4:P3

D'Ambrosio SM, Gibson-D'Ambrosio RE, Milo GE, Casto BC, Kelloff GJ, Steele VE (2000) Differential response of normal premalignant and malignant human oral epithelial cells to growth inhibition by chemopreventive agents. Anticancer Res 20:2273–2280

D'Ambrosio SM, Gibson-D'Ambrosio RE, Wani G, Casto BC, Milo GE, Kelloff GJ, Steele VE (2001) Modulation of Ki67, p53, RARβ expression in normal, premalignant, and malignant human oral epithelial cells by chemopreventive agents. Anticancer Res 21:3229–3235

Forastiere A, Koch W, Trotti A, Sidransky D (2001) Head and neck cancer. N Engl J Med 345:1890–1900

Garzino-Demo P, Dell'Acqua A, Dalmasso P, Fasolis M, La Terra Maggiore GM, Ramieri G, Berrone S, Rampino M, Schena M (2006) Clinico-pathological parameters and outcome of 245 patients operated for oral squamous cell carcinoma. J Craniomaxillofac Surg 34:344–350

Gillison ML, Koch WM, Capone RB, Spafford M, Westra WH, Wu L, Zahurak ML, Daniel RW, Viglione M, Symer DE, Shah KV, Sidransky D (2000) Evidence for a causal association between human papillomavirus and a subset of head and neck cancers. J Natl Cancer Inst 92:709–720

Gillison ML, Shah KV (2001) Human papillomavirus-associated head and neck squamous cell carcinoma: mounting evidence for an etiologic role for human papillomavirus in a subset of head and neck cancers. Curr Opin Oncol 13:183–188

Glade MJ (1999) Food, nutrition, and thc prevention of cancer: a global perspective. American Institute for Cancer Research/World Cancer Research Fund, American Institute for Cancer Research, 1997. Nutrition 15:523–526

Han C, Ding H, Casto B, Stoner GD, D'Ambrosio SM (2005) Inhibition of the growth of premalignant and malignant human oral cell lines by extracts and components of black raspberries. Nutr Cancer 51:207–217

He J, Wallace TC, Keatley KE, Failla ML, Giusti MM (2009) Stability of black raspberry anthocyanins in the digestive tract lumen and transport efficiency into gastric and small intestinal tissues in the rat. J Agric Food Chem 57:3141–3148

Hong WK, Spitz MR, Lippman SM (2000) Cancer chemoprevention in the 21st century: genetics, risk modeling, and molecular targets. J Clin Oncol 18(21 Suppl):9S–18S

Huang DW, Sherman BT, Lempicki RA (2009) Systematic and integrative analysis of large gene lists using DAVID Bioinformatics Resources. Nature Protoc 4:44–57

IARC Working Group on the Evaluation of Carcinogenic Risks to Humans (2004) IARC monographs on the evaluation of carcinogenic risks to humans, tobacco smoke and involuntary smoking, vol 83. IARC Press, Lyon, France

IARC working group on the evaluation of carcinogenic risks to humans (2007) IARC Monographs on the evaluation of carcinogenic risks to humans, human papillomaviruses, vol 90. IARC Press, Lyon

Jemal A, Tiwari RC, Murray T, Ghafoor A, Samuels A, Ward E, Feuer EJ, Thun MJ (2004) Cancer statistics, 2004. CA Cancer J Clin 54:8–29

Kanehisa M, Goto S, Furumichi M, Tanabe M, Hirakawa M (2010) KEGG for representation and analysis of molecular networks involving diseases and drugs. Nucleic Acids Res 38(Database issue):D355–D360

Kelloff GJ, Sigman CC, Greenwald P (1999) Cancer chemoprevention: progress and promise. Eur. J. Cancer 35:2031–2038

Knobloch TJ, Casto BC, Stoner GD, Weghorst CM (2003). Black raspberry extract-responsive genes in oral cancer cells (in vitro), unpublished

Knobloch TJ, Pearl DK, Huang K, Weghorst CM (2008). Analysis of lyophilized black raspberry extract-responsive genes in oral cancer, unpublished

Knobloch TJ, Pearl DK, Uhrig LK, Sardo CL, Warner BM, Ferguson JM, Agrawal A, Shuller DE, Clinton SK, Weghorst CM (2010). Interim analysis of black raspberry-responsive genes in oral cancer patients following short-term clinical exposures, unpublished

Kreimer AR, Clifford GM, Boyle P, Franceschi S (2005) Human papillomavirus types in head and neck squamous cell carcinomas worldwide: a systematic review. Cancer Epidemiol Biomarkers Prev 14:467–475

Kresty LA, Frankel WL, Hammond CD, Baird ME, Mele JM, Stoner GD, Fromkes JJ (2006) Transitioning from preclinical to clinical chemopreventive assessments of lyophilized black raspberries: interim results show berries modulate markers of oxidative stress in Barrett's esophagus patients. Nutr Cancer 54:148–156

Kresty LA, Morse MA, Morgan C, Carlton PS, Lu J, Gupta A, Blackwood M, Stoner GD (2001) Chemoprevention of esophageal tumorigenesis by dietary administration of lyophilized black raspberries. Cancer Res 61:6112–6119

Lang JC, Tobin EJ, Knobloch TJ, Schuller DE, Bartynski KJ, Mountain RE, Nicholson R, DeYoung BR, Weghorst CM (1998) Frequent mutation of p16 in squamous cell carcinoma of the head and neck. Laryngoscope 108:923–928

Lee H, Li D, Prior T, Casto B, Weghorst CM, Shuler CF, Milo GE (1997) Ineffectiveness of the presence of H-ras/p53 combination mutations in squamous cell carcinoma cells to induce the conversion of a nontumorigenic to a tumorigenic tumor type. Cell Biol Toxicol 13:419–434

Leon X, Quer M, Diez S, Orus C, Lopez-Pousa A, Burgues J (1999) Second neoplasm in patients with head and neck cancer. Head Neck 21:204–210

Li C, Wong WH (2001) Model-based analysis of oligonucleotide arrays: expression index computation and outlier detection. Proc Natl Acad Sci USA 98:31–36

Liang C, McClean MD, Marsit C, Christensen B, Peters E, Nelson HH, Kelsey KT (2009) A population-based case-control study of marijuana use and head and neck squamous cell carcinoma. Cancer Prev Res 2:759–768

Lippman SM, Sudbø J, Hong WK (2005) Oral cancer prevention and the evolution of molecular-targeted drug development. J Clin Oncol 23:346–356
Mao L, Hong WK, Papadimitrakopoulou VA (2004) Focus on head and neck cancer. Cancer Cell 5:311–316
Mashberg A, Boffetta P, Winkelman R, Garfinkel L (1993) Tobacco smoking, alcohol drinking and cancer of the oral cavity and oropharynx among US veterans. Cancer 72:1369–1375
Moyer RA, Hummer KE, Finn CE, Frei B, Wrolstad RE (2002) Anthocyanins, phenolics, and antioxidant capacity in diverse small fruits: *vaccinium*, *rubus*, and *ribes*. J Agric Food Chem 50:519–525
Orr IM (1933) Oral cancer in betel nut chewers in Travancore, its aetiology, pathology, and treatment. Lancet II:575–580
Papadimitrakopoulou V, Izzo J, Lippman SM, Lee JS, Fan YH, Clayman G, Ro JY, Hittelman WN, Lotan R, Hong WK, Mao L (1997) Frequent inactivation of p16INK4a in oral premalignant lesions. Oncogene 14:1799–1803
Parkin DM et al (eds) (2002) Cancer incidence in five continents, vol 8. IARC Scientific Publications No. 155, IARC, Lyon
Parkin DM, Bray F, Ferlay J, Pisani P (2005) Global cancer statistics, 2002. CA Cancer J Clin 55:74–108
Parmigiani G et al (eds) (2003) DNA-Chip Analyzer (dChip). In: The analysis of gene expression data: methods and software. Springer, New York, NY, pp 120–141
Pavia M, Pileggi C, Nobile CG, Angelillo IF (2006) Association between fruit and vegetable consumption and oral cancer: a meta-analysis of observational studies. Am J Clin Nutr 83:1126–1134
Reed AL, Califano J, Cairns P, Westra WH, Jones RM, Koch W, Ahrendt S, Eby Y, Sewell D, Nawroz H, Bartek J, Sidransky D (1996) High frequency of p16 (CDKN2/MTS-1/INK4A) inactivation in head and neck squamous cell carcinoma. Cancer Res 56:3630–3633
Reibel J (2003) Update on the evidence, with recommendations. Med Princ Pract 1(suppl 12): 22–32
Sasaki T, Moles DR, Imai Y, Speight PM (2005) Clinico-pathological features of squamous cell carcinoma of the oral cavity in patients <40 years of age. J Oral Pathol Med 34:129–133
Schwartz LH, Ozsahin M, Zhang GN, Touboul E, De Vataire F, Andolenko P, Lacau-Saint-Guily J, Laugier A, Schlienger M (1994) Synchronous and metachronous head and neck carcinomas. Cancer 74:1933–1938
Slaughter DP (1944) Multiplicity of origin of malignant tumors; collective review. Internat Abstr Surg 79:89–98
Slaughter DP (1946) Multicentric origin of intraoral carcinoma. Surgery 20:133–146
Slaughter DP, Southwick HW, Smejkal W (1953) "Field cancerization" in oral stratified squamous epithelium: clinical implications of multicentric origin. Cancer 6:963–968
Sobin LH, Gospodarowicz MK, Wittekind C (eds) (2009) TNM classification of malignant tumours, 7th edn. Wiley, Hoboken, NJ
Sporn MB (1976) Approaches to prevention of epithelial cancer during the preneoplastic period. Cancer Res 36:2699–2702
Sporn MB, Dunlop NM, Newton DL, Smith JM (1976) Prevention of chemical carcinogenesis by vitamin A and its synthetic analogs (retinoids). Fed Proc 35:1332–1338
Stocks P (1933). Cancer incidence in North Wales and Liverpool region in relation to habits and environment. British Empire Cancer Campaign 35th Annual Report (Suppl. to Part 2):1–127
Stoner GD (2009) Foodstuffs for preventing cancer: the preclinical and clinical development of berries. Cancer Prev Res 2:187–194
Stoner GD, Morse MA, Kelloff GJ (1997) Perspectives in cancer chemoprevention. Environ Health Perspect 105(Suppl 4):945–954
Stoner GD, Sardo C, Apseloff G, Mullet D, Wargo W, Pound V, Singh A, Sanders J, Aziz R, Casto B, Sun X (2005) Pharmacokinetics of anthocyanins and ellagic acid in healthy volunteers fed freeze-dried black raspberries daily for 7 days. J Clin Pharmacol 45:1153–1164

Tian Q, Giusti MM, Stoner GD, Schwartz SJ (2006) Urinary excretion of black raspberry (*Rubus occidentalis*) anthocyanins and their metabolites. J Agric Food Chem 54:1467–1472
U.S. Department of Health and Human Services (Nov 2000) Healthy people 2010: understanding and improving health, 2nd edn. US Government Printing Office, Washington, DC
U.S. Department of Health and Human Services. Common Terminology Criteria for Adverse Events (CTCAE): Version 4.02. [http://evs.nci.nih.gov/ftp1/CTCAE/CTCAE_4.02_2009-09-15_QuickReferenc e_8.5x11.pdf]
Vokes EE, Weichselbaum RR, Lippman SM, Hong WK (1993) Head and neck cancer. N Engl J Med 328:184–194
Wang SY, Lin HS (2000) Antioxidant activity in fruits and leaves of blackberry, raspberry, and strawberry varies with cultivar and developmental stage. J Agric Food Chem 48:140–146
Weghorst CM, Clinton SK, Agrawal A (2004). Chemopreventive agent-responsive genes in oral cancer, The Ohio State University, Internal Review Board Protocol OSU0497
Weghorst CM, Clinton SK, Agrawal A (2006). Chemoprevention of oral cancer in Appalachia, The Ohio State University, Internal Review Board Protocol OSU06132
Weghorst CM, Clinton SK, Agrawal A (2008). Food-based modulation of biomarkers in human tissues at high-risk for oral cancer, The Ohio State University, Internal Review Board Protocol OSU07085
Whitmore GA, Lee MLT, Knobloch TJ, Weghorst CM (2008). Interim analysis of oral cancer patients following short-term exposure to lyophilized black raspberries: affymetrix genechip expression profiling, unpublished
Wilson WR (1908) The natural history of cancer, with special reference to its causation and prevention. William Wood and Company, New York, NY
Wiseman M (2008) The second World Cancer Research Fund/American Institute for Cancer Research expert report. Food, nutrition, physical activity, and the prevention of cancer: a global perspective. Proc Nutr Soc 67:253–256
Wynder EL, Stellman SD (1977) Comparative epidemiology of tobacco-related cancers. Cancer Res 37:4608–4622
Xue H, Aziz RM, Sun N, Cassady JM, Kamendulis LM, Xu Y, Stoner GD, Klaunig JE (2001) Inhibition of cellular transformation by berry extracts. Carcinogenesis 22:351–356
Yeudall WA, Crawford RY, Ensley JF, Robbins KC (1994) MTS1/CDK4I is altered in cell lines derived from primary and metastatic oral squamous cell carcinoma. Carcinogenesis 15: 2683–2686
Zhang ZF, Morgenstern H, Spitz MR, Tashkin DP, Yu GP, Marshall JR, Hsu TC, Schantz SP (1999) Marijuana use and increased risk of squamous cell carcinoma of the head and neck. Cancer Epidemiol Biomarkers Prev 8:1071–1078

Chapter 15
Effects of Black Raspberries on Cellular and Epigenetic Biomarkers of Colon Cancer Development in Humans

Gary D. Stoner, Li-Shu Wang, Christine Sardo, Mark Arnold, Edward Martin, Wendy Frankel, and Dennis Pearl

Abstract Colorectal cancer (CRC) is the leading digestive tract cancer in the Western world, particularly in the United States where it accounts for approximately 10% of all cancer deaths. The multistage development of CRC is associated with chromosomal instability, DNA-repair defects, aberrant DNA methylation, and mutational events in oncogenes and tumor suppressor genes. Preclinical studies using cultured human colon tumor cells and animal models of colorectal cancer indicate that black raspberries (BRBs) and their constituent anthocyanins and ellagitannins elicit chemopreventive effects against CRC. A 7-day Phase I trial indicated that BRBs are well tolerated by humans and their component anthocyanins and ellagic acid are absorbed into blood. The results of a Phase Ib trial in which BRBs were administered daily to colorectal cancer patients from the time of diagnosis of the disease until surgical removal of the tumor (average = 3 weeks) are presented in this chapter. BRB treatment resulted in reduced proliferation and increased apoptosis of CRC cells. In addition, tumor angiogenesis was inhibited by berries. BRB treatment reduced ß-catenin expression and enhanced E-cadherin expression in CRC indicating a protective effect on the Wnt signaling pathway. DNA methylation assays showed that BRBs are capable of demethylating tumor suppressor genes associated with the Wnt pathway, in part, through inhibiting the expression of DNMT1, a DNA methyltransferase that is commonly overexpressed in CRC. These data suggest that BRBs should be further examined for chemopreventive effects against CRC.

Keywords Chemoprevention · Human · Colon · Cancer · Black raspberries · DNA methylation · Proliferation · Apoptosis · Angiogenesis

G.D. Stoner (✉)
Department of Medicine, Medical College of Wisconsin, Milwaukee, WI 53226, USA
e-mail: gstoner@mcw.edu

G.D. Stoner, N.P. Seeram (eds.), *Berries and Cancer Prevention*,
DOI 10.1007/978-1-4419-7554-6_15, © Springer Science+Business Media, LLC 2011

1 Introduction

1.1 Colon Cancer

Colorectal cancer (CRC) is the leading digestive tract cancer in the Western world, particularly in the United States where it accounts for approximately 10% of all cancer deaths (Jemal et al., 2009). Every year in the US, about 160,000 cases of CRC are diagnosed, and 57,000 patients die from the disease. The 5-year survival from CRC is 64% and declines to 57% at 10 years after diagnosis. However, for persons with distant metastases at the time of diagnosis, the 5-year survival is only 10%. CRC is a multi-stage disease, beginning as a benign adenomatous polyp, which develops into an advanced adenoma with high-grade dysplasia and then progresses to an invasive adenocarcinoma (Kinzler and Vogelstein, 2002). Between 24 and 47% of asymptomatic average-risk individuals over 50 years of age are estimated to have adenomatous polyps (Anderson et al., 2002). Thus, the prevention of colon cancer by routine colonoscopy to remove adenomatous polyps is an important strategy to reduce mortality from the disease. Chemoprevention is another approach for the prevention of CRC, and the present chapter is devoted to a discussion of the potential use of berries for this purpose.

Epidemiological studies have identified multiple risk factors for colon cancer. The disease is associated with a number of inherited cancer predisposition syndromes, including hereditary non-polyposis colon cancer [HNPCC] and familial adenomatous polyposis [FAP], as well as a family history of colorectal cancer and inflammatory bowel disease (Rowley, 2005). Other risk factors include physical inactivity, obesity, smoking, alcohol consumption, diets high in fat and red meats, and inadequate intake of dietary fiber, fruits and vegetables (Martinez, 2005). The higher occurrence of the disease amongst populations in the Western world has been attributed to a higher intake of high-fat, high-meat diets along with an inadequate consumption of vegetables and fruit (Norat et al., 2005). To prevent or reduce risk of CRC, therefore, international and national organizations promote dietary recommendations that emphasize a plant-based diet of fruits, vegetables, and whole grains, and dairy and meat products low in saturated and trans fatty acids, in addition to regular physical activity and avoidance of excess alcohol and weight gain (WHO, 2003).

The role of chemical carcinogens in the induction of CRC in humans has not been fully elucidated. However, certain food-borne carcinogens such as benzo(a)pyrene (BaP), a polycyclic aromatic hydrocarbon, and 2-amino-1-methyl-6-phenylimidazol[4,5-*b*]pyridine (PhIP), an aromatic amine, which are produced during the process of smoking and barbequing meats, are linked with the development of colon cancer (Sinha et al., 2005; Nakagama et al., 2002). The production of these carcinogens increases markedly with the extent of pyrolysis of the meat, so blackened meats tend to contain the highest amounts. Other carcinogens with the potential ability to induce colon cancer in animals and humans include certain nitrosamines, nitrosoureas, and nitrosoguanidines (Kuhnle and Bingham, 2007).

Some of these agents have been isolated from stomach contents and feces and they likely play a role in the development of CRC in humans. Polycyclic hydrocarbons and nitrosamines are also prominent carcinogens in tobacco smoke and they may be responsible for the higher occurrence of colon cancer amongst tobacco smokers (Chao et al., 2000).

2 Molecular Basis of Colon Cancer

As indicated above, the development of CRC is a multi-stage process. Vogelstein et al. (1988) first described the time-dependent accumulation of genetic mutations in colonic epithelium as it progresses from normal epithelium > dysplastic aberrant crypt foci (ACF) > early adenoma > late adenoma > cancer > metastatic cancer. These genetic mutations are caused by genomic instability which takes several forms in CRC including chromosomal instability, DNA-repair defects, and aberrant DNA methylation. Markowitz and Bertagnolli (Markowitz and Bertagnolli, 2009) have recently summarized the roles of these different forms of genomic instability in the causation of both sporadic and heritable colon cancers and these will be discussed briefly here.

2.1 Chromosomal Instability

This is the most common type of genomic instability in CRC, and it leads to changes in chromosomal copy number and structure. Chromosomal instability leads to a loss of wild-type copies of tumor suppressor genes such as *P53*, *adenomatous polyposis coli (APC),* deleted in colon cancer (*DCC*) and SMAD family member 4 (*SMAD4*), whose normal functions are to suppress the malignant phenotype. In CRC, there are numerous rare inactivating mutations in genes whose normal function is to maintain chromosome stability, and these mutations are responsible for a significant portion of the chromosomal instability in these tumors.

2.2 DNA-Repair Defects

In some CRCs, the DNA mismatch repair genes are inactivated. This inactivation can be inherited, such as in HNPCC, or acquired, as in tumors with methylation-associated silencing of genes that encode DNA mismatch repair proteins. In patients with HNPCC, germ-line defects in mismatch-repair genes (mainly *MLH1* and *MSH2*) result in a lifetime risk of CRC of about 80% (Lynch et al., 2008). In addition to germ-line defects, the loss of mismatch-repair function in HNPCC patients is caused by somatic mutation of the wild type allele of mismatch repair genes.

2.3 Aberrant DNA Methylation

DNA methylation in mammalian cells is regulated by a family of highly related DNA methyltransferase enzymes (DNMT1, DNMT3a and DNMT3b) which mediate the transfer of methyl groups from S-adenosylmethionine to the 5′ position of cytosine bases in the dinucleotide sequence CpG. Studies have shown that all three DNMTs are overly expressed in several tumor types, including CRC (Robertson et al., 1999). This can lead to aberrant methylation of the CpG-rich "CpG islands" in the promoter sequences of genes, resulting in loss of their expression; i.e., gene silencing. One gene that is silenced in sporadic colorectal cancers with microsatellite instability *is MLH1* (Issa, 2004). There is another set of genes that becomes aberrantly methylated as a group, a condition called the CpG island methylator phenotype (CIMP) (Toyota et al., 1999). In this chapter, we present evidence for the ability of berries to demethylate certain tumor suppressor genes associated with the Wnt signaling pathway which is altered in a high percentage of colorectal cancers (Goss and Groden, 2000).

2.4 Mutational Activation of Oncogenes

Several oncogenes are activated by mutation in colorectal cancer (Markowitz and Bertagnolli, 2009). Mutations in the *KRAS a*nd *BRAF* genes, which activate the mitogen-activated protein kinase (MAPK) signaling pathway, occur in about 40 and 15% of colorectal cancers, respectively. *BRAF* mutations appear to occur earlier in the process of colorectal cancer development than *KRAS* mutations because they are observed more frequently in hyperplastic polyps, serrated adenomas, and proximal colon cancers. About one-third of CRCs also exhibit activating somatic mutations in the *PI3KCA* gene, which encodes the catalytic subunit of phosphatidylinositol-3-kinase (*P13K*).

2.5 Mutational Inactivation of Tumor Suppressor Genes

A signaling pathway that is of great importance in the development of colorectal cancers is the Wnt pathway (Fig. 15.1). The activation of this pathway is regarded as the initiating event in colorectal cancer (Markowitz and Bertagnolli, 2009). Wnt signaling occurs when ß-catenin protein binds to members of the T-cell factor-lymphocyte enhancer family in the nucleus to produce a transcription factor that regulates genes involved in cell activation, including c-*MYC* and cyclin D1. In normal cells, a ß-catenin degradation complex regulates the amount of ß-catenin in the cytoplasm. A component of this complex is the APC protein which degrades ß-catenin and reduces its nuclear localization. In colorectal cancer cells, the APC gene is commonly mutated leading to the absence of a functional APC protein. In the absence of a functional APC protein, cellular levels of ß-catenin increase

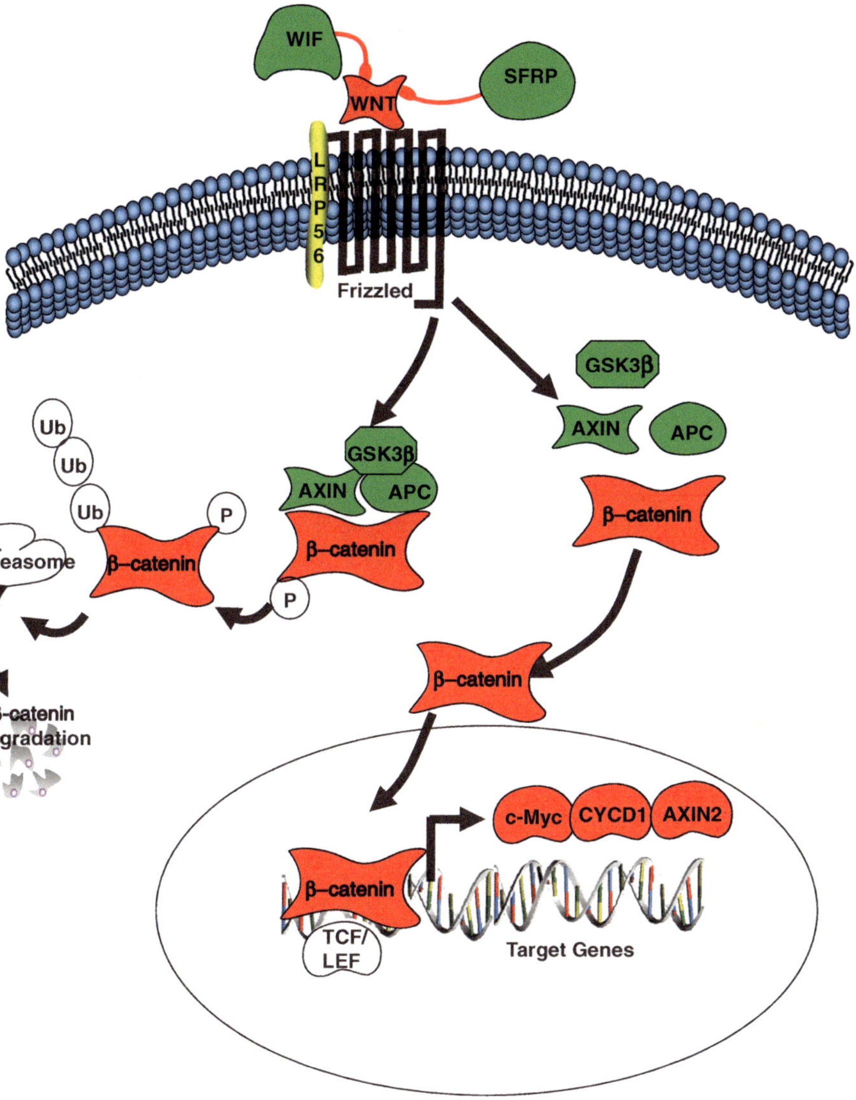

Fig. 15.1 Wnt signaling pathway. In the absence of Wnt protein binding to the Frizzled receptor, the AXIN/GSK3ß/APC protein complex is formed and this complex binds ß-catenin resulting in its phosphorylation. Phosphorylated ß-catenin is ubiquinated (Ub) and then undergoes proteosomal degradation. In this manner, normal cells regulate the level of cytoplasmin ß-catenin. When Wnt is highly activated by mutations in the APC and/or ß-catenin genes, Wnt protein binds to Frizzled and activates a cytoplasmic protein called Dishevelled. Dishevelled inhibits the activity of AXIN/GSK3ß/APC, such that the complex no longer binds to ß-catenin (*right side* of figure) leading to its accumulation in the cytoplasm. The excess ß-catenin then translocates into the nucleus and binds to members of the T-cell factor (TCF)/Lymphoid enhancing factor (LEF) family of DNA binding proteins leading to transcription of Wnt target genes such as c-Myc, cyclin D1 (CYCD1) and AXIN2. Activation of these genes leads to enhanced cell proliferation

and Wnt signaling is inappropriately activated. Somatic mutations and deletions that inactivate both copies of the APC gene are present in at least 70–80% of sporadic colorectal cancers (Kinzler and Vogelstein, 2002; Lynch et al., 2008; Goss and Groden, 2000). In addition, germ-line mutations in *APC* give rise to familial adenomatous polyposis (FAP) an inherited cancer-predispositon syndrome in which the risk for developing colorectal cancer by the age of 40 years is nearly 100% (Kinzler and Vogelstein, 2002; Lynch et al., 2008; Goss and Groden, 2000). Mutations in the ß-catenin gene itself are also found in a small percentage of colorectal cancers (Kinzler and Vogelstein, 2002; Goss and Groden, 2000). These mutations can render the protein resistant to the ß-catenin degradation complex and subsequent activation of Wnt signaling. The inactivation of the p53 pathway by mutation of *TP53* is the second most important genetic alteration in colorectal cancer. In most tumors, both alleles of *TP53* are inactivated, usually by a combination of a missense mutation that inactivates the transcriptional activity of p53 and a deletion on chromosome 17p that elimates the second allele of *TP53* (Kinzler and Vogelstein, 2002; Baker et al., 1990). Inactivation of *TP53* frequently coincides with the progression of large adenomas into invasive adenocarcinomas (Baker et al., 1990). Finally, the mutational inactivation of the TGF-ß signaling pathway is a third step in the progression to colorectal cancer (Grady and Markowitz, 2008). The *TGFBR2* gene can be inactivated by a variety of mechanisms, and its inactivation coincides with the transition from the adenoma stage to high-grade dysplasia or carcinoma.

2.6 Other Molecular Events

Additional molecular events involved in the development of colorectal cancer include alterations in growth factor and stem-cell pathways. One alteration of great interest to chemoprevention researchers is the activation of prostaglandin signaling during the development of colonic adenomas. Prostaglandin signaling can be induced by mitogen-associated upregulation of cyclooxygenase-2 (COX-2), an enzyme that mediates the synthesis of prostaglandin E_2 (PGE_2) from arachidonic acid, and by inflammation. PGE_2 activity can also be increased by the loss of 15-prostaglandin dehydrogenase (15-PDGH), the rate-limiting enzyme catalyzing the degradation of prostaglandin (Yan et al., 2004). Increased levels of COX-2 are present in about two-thirds of colorectal cancers, and there is loss of 15-PDGH in about 80% of these cancers. Numerous animal studies have shown that inhibition of COX-2 by chemopreventive agents reduces the development of colonic adenomas and carcinomas (Marnett and Dubois, 2002). Clinical trials have demonstrated that COX-2 inhibitors, especially certain non-steroidal anti-inflammatory drugs (NSAIDs), regress adenomas in FAP patients (Steinbach et al., 2000) and prevent recurrent adenomas in sporadic cases (Baron et al., 2003; Bertagnolli et al., 2006). The reader is referred to the review article of Markowitz and Bertagnolli (2009) for a more comprehensive discussion of molecular events involved in the development of colorectal cancer in humans.

3 Epidemiological Evidence for the Prevention of Colon Cancer with Berries

A high consumption of fruit and vegetables is thought to be associated with a reduced risk for colorectal cancer (Norat et al., 2005; Wirfalt et al., 2009). However, a recent review by an international panel of experts concluded that the evidence in support of this is limited (World Cancer Research Fund/American Institute for Cancer Research, 2007). In view of this, it is not surprising that it has been difficult to confirm a role for berries, as a single type of fruit, in the prevention of colorectal cancer. One study examined the effect of fruit and vegetable consumption, including strawberries and blueberries, on the incidence of colon and rectal cancers in the Nurses' Health Study (88,764 women) and the Health Professionals' Follow-up Study (47, 325 men) and concluded that the frequent consumption of all fruits (including berries) and vegetables examined did not confer protection from either colon or rectal cancer (Michels et al., 2000). Another study investigated the association between colorectal adenoma growth and fruit and berry consumption in Norway (Almendingen et al., 2004). A weakly positive association was found; however, the types and amounts of berries consumed were not discussed. A major difficulty in making definitive conclusions regarding the relationship between berry use and risk for human cancer is that of separating berry consumption from that of other fruits in epidemiological studies. In addition, the seasonal use of many berry types during the year compromises the acquisition of accurate consumption data.

4 Preclinical Studies with BRBs and Colon Cancer

4.1 Cell Culture Studies

There are numerous reports of the effects of extracts from different berry types, including red raspberries, on proliferation, cell cycle, apoptosis, and invasive potential of human colon cancer cells. Relatively few studies, however, have been reported using extracts from black raspberry. Seeram et al. (2006) examined the inhibitory effects of extracts from multiple berry types, including black raspberries (BRBs), on proliferation and apoptosis of human HT-29 colon cancer cells. All berry extracts were effective in reducing proliferation of HT-29 cells, but only black raspberry and strawberry extracts stimulated apoptosis. In a recent report from Ohio State University, 25 black raspberry samples that varied in their degree of ripeness, growing location within Ohio, and cultivar (Bristol, Jewel, MacBlack) were extracted and tested for their effects on growth of HT-29 colon cancer cells (Johnson, 2009). All extracts inhibited proliferation, and the extent of inhibition ranged from 33 to 118%, with values higher than 100% indicating cytotoxic effects. The effects of BRB extracts on proliferation, apoptosis, gene expression, and differentiation of other cultured epithelial cell types, such as mouse epidermal cells, human oral keratinocytes, and rat esophageal epithelial cells, are discussed in other chapters of this volume.

4.2 *Animal Bioassays*

Harris et al. (2001) reported on the ability of freeze-dried black raspberry powder to inhibit colon cancer produced in Fisher-344 rats with the carcinogen, azoxymethane (AOM). When fed at 2.5, 5.0 and 10% of the diet, BRBs reduced the total tumor (adenoma + adenocarcinoma) multiplicity by 42, 45 and 71% ($P<0.05$ in all groups), respectively, relative to AOM controls. Studies were not done to determine the mechanism(s) of tumor inhibition by BRBs; however, berry treatment reduced urinary levels of the oxidative DNA adduct, 8-hydroxy-2′-deoxyguanosine (8-OH-dG), in AOM-treated animals indicating a protective effect against oxidative stress. Recently, Bi et al. (2010) reported that the inclusion of 10% freeze-dried BRBs in the diets of Apc+/– Min mice and Muc2–/– mice for 12 weeks significantly inhibited spontaneous intestinal tumor formation in both models. Mechanistic studies revealed that the berries inhibited tumor development in Apc+/– mice by suppressing Wnt (ß-catenin) signaling and in Muc2–/– mice by reducing chronic inflammation. Intestinal cell proliferation was reduced by BRBs in both models; however, the berries had no effect on mucus differentiation of intestinal epithelial cells.

Ulcerative colitis, a chronic inflammatory disease of the colonic mucosa, can predispose to colon cancer. This disease can be produced in mice and rats by the administration of dextran sodium sulfate (DSS) in the drinking water. Montrose et al. (2010) added 3% DSS to the drinking water of C57BL/6 mice fed either a control diet or a diet containing 5.0 or 10% BRB powder for 7–14 days. Treatment with the berries resulted in a marked reduction in DSS-induced acute injury to the colonic epithelium. In addition, BRB treatment modestly suppressed colon tissue levels of several pro-inflammatory cytokines including interleukin-1ß (IL-1ß) and tumor necrosis factor-α (TNF-α). COX-2 levels in the colon were dramatically reduced with a concomitant reduction in the plasma levels of PGE_2. These findings demonstrate a potent anti-inflammatory effect of BRBs during DSS-induced colonic injury, suggesting that BRBs may have a therapeutic role in the pathogenesis of ulcerative colitis.

5 Human Clinical Trials

5.1 *Phase Ia Clinical Trial*

Phase I clinical trials are undertaken to determine the safety/tolerability of agents as well as their pharmacokinetics of up-take and distribution. The results of a Phase Ia clinical trial of BRB powder taken orally for a period of 7 days have been published (Stoner et al., 2005). Briefly, eleven (10 male, 1 female) healthy subjects ranging from 20 to 49 years of age were enrolled in the trial to determine the safety/tolerability of freeze-dried BRBs following oral administration and plasma levels of the four BRB anthocyanins (cyanidin-3-glucoside, cyanidin-3-sambubioside, cyanidin-3- rutinoside, and cyanidin-3-xylosylrutinoside), as well as ellagic acid. Subjects consumed 45 g of freeze-dried BRB powder daily in a slurry of water for 7 days. Forty five grams of BRB powder is equivalent to about one pound of fresh BRBs. It is also equivalent to an animal diet containing 5% BRB powder – a diet that has proven chemopreventive potential in numerous animal models including the mouse intestine and rat colon. During berry treatment, subjects refrained from consuming beverages and foods that are high in phenols. Blood samples were collected pre-dose on days 1 and 7 and at 10 time intervals post-dose. Urine was collected for 12 h pre-dose on days 1 and 7 and at three 4-h intervals post-dose.

The results of this study indicated that the BRB treatment was well tolerated. All 11 subjects completed the study. Four subjects reported a total of 5 adverse events. These included 3 different types of adverse events: (a) constipation, mild to moderate and possibly or probably related to consumption of the freeze-dried black raspberry powder; (b) dark stools, mild and also probably related to consumption of the freeze-dried black raspberry powder; and (c) hematoma at venipuncture site, mild and not related to the consumption of freeze-dried black raspberry powder. Maximum concentrations of the anthocyanins and ellagic acid in plasma occurred at 1–2 h and maximum quantities in urine appeared from 0 to 4 h. Overall, less than 1% of the administered dose of all four anthocyanins and ellagic acid were absorbed into plasma and excreted in urine. These results are in agreement with animal studies showing minimal up-take of anthocyanins and ellagitannins into serum or plasma (He et al., 2006). Anthocyanin and ellagic acid levels in urine were several-fold higher than in plasma, suggesting that the up-take of these compounds into plasma may have been underestimated by measuring only the free and not the protein-bound compounds. None of the pharmacokinetic parameters changed significantly between days 1 and 7. In another study involving 10 subjects, we observed that the oral consumption daily of 90 g of BRB powder in water for a period of 14 days was also well tolerated (unpublished data). No pharmacokinetic studies were undertaken in this trial.

5.2 Phase Ib Clinical Trial in Patients with Colorectal Cancer

After demonstrating in the above Phase I trial that black raspberries are well tolerated by humans when consumed orally, we and our colleagues embarked on a series of pilot Phase Ib trials to determine whether the treatment of small cohorts of at-risk patients with BRBs might elicit chemopreventive effects. The first two trials, one in 20 patients with Barrett's esophagus (Kresty et al., 2006) and another in 17 patients with oral dysplasia (Shumway et al., 2008), are discussed in other chapters of this volume. With respect to colon cancer, our initial trial was conducted in patients with CRC to determine if the short-term oral administration of BRBs would modify biomarkers of cell proliferation, apoptosis, and angiogenesis in colorectal tumors and in adjacent normal tissues. In addition, we determined whether the berries might have the capability of demethylating tumor suppressor genes involved in the development of colorectal cancer. The results of this trial will be described in detail here. It should be emphasized at the beginning that we did not conduct this study to determine if BRBs might serve as an alternative to standard-of-care (surgery, chemotherapy, and radiotherapy) treatment of CRC. Rather, we took advantage of a short-term treatment model in CRC patients to determine if BRBs might influence biomarkers of colon cancer development. Ultimately, we plan to evaluate the ability of BRBs to regress and prevent the recurrence of adenomas in at-risk patients.

5.2.1 Black Raspberry Powder

Fresh frozen BRBs (Jewel variety, 2004 harvest) were grown on an Ohio farm, mechanically harvested when ripe, and washed and frozen at –20°C on the farm within 2 h of the time of harvest. The berries were shipped frozen to Van Drunen Farms in Momence, Illinois for freeze-drying as described (Stoner, 2009). The dried berries were pulverized into a fine powder and the powder shipped frozen to the Ohio State University where it was kept at –20°C until packaged for use in the trial. The nutrient content (Table 15.1) of the powder was determined by Covance Laboratories in Madison, Wisconsin. Covance also analyzed the powder for contamination with pesticides, herbicides, and fungicides and only a very low level of one fungicide was found. The anthocyanin content of the berries was determined in the laboratory of Dr. Steven Schwartz of the Department of Food Technology at the Ohio State University. The variation in the content of most of the nutrients listed in Table 15.1 is not greater than 20–25% from one crop year to the next when the berries are handled as described (Stoner, 2009).

The BRB powder was vacuum packed and sealed in 20 g quantities in bags composed of layered nylon, linear low-density polyethylene and aluminum by Central Compounding Pharmacy in Worthington, Ohio. This composition provides a barrier to moisture and oxygen while maintaining flexibility. The bags were taken to the Ohio State University Comprehensive Cancer Center where they were kept frozen until distributed to patients accrued to the trial. Patients were instructed to keep the berry powder in their freezer at home during use in the trial.

5.2.2 Patient Population and Clinical Trial Procedures

The protocol for this trial was approved by the Institutional Review Boards of the Ohio State University Comprehensive Cancer Center and the University of Texas, San Antonio. UT-San Antonio treated five of the 25 patients in this study. Written informed consent was obtained from all patients before participation in the trial.

Table 15.1 Some potential chemopreventive agents in BRBs[a]

Components	mg/100 g dry weight[b]
Minerals	
calcium	217.00
selenium	<3.00
Zinc	2.40
Vitamins	
vitamin A from carotene	98.95
vitamin E nature	16.00
β-carotene	0.06
α-tocopherol	10.48
γ-tocopherol	11.05
folate	0.15
Sterols	
β-sitosterol	102.00
campesterol	5.50
Simple phenols	
ellagic acid	100.00
ferulic acid	5.00
ρ-coumaric acid	8.34
quercetin	42.45
Anthocyanins (complex phenols)	
cyanidin-3-glucoside	200.00
cyanidin-3-sambubioside	180.00
cyanidin-3-rutinoside	2,002.00
cyanidin-3-xylosylrutinoside	400.00

[a]Data from crop year 2004.
[b]Components reported in mg/100 g dry weight, except selenium in μg/100 g, and vitamin A from carotene and vitamin E nature in IU/100 g.

Inclusion Criteria

Patients accrued to the trial had one of the following: (a) a pathologic diagnosis of early stage CRC (primary or recurrent) and were considered as candidates for colorectal surgery; (b) a diagnosis of stage IV CRC with metastatic lesions in the liver or abdomen, and for whom surgery to resect the colorectal lesion was planned; (c) rectal cancer and were eligible for berry treatment prior to proceeding with chemoradiation or surgery if they did not have obstructive lesions or obstructive symptoms; and (d) a high likelihood for colorectal malignancy based upon prior conditions such as rectal bleeding, weight loss, anemia, changes in bowel movement habits, X-ray evidence of colorectal mass, etc.

Exclusion Criteria

Patients who had one of the following were excluded from the trial:(a) obstructive rectal cancer or symptoms which led them to be considered as candidates for immediate neoadjuvant chemo-radiation treatment or surgery; (b) clinical symptoms of obstruction or bleeding and who were candidates for immediate surgery; (c) were currently receiving radiation therapy or chemotherapy (must have been > 4 weeks since last chemotherapy and > 3 weeks after radiation treatment); (d) were taking NSAIDs and could not be taken off NSAIDs due to their clinical condition; (e) were pregnant or lactating; or (f) uncontrolled, uncompensated cardiac, hepatic or pulmonary diseases, or uncontrolled infectious diseases or diabetes mellitus.

Treatment with Black Raspberry Powder

Twenty five patients were enrolled into the trial. Each patient received 60 g of BRB powder daily from the time of initial accrual to the trial until the day before colorectal cancer surgery. Because the pharmacokinetic data showed that BRB anthocyanins and ellagic acid are rapidly absorbed and removed from the blood within approximately 4 h, patients took the berries in 20 g quantities in about 100 mL of water three times daily (morning, mid-day and evening). Sixty grams of berry powder approximates 1.3 lb of fresh BRBs per day and is equivalent to a rodent diet of ~7% berry powder. BRB powder was found to be chemopreventive in the rat colon and in mouse intestine when provided in the diet at concentrations of 5–10% (Bi et al., 2010; Harris et al., 2001; Montrose et al., 2010).

Evaluations Before, During and After Berry Treatment

Initially, all 25 patients were given a physical examination. Their medical/surgical history was obtained, and laboratory tests for lactic dehydrogenase (LDH), alkaline phosphatase (ALP), alanine aminotransferase/aspartate aminotransferase (ALT/AST), carcinoembryonic antigen (CEA), cell blood counts (CBC), and a complete metabolic panel were completed. Patients then participated in a 24 h verbal food recall to establish consumption patterns of phenol-rich foods, including berry products, before being treated with BRB powder. During berry treatment, patients were contacted either by phone or in the clinic to monitor for compliance and potential adverse event(s). Patients were requested to avoid consumption of berry types other than the BRB powder during the trial.

Tissue and Urine Collection

All 25 patients accrued to this trial had a diagnosis of CRC. Because the tissues taken for initial diagnosis were not available for study, it was necessary to obtain additional tissue specimens before treatment of the patients with BRBs. Initially, patients signed the consent form, after which they discontinued any use of NSAIDs. After about 5 days, three biopsies each of adjacent normal (<2 cm from tumors) and colorectal tumor tissues were taken from each patient. One-half of each biopsy was frozen in liquid nitrogen and the other half placed in 10% buffered formalin. Within 24 h after fixation in formalin, the formalin was removed and replaced with phosphate buffered saline (PBS). Patients began taking BRB powder approximately

24 h after the biopsies were taken and then daily until approximately 12–36 h before colorectal cancer surgery. At surgery, an additional three biopsies each of adjacent normal and tumor tissue were taken from each patient and placed in buffered formalin or frozen as described for the pre-treatment biopsies. All tissue specimens were classified histopathologically as either normal or tumor by Dr. Wendy Frankel, a medical pathologist. All tumors were adenocarcinomas. Pre- and post-treatment urine specimens (~50 mL each) were collected at baseline and after berry treatment. To insure the stability of berry anthocyanins, the specimens were stored at –80°C after adding 5% trifluoroacetic acid (TFA) to reduce the pH to acidity. The anthocyanins and other phenols in BRBs are more stabile in acid pH.

5.3 Laboratory Analyses

5.3.1 Measurement of Berry Anthocyanins in Colorectal Tissues and Urine

The procedures for extraction of BRB anthocyanins from the colorectal tissues and urine specimens have been described in detail (Tian et al., 2005). Separation of tissue and urinary anthocyanins was conducted on a Symmetry C18 column (4.6 × 75 mm, 3.5 μm; Waters Corp.) using an Alliance 2695 HPLC system coupled with a Quattro Ultima triple quadrupole mass spectrometer (Waters Corp.) via an electrospray probe operated in positive mode as described (Tian et al., 2005). Monitored anthocyanins were *m/z* 595 → 287 (cyanidin-3-rutinoside), *m/z* 727 → 287 (cyanidin-3-xylosylrutinoside), *m/z* 449 → 287 (cyanidin-3-glucoside) and *m/z* 581 → 287 (cyanidin-3-sambubioside). Cyanidin-3-glucoside obtained from Indofine Chemical Co., Inc. was used as the standard for quantification. All levels of anthocyanins analyzed in tissue and urine samples fell within the standard curve range and were expressed as cyanidin glucoside equivalents in pmol/mL urine or fmol/mg tissue. Total anthocyanins recovered from urine samples were calculated by summing the concentrations of individual anthocyanin peaks.

5.3.2 Analysis of DNA Methylation

DNA Extraction and Bisulfite Conversion

Adjacent normal and tumor tissues were used for extraction of genomic DNA. Paraffin-embedded tissues were cut into 10 μm sections and DNA was extracted using a PicoPure DNA kit (MDS Analytical Technologies). Extracted DNA was purified using the QIAquick PCR purification kit (Qiagen). 500 ng of extracted DNA was bisulfite-converted using the EZ DNA Methylation kit (Zymo Research) according to the manufacturer's instructions.

Mass array

High-throughput MassARRAY was used to quantify methylation levels of the CpG islands of the tumor suppressor genes, *p16*, *PAX6a*, *SFRP2*, *SFRP5*, and *WIF1* as described (Huang et al., 2009). Briefly, bisulfite-converted DNA was amplified with primers, the PCR products spotted on a 384-pad SpectroCHIP (Sequenom), and spectrally acquisited on a MassARRAY analyzer. Methylation data of individual units (1–4 CpG sites per unit) were generated by EpiTyper software (Sequenom).

Pyrosequencing

The LINE-1 repetitive element bisulfite/pyrosequencing assay was used to estimate global methylation (Issa et al., 2001). Bisulfite-converted DNA was amplified and sequenced using PyroMark LINE-1 kit (Qiagen) which contains PCR primers and a sequencing primer provided by the company. PCR cycling conditions were 95°C (30 s), 50°C (30 s), and 72°C (30 s) for 35 cycles. The PCR product was purified and methylation quantified using the PSQ HS 96 Pyrosequencing System (Pyrosequencing Inc, Westborough, MA).

Immunohistochemical Staining and Computer-Assisted Image Analysis

Procedures for immunohistochemical staining for ß-catenin, E-cadherin, c-Myc, Ki-67, TUNEL, p16, CD105 or DNMT1 have been described in detail (Wang et al., 2009). Stained tissue was viewed and photographed at 200× magnification with a bright-field microscope mounted with a high-resolution spot camera. The camera was interfaced with a computer containing a matrix frame grabber board and image analysis software (Simple PCI Imaging Systems, Compix Inc.). For all antigens, up to 30 whole crypts of normal epithelium and 30 fields of tumor from the three pieces of adjacent normal and tumor biopsies collected at each time point per patient were analyzed and the staining intensities quantified by image analysis software. Quantification of Ki-67 staining in normal crypts was done in the proliferative region, approximately the lower 1/3rd of each crypt. Nuclear but not cytoplasmic ß-catenin was quantified.

5.3.3 Statistics

Methylation and immunohistochemical staining data were quantified by determining the percent change of each variable from baseline. Differences in mean percent change and anthocyanin levels were compared by Student t test. All analyses were two-sided, and a p value of less than 0.05 was considered to be significant. Linear regression was used to determine the correlation between the percent change of methylation and the percent change of DNMT1 expression.

5.4 Results

5.4.1 Patient Characteristics

Although 25 patients were entered into the trial, complete laboratory data could be obtained from only 20. Biopsies collected from 5 patients were too small for

Table 15.2 Characteristics of colorectal cancer patients in this study

	No. of patients (%)
Gender	
Female	3 (15)
Male	17 (85)
Age	
<45	2 (10)
45–60	8 (40)
>60	10 (50)
Average 59	
Tumor location	
Transverse, descending, and sigmoid colon	3 (15)
Cecum and ascending colon	3 (15)
Rectum	14 (70)
Metastatic disease	
Lymph node involved	2 (10)
No evidence	18 (90)
Berry treatment (weeks)	
≤ 3	11 (55)
3–4	6 (30)
> 4	3 (15)
Average 3	
Berry doses (20 g/dose, 3 doses/day)	
≤ 50	8 (40)
50–100	10 (50)
>100	2 (10)
Average 67	
Compliance (%)	
80–90	1 (5)
90–100	8 (40)
100	11 (55)
Toxicities reported	
Diarrhea	3 (15)
Constipation	4 (20)
None	13 (65)
Improved bowel movements	15 (75)

the complete panel of studies undertaken. The characteristics of the 20 patients are summarized in Table 15.2. Seventeen of the 20 patients were accrued at the Ohio State University and 3 at the University of Texas, San Antonio. The average age of the study population was 65. Seventeen of the 20 patients were male. Six patients had colon cancer (30%) and the other 14 (70%) had rectal cancer. Two patients presented with metastatic disease.

5.4.2 Berry Treatment and Compliance Data

Patients were treated with BRB powder for an average of 3 weeks (range 1–9 weeks) (Table 15.2). Patient compliance was excellent with each patient consuming >90% of the stipulated daily doses of berry powder, based upon self-reporting and return of empty bags. The berry powder was generally well-tolerated with 7 patients reporting mild disturbances of the gastrointestinal tract; i.e., diarrhea or constipation that resolved within 2–3 days. Patient LDH, ALP, ALT/AST, CEA, CBC, and metabolic profiles were not influenced by BRB treatment. Several patients remarked that treatment with berries improved regularity in bowel movements.

5.4.3 Anthocyanins in Urine and Colorectal Tissue

Anthocyanins could not be detected in the urine of any patient before treatment with BRB powder. In contrast, all four anthocyanins were detected in the urine of all 20 patients following berry treatment. The amounts of the four anthocyanins in the urine of all patients ranged from 56 to 1,822 pmol/mL. The four anthocyanins were detected in colorectal tissues from 18 of the 20 patients; however, the amounts were much lower than those in the urine, ranging from 1.7 to 2,011.5 fmol/mg tissue. The levels of total anthocyanins in adjacent normal tissue versus tumor tissue were 299.9 ± 754.9 and 55.4 ± 60.8 fmol/mg tissue (mean $\pm$ S.D.), respectively. The levels in adjacent normal tissue were not significantly different from those in tumor tissue (p=0.21).

5.4.4 BRBs Cause Promoter Demethylation of Tumor Suppressor Genes in Wnt Pathway

As indicated above, tumor suppressor genes can be silenced by hypermethylation of their promoter sequences. This usually occurs due to increased activity of DNA methyltransferases in tumors. In initial studies using tissues from all 20 patients, the *SFRP2*, *PAX6a,* and *WIF1* tumor suppressor genes in the Wnt pathway (Fig. 15.1) were found to be methylated to greater extents in colorectal tumor tissues than in adjacent normal tissues both before and after berry treatment (data not shown). However, preliminary analysis of combined methylation data from all 20 patients showed that BRB treatment for different periods of time (1–9 weeks) produced no significant effects on promoter demethylation of these genes in either adjacent normal or colorectal tumor tissues Wang et al. (2010).

Significant differences in promoter demethylation of these genes were observed; however, when the patients were divided into two groups based upon: (a) the number of BRB doses taken and (b) the extent of changes in the expression of the methyltransferse enzyme, DNMT1. Data from analyses of adjacent normal tissues are shown in Fig. 15.2. N1 and N2 refer to adjacent normal tissues taken from patients that had received an average of either 83 or 52 berry doses, respectively. Significant decreases in percent methylation change from baseline of the *SFRP2* and *PAX6a* tumor suppressor genes, as well as DNMT1 protein expression, were

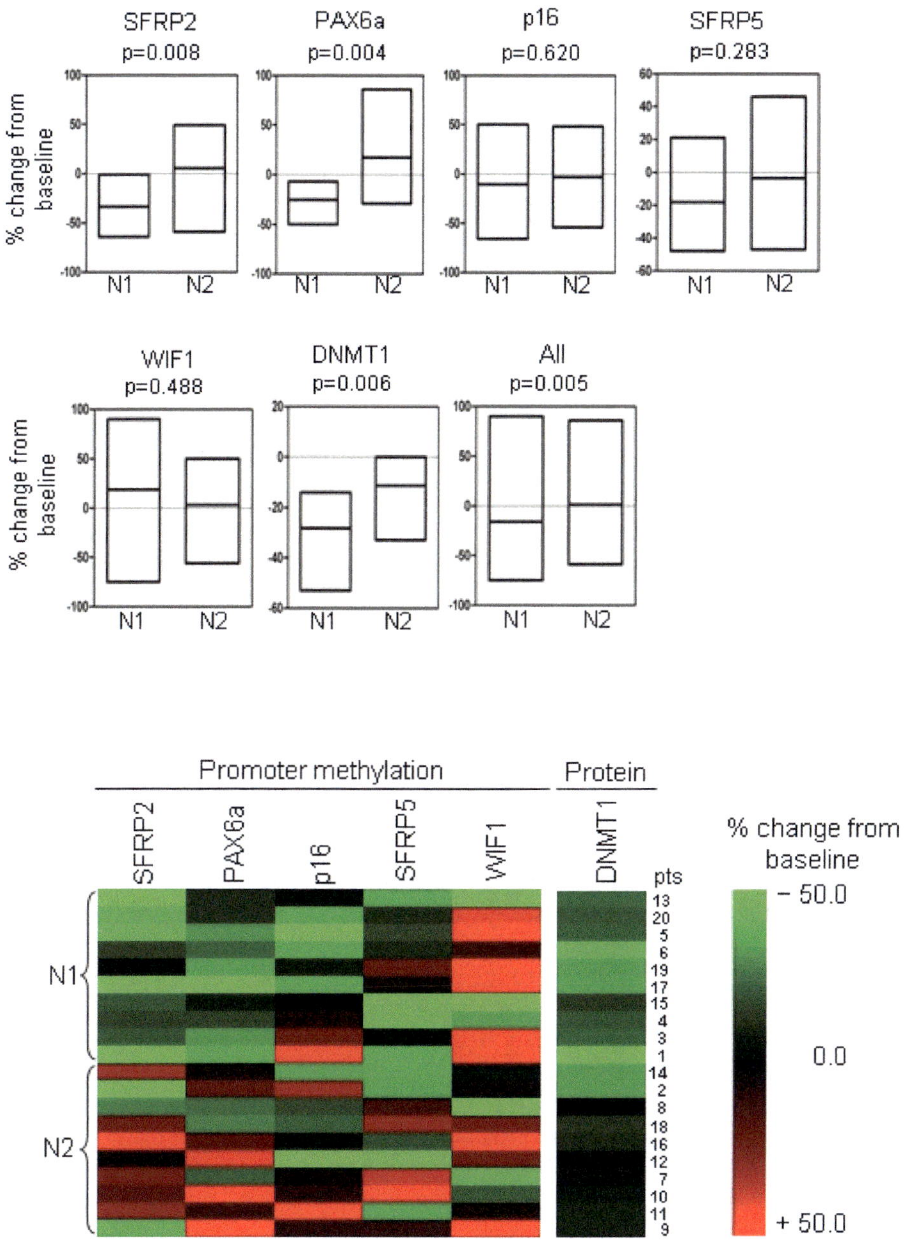

Fig. 15.2 Percent change from baseline in methylation, including promoter and global methylation, and DNMT1 protein expression in adjacent normal tissues from 20 colorectal cancer patients who consumed freeze-dried black raspberry powder daily for an average of 3 weeks. Significant decreases from baseline were found in promoter methylation of *SFRP2*, *PAX6a* and all 5 genes combined (combination of changes from *SFRP2*, *PAX6a*, *p16*, *SFRP5* and *WIF1*) in N1 versus N2 groups ($p<0.05$). This is associated with decreased DNMT1 protein expression, and longer berry treatment (83 vs. 52 doses). In the heat map, *red color* depicts increased gene methylation from normal and *green color* depicts decreased gene methylation

observed in N1 versus N2 tissues. The box labeled "All" indicates that the reduction in methylation of all five tumor suppressor genes (*SFRP2*, *PAX6a*, *p16*, *SFRP5*, and *WIF1*) combined was significant in the N1 group versus the N2 group. Comparing heat-maps in Figs. 15.2 and 15.3, it is apparent that adjacent normal colorectal tissues generally responded more favorably to berry-induced promoter demethylation than colorectal adenocarcinomas as evidenced by the relative amount of green color which depicts reduced gene methylation.

Figure 15.3 illustrates data from methylation analyses of colorectal adenocarcinomas. Ta and Tb refer to adenocarcinomas taken from patients that had received an average of either 85 berry doses or 51 berry doses, respectively. Significant decreases in percent methylation change from baseline of the *SFRP2*, *PAX6a*, and *WIF1* genes, as well as DNMT1 protein expression, were observed in Ta versus Tb group adenocarcinomas. When promoter methylation data from all five suppressor genes were combined, the Ta tumor data were significantly different from the Tb tumor data. These results suggest that the degree of change in promoter methylation of tumor suppressor genes and in DNMT1 protein expression was influenced by the total dose of BRB powder consumed.

There was a positive correlation between changes in DNMT1 protein expression and in promoter methylation (Fig. 15.2c, $p=0.006$, $R^2 = 0.181$) (data not shown). Lastly, berry treatment did not cause significant changes from baseline in global methylation in either adjacent normal colon or in colorectal adenocarcinomas from the high and low berry dose groups as measured by the LINE-1 repetitive element bisulfite/pyrosequencing assay (data not shown).

5.4.5 Wnt Signaling, Cell Proliferation, Apoptosis and Angiogenesis

Because the above data indicated that, in some patients, BRB treatment led to demethylation of tumor suppressor genes upstream of the Wnt pathway, we used quantitative immunohistochemistry to determine if BRB treatment also affected the expression of genes downstream of the pathway (i.e., ß-catenin, E-cadherin and c-Myc). Representative staining of each antigen is shown in Fig. 15.4a. In adjacent normal tissues from the high dose (N1) berry group, BRB treatment led to a decrease in ß-catenin expression and an increase in E-cadherin expression when compared to the low dose (N2) group ($p<0.05$, Fig. 15.4b). This was accompanied by a decrease in Ki-67 protein expression and an increase in TUNEL staining in the N1 as compared to the N2 group ($p<0.05$). CD105 was decreased and p16 was increased in both N1 and N2 groups but the differences between groups were not significant ($p>0.05$).

In the adenocarcinomas, BRB treatment led to reductions in the protein expression levels of ß-catenin, Ki-67 and CD105 and increases in the expression of TUNEL, and p16 in Ta tissues from the high dose group versus Tb tissues from the low dose group (Fig. 15.4c). Again, these data suggest that the responses to BRBs are related to berry dose and treatment time.

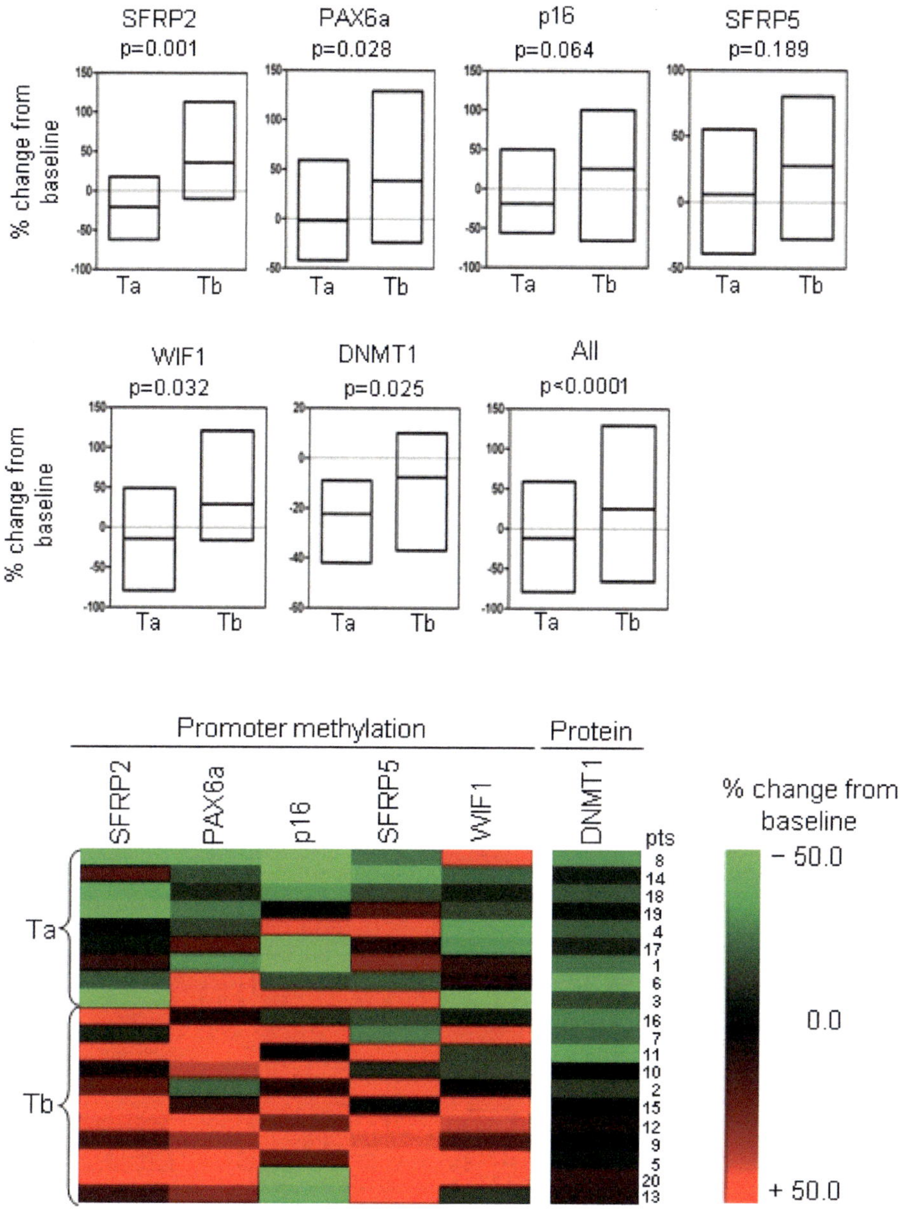

Fig. 15.3 This figure depicts the percent change from baseline in methylation, including promoter and global methylation, and DNMT1 expression in the adenocarcinomas. Significant decreases from baseline were found in promoter methylation of *SFRP2*, *PAX6a* and *WIF1* and all 5 genes combined in Ta versus Tb groups ($p<0.05$). This is associated with decreased DNMT1 protein expression and longer berry treatment (85 vs. 51 doses). The meaning of the colors (*red* and *green*) in the heat map is described in Fig. 15.2

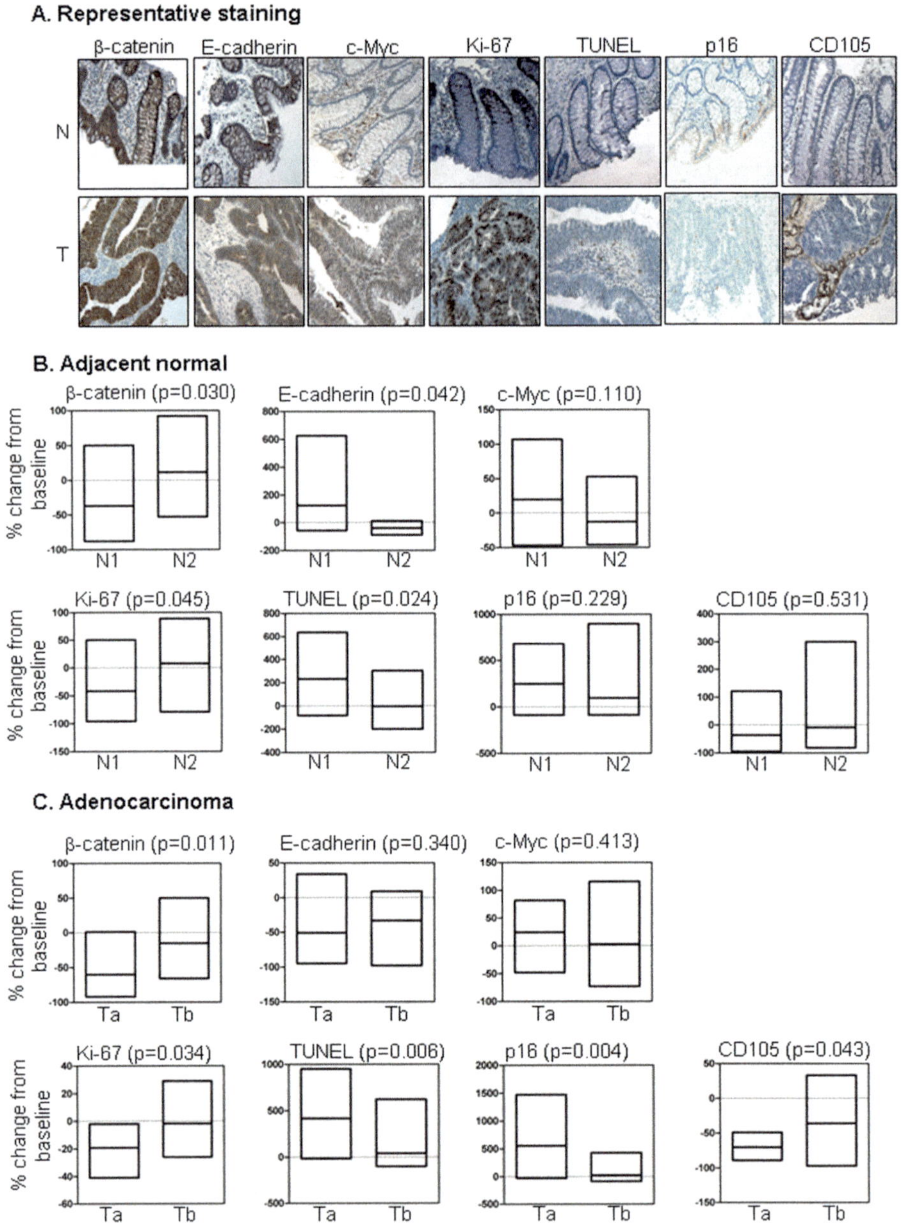

Fig. 15.4 Percent change from baseline in expression of proteins (ß-catenin, E-cadherin, and c-Myc) downstream of the Wnt signaling pathway as well as biomarkers of cell proliferation (Ki-67), apoptosis (TUNEL), and angiogenesis (CD105) after berry treatment as determined by quantitative immunohistochemistry. (**a**) Representative staining of β-catenin, E-cadherin, c-Myc, Ki-67, TUNEL, p16, and CD105. (**b**) In adjacent normal tissue, nuclear β-catenin and Ki-67 staining were decreased significantly in the N1 versus N2 group, whereas, E-cadherin and TUNEL staining were significantly increased in N1 versus N2. (**c**) In adenocarcinomas, β-catenin, Ki-67, TUNEL, p16 and CD105 are positively modulated by BRB treatment to a greater extent in tumors from the Ta group than those in the Tb group

6 Summary and Conclusions

Colorectal cancer (CRC) is the leading cause of digestive tract cancer in the Western world. The development of CRC is a multistage process, beginning as a benign adenomatous polyp which develops into an advanced adenoma with high-grade dysplasia and then progresses to invasive adenocarcinoma. Genomic instability that leads to mutational events in key genes is responsible for the development of the disease. One type of genomic instability is aberrant DNA methylation in the promoter sequences of tumor suppressor genes leading to their silencing. Preclinical studies in our laboratory and others showed that black raspberries elicit chemopreventive effects in cultured human colon cancer cells and in animal model systems of colorectal cancer and ulcerative colitis. Based upon this data, we decided to evaluate the potential efficacy of BRBs in the prevention of colorectal cancer in humans.

Initially, a Phase I clinical trial was conducted in a small cohort of individuals. The results of this trial indicated that BRBs are well tolerated by humans when consumed orally in a slurry of water. The uptake of berry anthocyanins and ellagic acid into blood was maximal at 1–2 h and urinary levels of these compounds were maximal at 4 h. Overall up-take of these compounds was less than 1% of the administered dose. Based upon these results in the Phase I trial, a Phase 1b trial was undertaken in a small cohort of 20 colorectal cancer patients to determine if short-term BRB treatment might influence biomarkers of CRC. BRBs were administered orally to the patients from the time of initial diagnosis of the disease until surgical removal of the tumor (average treatment time = 3 weeks). Quantitative immunohistochemical analysis of tumor and adjacent normal tissues collected before berry treatment and at surgery indicated that the berries inhibited the proliferation of both adjacent normal and colorectal tumor cells, and stimulated apoptosis of tumor cells. The berries inhibited the development of new blood vessels in the tumors (angiogenesis) as indicated by staining for CD105. BRB treatment also positively influenced the expression levels of ß-catenin and E-cadherin in the Wnt signaling pathway. Finally, we present the first evidence of the ability of BRBs to demethylate the promoter regions of the tumor suppressor genes *SFRP2*, *PAX6a*, *SFRP5*, and *WIF*1 in the Wnt signaling pathway, and also the *P16* tumor suppressor gene which is inactivated in a high percentage of colorectal tumors. Collectively, these data suggest that short-term treatment of patients with colorectal cancer led to significant protective effects on multiple biomarkers of tumor development and provide a strong basis for additional human trials to evaluate the chemopreventive effects of BRBs for colorectal cancer.

References

Almendingen K, Hofstad B, Morten HV (2004) Dietary habits and growth and recurrence of colorectal adenomas: results from a three-year endoscopic follow-up study. Nutr Cancer 49:131–138

Anderson WF, Guyton KZ, Hiatt RA et al (2002) Colorectal cancer screening for persons at average risk. J Natl Cancer Inst 94:1126–1133

Baker SJ, Markowitz S, Fearon ER et al (1990) Suppression of human colorectal carcinoma cell growth by wild-type p53. Science 249:1233–1238

Baker SJ, Preisinger AC, Jessup JM et al (1990) p53 Gene mutations occur in combination with 17p allelic deletions as late events in colorectal tumorigenesis. Cancer Res 50:7717–7722

Baron J, Cole BF, Sandler RS (2003) A randomized trial of aspirin to prevent colorectal adenomas. N Engl J Med 348:891–899

Bertagnolli MM, Eagle CJ, Zauber AG et al (2006) Celecoxib for the prevention of sporadic colorectal adenomas. N Engl J Med 355:873–884

Bi X, Fang W, Wang L-S et al (2010) Black raspberries inhibit intestinal tumorigenesis in *Apc+/–* and *Muc2–/–* mouse models of colorectal cancer (in press, Cancer Prevention Research)

Chao A, Thun MJ, Jacobs EJ et al (2000) Cigarette smoking and colorectal cancer mortality in the cancer prevention study II. J Natl Cancer Inst 92:1888–1896

Goss KH, Groden J (2000) Biology of the adenomatous polyposis coli tumor suppressor. J Clin Oncol 18:1967–1979

Grady WM, Markowitz SD (2008) TGF-ß signaling pathway and tumor suppression. In: Derynck R, Miyazano K (eds) The TGF-ß family. Cold Spring Harbor Laboratory Press, Cold Spring Harbor, NY

Harris GK, Gupta A, Nines RG et al (2001) Effects of lyophilized black raspberries on azoxymethane-induced colon cancer and 8-hydroxy-2′-deoxyguanosine levels in the Fischer 344 rat. Nutr Cancer 40:125–133

He J, Magnuson BA, Lala G et al (2006) Intact anthocyanins and metabolites in rat urine and plasma after 3 months of anthocyanin supplementation. Nutr Cancer 54:3–12

Huang Y-W, Liu JC, Deatherage DEet al (2009) Epigenetic repression of microRNA-129-2 leads to overexpression of SOX4 oncogene in endometrial cancer. Cancer Res 69:9038–9046

Issa J-PJ, Ahuja N, Toyota Met al (2001) Accelerated age-related CpG island methylation in ulcerative colitis. Cancer Res 61:3573–3577

Issa JP (2004) CpG island methylator phenotype in cancer. Nat Rev Cancer 4:988–993

Jemal A, Siegel R, Ward E et al (2009) Cancer statistics. CA Cancer J Clin 59:225–249

Johnson JL (2009) Effect of black raspberry extracts on colon cancer cell proliferation. Master's Thesis. etd. ohiolink.edu/sendpdf.cgi/Johnson

Kinzler KW, Vogelstein B (2002) Colorectal tumors. In: Vogelstein B, Kinsler KW (eds) The genetic basis of human cancer, 2nd edn. McGraw-Hill, New York, NY

Kresty LA, Frankel W, Hammond C et al (2006) Transitioning from preclinical to clinical chemopreventive assessments of lyophilized black raspberries: interim results show berries modulate markers of oxidative stress in Barrett's esophagus patients. Nutr Cancer 54:148–156

Kuhnle GGC, Bingham SA (2007) Dietary meat, endogenous nitrosation and colorectal cancer. Biochem Soc Trans 35:1355–1357

Lynch HT, Lynch JF, Lynch PM et al (2008) Hereditary colorectal cancer syndromes: molecular genetics, genetic counseling, diagnosis and management. Fam Cancer 7:27–39

Markowitz SD, Bertagnolli MM (2009) Molecular basis of colorectal cancer. N Engl J Med 361:2449–2460

Marnett LJ, Dubois RN (2002) COX-2, a target for colon cancer prevention. Annu Rev Pharmacol Toxicol 2:55–80

Martinez ME (2005) Primary prevention of colorectal cancer: lifestyle, nutrition, exercise. Recent Results Cancer Res 166:177–211

Michels KB, Giovannucci E, Joshipura KJ et al (2000) Prospective study of fruit and vegetable consumption and incidence of colon and rectal cancers. J Natl Cancer Inst 92:1740–1752

Montrose DC, Horelik NA, Madigan J et al (2010) Anti-inflammatory effects of lyophilized black raspberry powder in ulcerative colitis (in press, Carcinogenesis)

Nakagama H, Ochiai M, Ubafai T et al (2002) A rat colon cancer model induced by 2-amino-1-methyl-6-phenylimidazo[4,5-b]pyridine, PhIP. Mutat Res 506:137–144

Norat T, Bingham S, Ferrari P et al (2005) Meat, fish, and colorectal cancer risk: the European prospective investigation into cancer and nutrition. J Natl Cancer Inst 97:906–916

Robertson KD, Uzvolgyi E, Liang G et al (1999) The human DNA methyltransferases (DNMTs) 1, 3a and 3b: coordinate mRNA expression in normal tissues and overexpression in tumors. Nucleic Acids Res 27:2291–2298

Rowley PT (2005) Inherited susceptibility to colorectal cancer. Annu Rev Med 56:539–554

Seeram NP, Adams LS, Zhang Y et al (2006) Blackberry, black raspberry, blueberry, cranberry, red raspberry, and strawberry extracts inhibit growth and stimulate apoptosis of human cancer cells in vitro. J Agric Food Chem 54:9329–9339

Shumway BS, Kresty LA, Larson PE et al (2008) Effects of a topically applied bioadhesive berry gel on loss of heterozygosity indices in premalignant oral lesions. Cancer Res 14:2412–2430

Sinha R, Kulldorff M, Gunter MJ et al (2005) Dietary benzo(a)pyrene intake and risk of colorectal adenoma. Cancer Epidemiol Biomark Prev 14:2030–2034

Steinbach G, Lynch PM, Phillips RKS et al (2000) The effect of celecoxib, a cyclooxygenase-2 inhibitor, in familial adenomatous polyposis. N Engl J Med 342:1946–1952

Stoner GD (2009) Foodstuffs for cancer prevention: the preclinical and clinical development of berries. Cancer Prev Res 2:187–192

Stoner GD, Sardo C, Apseloff G et al (2005) Pharmacokinetics of anthocyanins and ellagic acid in healthy volunteers fed freeze-dried black raspberries daily for 7 days. J Clin Pharm 45:1153–1164

Tian Q, Aziz RM, Stoner GDet al (2005) Anthocyanin determination in black raspberry (*Rubus occidentalis*) and biological specimens using liquid chromatography-electrospray ionization tandem mass spectrometry. J Food Sci 70:C43–C47

Toyota M, Ahuja N, Ohe-Toyota M et al (1999) CpG island methylator phenotype in colorectal cancer. Proc Natl Acad Sci USA 96:8681–8686

Vogelstein B, Fearon ER, Hamilton SR et al (1988) Genetic alterations during colorectal-tumor development. N Engl J Med 319:525–532

WHO (2003) Joint WHO FAO expert report on diet, nutrition, and the prevention of chronic disease. WHO, Geneva

Wang L-S, Arnold M, Huang Y-W et al (2010) Modulation of genetic and epigenetic biomarkers of colon cancer in humans by black raspberries: a phase I pilot study (in press, Clin Cancer Res)

Wang L-S, Hecht SS, Carmella SG et al (2009) Anthocyanins in black raspberries prevent esophageal tumors in rats. Cancer Prev Res 2:187–191

Wirfalt E, Midthune D, Reedy J et al (2009) Associations between food patterns defined by cluster analysis and colorectal cancer incidence in the NIH-AARP diet and health study. Eur J Clin Nutr 63:7–7–717

World Cancer Research Fund/American Institute for Cancer Research (2007) Food, nutrition, physical activity, and the prevention of cancer: a global perspective. AICR, Washington, DC

Yan M, Rerko RM, Platzer P et al (2004) 15-Hydroxyprostaglandin dehydrogenase, a COX-2 oncogene antagonist, is a TGF-ß-induced suppressor of human gastrointestinal cancers. Proc Natl Acad Sci 101:17468–17473

Index

G.D. Stoner, N.P. Seeram (eds.), *Berries and Cancer Prevention*,
DOI 10.1007/978-1-4419-7554-6, © Springer Science+Business Media, LLC 2011

Printed by Printforce, the Netherlands